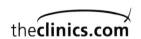

SURGICAL ONCOLOGY CLINICS OF NORTH AMERICA

Advances in the Management of Thyroid Cancer

GUEST EDITOR
Robert L. Witt, MD

CONSULTING EDITOR
Nicholas J. Petrelli, MD

January 2008 • Volume 17 • Number 1

SAUNDERS

An Imprint of Elsevier, Inc.
PHILADELPHIA   LONDON   TORONTO   MONTREAL   SYDNEY   TOKYO

W.B. SAUNDERS COMPANY
A Division of Elsevier Inc.

1600 John F. Kennedy Boulevard, Suite 1800 • Philadelphia, PA 19103-2899

http://www.theclinics.com

SURGICAL ONCOLOGY CLINICS	Volume 17, Number 1
OF NORTH AMERICA	ISSN 1055-3207
January 2008	ISBN-13: 978-1-4160-5807-6
Editor: Catherine Bewick	ISBN-10: 1-4160-5807-9

The ideas and opinions expressed in the *Surgical Oncology Clinics of North America* do not necessarily reflect those of the Publisher. The Publisher does not assume any responsibility for any injury and/or damage to persons or property arising out of or related to any use of the material contained in this periodical. The reader is advised to check the appropriate medical literature and the product information currently provided by the manufacturer of each drug to be administered to verify the dosage, the method and duration of administration, or contra-indications. It is the responsibility of the treating physician or other health care professional, relying on independent experience and knowledge of the patient, to determine drug dosages and the best treatment for the patient. Mention of any product in this issue should not be construed as endorsement by the contributors, editors, or the Publisher of the product or manufacturers' claims.

Surgical Oncology Clinics of North America (ISSN 1055-3207) is published quarterly by Elsevier Inc., 360 Park Avenue South, New York, NY 10010-1710. Months of publication are January, April, July, and October. Business and editorial offices: 1600 John F. Kennedy Boulevard, Suite 1800, Philadelphia, PA 19103-2899. Customer service office: 6277 Sea Harbor Drive, Orlando, FL 32887–4800. Periodicals postage paid at New York, NY, and additional mailing offices. Subscription prices are $202.00 per year (US individuals), $308.00 (US institutions) $102.00 (US student/resident), $232.00 (Canadian individuals), $375.00 (Canadian institutions), $137.00 (Canadian student/resident), $272.00 (foreign individuals), $375.00 (foreign institutions), and $137.00 (foreign student/resident). Foreign air speed delivery is included in all *Clinics* subscription prices. All prices are subject to change without notice. POST-MASTER: Send address changes to *Surgical Oncology Clinics of North America*, Elsevier Periodicals Customer Service, 6277 Sea Harbor Drive, Orlando, FL 32887–4800. **Customer Service: 1-800-654-2452 (US). From outside the United States, call 1-407-345-4000. E-mail: hhspcs@wbsaunders.com.**

Reprints. For copies of 100 or more, of articles in this publication, please contact the Commercial Reprints Department, Elsevier Inc., 360 Park Avenue South, New York, New York 10010-1710. Tel. (212) 633-3813 Fax: (212) 462-1935 email: reprints@elsevier.com.

Surgical Oncology Clinics of North America is covered in *Index Medicus* and *EMBASE/Excerpta Medica, Current Contents/Clinical Medicine, and ISI/BIOMED.*

Printed in the United States of America.

CONSULTING EDITOR

NICHOLAS J. PETRELLI, MD, Bank of America Endowed Medical Director,
Helen F. Graham Cancer Center at Christiana Care Health System, Newark,
Delaware; and Professor of Surgery, Thomas Jefferson University,
Philadelphia, Pennsylvania

GUEST EDITOR

ROBERT L. WITT, MD, FACS, Chief, Head and Neck Oncology, Helen F. Graham Cancer
Center, Christiana Care Health System; and Adjunct Scientist, Center for Translational
Cancer Research, University of Delaware, Newark, Delaware; Associate Professor
of Otolaryngology, Department of Otolaryngology, Jefferson Medical College,
Philadelphia, Pennsylvania

CONTRIBUTORS

NEBIL ARK, MD, Department of Head and Neck Surgery, The University of Texas M.D.
Anderson Cancer Center, Houston, Texas

ADAM M. BECKER, MD, Chief Resident, Department of Otolaryngology-Head and Neck
Surgery, Medical College of Georgia, Augusta, Georgia

DAVID M. COGNETTI, MD, Fellow, Head and Neck Surgery, Department
of Otolaryngology-Head and Neck Surgery, University of Pittsburgh Medical Center,
Pittsburgh, Pennsylvania

MARC D. COLTRERA, MD, Professor and Vice-Chairman, Department
of Otolaryngology-Head and Neck Surgery, University of Washington, Seattle,
Washington

MARY F. CUNNANE, MD, Associate Professor of Pathology, Department of Pathology,
Anatomy, and Cell Biology, Jefferson Medical College; and Attending Pathologist,
Jefferson University Hospital, Philadelphia, Pennsylvania

HUNG Q. DAM, MD, Section of Nuclear Medicine, Department of Medicine,
Helen F. Graham Cancer Center, Christiana Care Health System, Newark; and Nuclear
Medicine Service, Department of Medicine, Wilmington Veterans' Affairs Medical
Center, Wilmington, Delaware; Clinical Instructor, Division of Nuclear Medicine,
Department of Radiology, Thomas Jefferson University, Philadelphia, Pennsylvania

ZIV GIL, MD, PhD, Senior Fellow, Head and Neck Service, Department of Surgery,
Memorial Sloan-Kettering Cancer Center, New York, New York

CHRISTINE G. GOURIN, MD, FACS, Associate Professor, Johns Hopkins University School of Medicine, Baltimore, Maryland

F. CHRISTOPHER HOLSINGER, MD, FACS, Department of Head and Neck Surgery, The University of Texas M.D. Anderson Cancer Center, Houston, Texas

CHARLES M. INTENZO, MD, Professor of Radiology and Director, Division of Nuclear Medicine and PET, Department of Radiology, Thomas Jefferson University, Philadelphia, Pennsylvania

WILLIAM M. KEANE, MD, Professor and Chairman, Department of Otolaryngology-Head and Neck Surgery, Thomas Jefferson University, Philadelphia, Pennsylvania

CHRIS KOPROWSKI, MD, Chairman, Department of Radiation Oncology, Helen F. Graham Cancer Center, Christiana Health Care System, Newark, Delaware

KELLY M. MALLOY, MD, Clinical Lecturer, Department of Otolaryngology/Head and Neck Surgery, University of Michigan, Ann Arbor, Michigan

TIMOTHY A. MANZONE, MD, JD, Associate Medical Director, Section of Nuclear Medicine, Department of Medicine, Helen F. Graham Cancer Center, Christiana Care Health System, Newark, Delaware

MATTHEW C. MILLER, MD, Chief Resident, Department of Otolaryngology-Head and Neck Surgery, Thomas Jefferson University, Philadelphia, Pennsylvania

DAVID NOLEN, BA, Department of Head and Neck Surgery, The University of Texas M.D. Anderson Cancer Center, Houston, Texas

SNEHAL G. PATEL, MD, Assistant Attending Surgeon, Head and Neck Service, Department of Surgery, Memorial Sloan-Kettering Cancer Center; and Assistant Professor of Surgery, Weill Medical College of Cornell University, New York, New York

EDMUND A. PRIBITKIN, MD, Professor and Academic Vice-Chairman, Department of Otolaryngology-Head and Neck Surgery, Thomas Jefferson University, Philadelphia, Pennsylvania

ADAM RABEN, MD, Clinical Attending, Department of Radiation Oncology, Helen F. Graham Cancer Center, Christiana Health Care System, Newark, Delaware

ADAM D. RUBIN, MD, Director, Lakeshore Professional Voice Center, Lakeshore Ear, Nose, and Throat Center, St. Clair Shores; and Adjunct Assistant Professor, Department of Otolaryngology, University of Michigan, Ann Arbor, Michigan

VIDYA V. SAGAR, MD, Medical Director, Section of Nuclear Medicine, Department of Medicine, Helen F. Graham Cancer Center, Christiana Care Health System, Newark, Delaware

ROBERT T. SATALOFF, MD, DMA, Professor and Chairman, Department of Otolaryngology-Head and Neck Surgery, Drexel University College of Medicine, Philadelphia, Pennsylvania

CHARLES J. SCHNEIDER, MD, Section of Oncology, Department of Medicine, Helen F. Graham Cancer Center, Christiana Care Health System, Newark, Delaware; Clinical Associate Professor, Department of Medicine, Thomas Jefferson University, Philadelphia, Pennsylvania

PRAKASH SESHADRI, MD, Section of Endocrinology, Department of Medicine, Diabetes and Metabolic Diseases Center at Christiana, Christiana Health Care System, Wilmington, Delaware

BHUVANESH SINGH, MD, PhD, Head and Neck Service, Department of Surgery, Memorial Sloan-Kettering Cancer Center, New York, New York

JOSEPH R. SPIEGEL, MD, Associate Professor and Director, Jefferson Center for Voice and Swallowing, Department of Otolaryngology-Head and Neck Surgery, Thomas Jefferson University, Philadelphia, Pennsylvania

JON F. STRASSER, MD, Clinical Attending, Department of Radiation Oncology, Helen F. Graham Cancer Center, Christiana Health Care System, Newark, Delaware

RANDAL S. WEBER, MD, FACS, Department of Head and Neck Surgery, The University of Texas M.D. Anderson Cancer Center, Houston, Texas

ROBERT L. WITT, MD, FACS, Chief, Head and Neck Oncology, Helen F. Graham Cancer Center, Christiana Care Health System; and Adjunct Scientist, Center for Translational Cancer Research, University of Delaware, Newark, Delaware; Associate Professor of Otolaryngology, Department of Otolaryngology, Jefferson Medical College, Philadelphia, Pennsylvania

VOLKERT B. WREESMAN, MD, PhD, Head and Neck Service, Department of Surgery, Memorial Sloan-Kettering Cancer Center, New York, New York; Department of Otolaryngology-Head and Neck Surgery, Academic Medical Center at the University of Amsterdam and Netherlands Cancer Institute, Amsterdam, the Netherlands

SESSUNU ZEMO, BA, Department of Head and Neck Surgery, The University of Texas M.D. Anderson Cancer Center, Houston, Texas

CONTENTS

Foreword   xiii
Nicholas J. Petrelli

Preface   xv
Robert L. Witt

**Clinical Impact of Molecular Analysis of Thyroid Cancer
Management**   1
Volkert B. Wreesmann and Bhuvanesh Singh

> Thyroid cancer constitutes a progressive continuum of disease
> ranging from indolent well-differentiated carcinomas to aggressive
> poorly differentiated carcinomas and universally fatal anaplastic
> carcinomas. The wide divergence in clinical behavior is poorly
> predicted for by current clinicopathological factors. Moreover,
> therapeutic armamentarium against aggressive thyroid cancers
> remains limited. Recent studies have identified a range of
> molecular alterations in thyroid cancers. Clinical implications of
> the molecular alterations include their utility in diagnostic
> evaluation, staging and targeted treatment. Continued molecular
> analysis of thyroid cancers promises to increase our understanding
> of its biologic behavior and is expected to have further impact on
> its clinical management.

Evaluation and Imaging of a Thyroid Nodule   37
Marc D. Coltrera

> The approach to the thyroid nodule has been incrementally
> modified over the past decade. The widespread adoption of fine
> needle aspiration in the 1980s, coupled with increased use of serial
> ultrasound monitoring, arguably led to the biggest changes in
> recommendations for surgical intervention during the past 50
> years. For the office-based practitioner, thyroid nodule presentation

patterns are changing with discoveries of more thyroid "incidentalomas" and with new risk assessment challenges associated with small (<1 cm) nodules. At the same time, improved primary evaluation techniques, most notably the increasing use of small, portable ultrasound imaging units, are making many clinicians more comfortable in recommending less invasive follow-up.

Pathology and Cytologic Features of Thyroid Neoplasms   57
Kelly M. Malloy and Mary F. Cunnane

Most thyroid neoplasms arise from follicular cells and are well differentiated. Anaplastic and poorly differentiated carcinomas are rare and have a high mortality. Five percent of tumors are of C-cell origin, and 20% to 25% of these are hereditary. Thyroid lymphoma is rare and occurs in the setting of Hashimoto's thyroiditis. Fine needle aspiration biopsy is the best diagnostic tool to classify thyroid neoplasms.

Initial Surgical Management of Thyroid Cancer   71
Robert L. Witt

The rapid increase in the rate of papillary thyroid cancer is likely caused by improved surveillance. A significant trend toward total thyroidectomy for low-risk differentiated thyroid cancer is present in the United States after a paradigm shift from treatment of macroscopic disease to the treatment of macroscopic and microscopic disease by increasingly sensitive tests. Compelling arguments for thyroid lobectomy and total thyroidectomy for low-risk thyroid cancer remain. The relatively small number of deaths from thyroid cancer, the small number of clinical thyroid cancers, and the huge number of incidental thyroid cancers are indicative of how little we understand the biology of this disease. Clinical medicine awaits biologic markers to refine treatment recommendations.

Surgery for Thyroid Cancer   93
Ziv Gil and Snehal G. Patel

A technique of thyroidectomy that facilitates resection of the thyroid, preserves the parathyroid glands with their blood supply, and preserves the recurrent and the superior laryngeal nerves is described. This technique provides a simple and versatile means of complete extracapsular thyroidectomy for lesions of the thyroid gland and minimizes postoperative complications.

Identification and Monitoring of the Recurrent Laryngeal Nerve During Thyroidectomy   121
Matthew C. Miller and Joseph R. Spiegel

Careful dissection of the recurrent laryngeal nerve (RLN) represents perhaps the most critical component of thyroidectomy. It long has been established that routine identification of the nerve reduces the risk of iatrogenic injury. In recent years, much attention has been paid to the role that functional monitoring plays in identification and preservation of the RLN. This article explores methods for detecting and identifying the RLN. It then examines the evolution of functional RLN monitoring, its potential advantages and disadvantages, statistical validity, and its role in the current medicolegal climate.

Management of Locally Invasive Well-Differentiated Thyroid Cancer 145

Nebil Ark, Sessunu Zemo, David Nolen, F. Christopher Holsinger, and Randal S. Weber

Thyroid carcinoma invasion of the aerodigestive tract and recurrent laryngeal nerve (RLN) are important factors with increase in morbidity and mortality. Primary treatment is surgery; the decision about the extent of surgery is difficult, because preserving function is as essential as removal of the tumor. This article discusses the literature relating to the assessment of disease, surgical management, and adjuvant therapy for invasive thyroid cancer of the aerodigestive tract and RLN and makes suggestions based on the authors' experience.

Management of the Neck in Differentiated Thyroid Cancer 157

David M. Cognetti, Edmund A. Pribitkin, and William M. Keane

Differentiated thyroid cancer is characterized by an excellent long-term prognosis, which unlike other head and neck carcinomas, is not influenced definitively by regional lymph node metastasis. The relative rarity of the disease, together with its tendency for delayed metastasis and its low mortality, makes a prospective randomized trial comparing treatment outcomes difficult. As a result, the effect of cervical lymph node metastases on survival is unclear, making meaningful recommendations for their management somewhat subjective. This article discusses guidelines for the management of the neck in differentiated.

Vocal Fold Paresis and Paralysis: What the Thyroid Surgeon Should Know 175

Adam D. Rubin and Robert T. Sataloff

The thyroid surgeon must have a thorough understanding of laryngeal neuroanatomy and be able to recognize symptoms of vocal fold paresis and paralysis. Neuropraxia may occur even with excellent surgical technique. Patients should be counseled appropriately, particularly if they are professional voice users. Preoperative or early postoperative changes in voice, swallowing, and airway function should prompt immediate referral to an otolaryngologist. Early recognition and treatment may avoid the development of complications and improve patient quality of life.

Postoperative Management of Thyroid Carcinoma   197

Timothy A. Manzone, Hung Q. Dam, Charles M. Intenzo,
Vidya V. Sagar, Charles J. Schneider, and Prakash Seshadri

Survival from differentiated thyroid carcinoma is generally good, but postoperative management plays an important role in minimizing the likelihood of disease recurrence. Postoperative management is generally performed by endocrinologists and nuclear medicine physicians, who exploit thyroid cells' inherent iodineavidity and sensitivity to hormonal manipulation in a unique cancer management paradigm. Endocrinologists manage thyroid hormone replacement/thyroid stimulating hormone suppression and coordinate surveillance. Nuclear physicians administer targeted therapy with radioactive iodine and perform imaging studies to assess disease status. This article provides an overview of the postoperative assessment, treatment, and follow-up of patients who have thyroid carcinoma.

**The Role of Radiation Therapy in the Management
of Thyroid Cancer**   219

Jon F. Strasser, Adam Raben, and Chris Koprowski

The goal of this article is to review the various indications for the application of external beam radiotherapy in the management of thyroid cancer. This article includes a discussion of published literature to define risk variables that increase the risk of recurrence after surgery that might be mitigated by the use of radiation therapy. Clinical outcomes, recent technologic advances in treatment planning and radiation delivery, and potential morbidity associated with treatment are also reviewed.

New Technologies in Thyroid Surgery   233

Adam M. Becker and Christine G. Gourin

Recent technological innovations are facilitating new approaches to surgery of the thyroid gland, including minimally invasive approaches that have the added advantage of allowing the surgeon to avoid drains, thus enabling outpatient surgery. Laryngeal nerve monitoring may be a useful adjunct in identification of the recurrent laryngeal nerve, particularly for the low-volume endocrine surgeon. Endoscopic surgical techniques allow improved visualization and permit thyroidectomy to be performed through small incisions, often less than 3 cm, which may improve cosmetic outcomes. Finally, surgical robotics, with the promise of further enhanced visualization and surgical dexterity better than that possible with traditional endoscopic approaches, may have future applications to thyroid surgery.

Index   249

FORTHCOMING ISSUES

April 2008

Translational Research in Surgical Oncology
Ben Li, MD, *Guest Editor*

July 2008

Update on Surgical Oncology in Europe
Bernard Nordlinger, MD, *Guest Editor*

October 2008

Regional Chemotherapy
Harold J. Wanebo, MD, *Guest Editor*

RECENT ISSUES

October 2007

**Tumor Immunology for the Practicing
Surgeon**
Robert P. Sticca, MD, *Guest Editor*

July 2007

Metastasectomy and Cytoreductive Surgery
Pascal Fuchshuber, MD, PhD, *Guest Editor*

April 2007

**Pre and Postoperative Cancer Imaging:
Practical and Innovative Approaches**
Scott H. Kurtzman, MD, *Guest Editor*

Surg Oncol Clin N Am
17 (2008) xiii–xiv

SURGICAL
ONCOLOGY CLINICS
OF NORTH AMERICA

Foreword

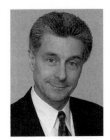

Nicholas J. Petrelli, MD
Consulting Editor

This issue of the *Surgical Oncology Clinics of North America* is devoted to thyroid cancer, a subject matter that was certainly overdue to review. The guest editor is Robert L. Witt, MD, Director of the Head and Neck Multidisciplinary Disease Site Center at the Helen F. Graham Cancer Center at Christiana Care, Newark, Delaware, and Associate Professor of Otolaryngology, Department of Otolaryngology, Jefferson Medical College, Thomas Jefferson University, Philadelphia, Pennsylvania. He is more than qualified to guest edit this issue.

As the readers can see from the Table of Contents of this issue of the *Surgical Oncology Clinics of North America*, Dr. Witt has assembled an experienced group of individuals in the field of thyroid cancer inclusive of basic science, clinical medicine, pathology, surgery, and technology. The discussions in these articles are practical and up-to-date.

In 2007, there were 559,650 Americans who died from cancer, which are more than 1500 people a day. It is known that cancer is the second most common cause of death in the United States, exceeded only by heart disease. In the United States, cancer accounts for one of every four deaths. In 2007, there were 33,550 new thyroid cancer cases in the United States, of whom 8070 were in males and 25,480 in females. As stated by Dr. Witt in his preface, the incidence of thyroid cancer is increasing and "the underlying causes are explored in the context of the prevailing pathology" in this issue of the *Surgical Oncology Clinics of North America*. Also in 2007, there were a total of 1530 deaths from thyroid cancer, 650 in males and 880 in females. On the other side of the coin, in 2007, there were more than 10 million American cancer survivors, illustrating that progress is definetly being made, although we still have several barriers to overcome.

Readers will enjoy the variety of articles dealing with thyroid cancer in this issue of the *Surgical Oncology Clinics of North America*. I congratulate Dr. Robert Witt for this issue and encourage my colleagues to share this knowledge with their trainees in surgical, medical, and radiation oncology.

Nicholas J. Petrelli, MD
Helen F. Graham Cancer Center
Christiana Care Health System
4701 Ogletown-Stanton Road
Suite 1213
Newark, DE 19713, USA

Department of Surgery
Thomas Jefferson University
College Building
1025 Walnut Street
Philadelphia, PA 19107, USA

E-mail address: npetrelli@christianacare.org

ELSEVIER
SAUNDERS

Surg Oncol Clin N Am
17 (2008) xv–xvi

SURGICAL
ONCOLOGY CLINICS
OF NORTH AMERICA

Preface

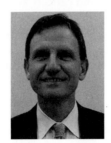

Robert L. Witt, MD, FACS
Guest Editor

Thyroid cancer and its management is a rapidly evolving subject. The goal of this issue is to focus on what is new from a scientific and practical standpoint.

The opening article is a detailed study of the underlying basic science concepts that provide a present foundation and a clear vision of how practice will progress in the near future. The preoperative work up is developing, and the germane topic of surgeon-performed in-office thyroid ultrasonography is outlined.

The incidence of thyroid cancer is, by all accounts, exploding. Underlying causes are explored in the context of the prevailing pathology. A clear trend toward more aggressive surgery is noted. Safe surgical practice is detailed, followed by a careful look at the role of nerve integrity monitors. New technologies for hemostasis, endoscopic techniques with smaller incisions, and robotic surgery have arrived. Management of the aggressive tumor with extra-thyroidal spread and neck metastasis is difficult because preserving function is as essential as removal of the tumor.

Survival from differentiated thyroid carcinoma is generally good, but postoperative management plays an important role in minimizing the likelihood of disease recurrence. Risk variables that increase the threat of recurrence after surgery and that might be mitigated by the use of radiation therapy in light of clinical outcomes, recent technological advances in treatment planning and radiation delivery, and potential morbidity associated with treatment are reviewed.

doi:10.1016/j.soc.2007.10.004

The thyroid surgeon must have a thorough understanding of laryngeal neuroanatomy and be able to recognize symptoms of vocal fold paresis and paralysis. Neuropraxia may occur even with excellent surgical technique. Improvements in the management of vocal immobility are updated.

Finally, the sobering thought that the relatively small number of deaths from thyroid cancer, the small number of clinical thyroid cancers, and the huge number of incidental thyroid cancers are indicative of how much more we need to understand regarding the biology of this disease. Clinical medicine awaits biological markers to refine treatment recommendations.

I am grateful for the opportunity to edit this issue of *Surgical Oncology Clinics of North America* and I thank the article contributors for their expertise on this subject.

Robert L. Witt, MD, FACS
Head and Neck Multidisciplinary Disease Site Center
Helen F. Graham Cancer Center
Christiana Care Health System
Medical Arts Pavilion #1, #112
4745 Stanton-Ogletown Road
Newark, DE 19713, USA

Department of Otolaryngology
Jefferson Medical College
Thomas Jefferson University
925 Chestnut Street
6th Floor
Philadelphia, PA 19107, USA

E-mail address: RobertLWitt@aol.com

ELSEVIER
SAUNDERS

Surg Oncol Clin N Am
17 (2008) 1–35

SURGICAL
ONCOLOGY CLINICS
OF NORTH AMERICA

Clinical Impact of Molecular Analysis on Thyroid Cancer Management

Volkert B. Wreesmann, MD, PhD[a,b],
Bhuvanesh Singh, MD, PhD[a,*]

[a]*Head and Neck Service, Department of Surgery, Memorial Sloan-Kettering Cancer Center, 1275 York Avenue, New York, NY 10021, USA*
[b]*Department of Otolaryngology-Head and Neck Surgery, Academic Medical Center at the University of Amsterdam and Netherlands Cancer Institute, Amsterdam, the Netherlands*

Thyroid cancers represent the most common malignancy of the endocrine system and the second most common malignancy in the head and neck region (excluding skin cancers) (Table 1) [1]. The majority of thyroid cancers (95%) are derived from the thyroid follicular cell. The remaining develop from parafollicular C cells (medullary thyroid cancer), soft tissue, or the lymphoreticular system within the thyroid gland (outside the scope of this review). Although they originate from a common progenitor cell, follicular cell–derived thyroid cancers represent a wide spectrum of disease with highly heterogeneous clinical behavior (Table 2). Thyroid tumors characterize a progressive disease continuum ranging from indolent well-differentiated papillary thyroid carcinoma (PTC) and follicular thyroid carcinoma (FTC) (20-year survival 90%–99%) to poorly differentiated thyroid cancers (PDTC) (20-year survival 20%–40%) to anaplastic thyroid carcinoma (ATC) (1-year survival <5%) [2]. The prevalence of individual subtypes of thyroid cancers is inversely proportional to their aggressiveness, with well-differentiated PTC (70%–85% of cases) and FTC (15%) the most common followed by PDTC (5%) and ATC (5%) (see Table 2).

Several lines of evidence suggest that genetic factors play a vital role in the pathogenesis and clinical behavior of thyroid cancer. Vital support for germline pathogenetic influences on thyroid cancer development includes the increased thyroid cancer incidence among families who have inherited genetic syndromes. Well-characterized examples include Gardner's

---

* Corresponding author.
E-mail address: singhb@mskcc.org (B. Singh).

1055-3207/08/$ - see front matter © 2008 Elsevier Inc. All rights reserved.
doi:10.1016/j.soc.2007.10.013   *surgonc.theclinics.com*

Table 1
Most common (nonskin) tumors of the head and neck region

Head and neck cancers	Relative frequency
Upper aerodigestive tract	80%–85%
Squamous cell carcinoma	80%
Adenocarcinoma	5%
Undifferentiated carcinoma	5%
Melanoma	10%
Thyroid	10%–15%
Papillary carcinoma	70%
Follicular carcinoma	10%
Medullary carcinoma	5%
Poorly differentiated (insular carcinoma)	5%
Anaplasti carcinoma	5%
Hürthle cell carcinoma	<5%
Lymphoma	<1%
Squamous cell carcinoma	<1%
Sarcoma	<1%
Parathyroid	<1%
Adenocarcinoma	
Soft tissue (mesenchymal)	
Liposarcoma	
Fibrosarcoma	
Dermatofibrosarcoma protuberans	
Malignant fibrous histiocytoma	
Angiosarcoma	
Kaposi's sarcoma	
Rhabdomyosarcoma	
Synovial sarcoma	
Odontogenic carcinoma and sarcoma	
Bone	<1%
Osteosarcoma	
Chondrosarcoma	
Ewing's sarcoma	
Odontogenic sarcoma/carcinoma	
Salivary glands	5%
Mucoepidermoid carcinoma	
Adenoid cystic carcinoma	
Acinic cell carcinoma	
Adenocarcinoma	
Neurovascular	<1%
Paraganglioma	
Olfactory neuroblastoma	
Neuroendocrine carcinoma	
Malignant schwannoma	
Hemangiopericytoma	

(adenomatous polyposis coli [APC]) [3], Cowden's (phosphatase and tensin homolog [PTEN]) [4], Carney's (protein kinase, cyclic adenosine monophasphate [cAMP]-dependent, regulatory, type I, alpha [PRKAR1A]) [5], and Werner syndromes (RECQL2) [6], all of which are linked to

Table 2
Clinicopathologic and genetic features of most common thyroid cancer subtypes

	Papillary carcinoma				Follicular tumors				Anaplastic carcinoma
	CPTC	FVPTC	TCV	PDPTC	FTA	MIFTC	WIFTC	PDFTC	UTC
Empty nuclei[a]	+	+	+	+	−	−	−	−	−
Papillary growth	+	−	+	+	−	−	−	−	−
Follicular growth	±	+	±	±	+	+	+	±	−
Mitotic activity	−	−	−	++	−	−	−	++	+++++
Necrosis	−	−	−	++	−	−	−	++	+++++
Nuclear polymorphism	−	−	−	++	−	−	−	++	+++++
Encapsulation	−	+	−	−	+	+	+	−	−
Capsular invasion	−	±	−	−	−	+	+++	−	−
Vascular invasion	±	±	−	+	−	+	+++	+	+
Multicentricity	+	−	+	−	−	−	−	−	−
Lymphatic metastasis	++	−	++	++	−	−	−	+	+++
Hematogenous metastasis	−	−	++	++	−	±	++	+++	+++++
Recurrence	10%	10%	40%	50%	0%	10%	40%	60%	100%
Death of disease	5%	5%	25%	40%	0%	10%	40%	60%	100%
RET/PTC	30%	<5%	30%	10%	0%	0%	0%	0%	0%
BRAF	40%	<5%	60%	70%	0%	0%	0%	0%	60%
RAS	<5%	40%	UNK	50%	30%	40%	50%	60%	70%
P53	<5%	<5%	30%	40%	0%	<5%	<5%	40%	80%
CTNNB1	<5%	<5%	UNK	25%	0%	0%	0%	25%	65%
PI3K-AKT-PTEN	24%	24%	24%	UNK	31%	55%	55%	UNK	58%
PPARγ	0%	30%	UNK	UNK	30%	40%	40%	UNK	0%

[a] Including optically clear nuclei, nuclear overlap, nuclear enlargement, irregularly shaped nuclei, nuclear grooves, and nuclear pseudoinclusions.

Abbreviations: CPTC, classical PTC; MIFTC, minimially invasive FTC; PDFTC, poorly differentiated FTC; PDPTC, poorly differentiated PTC; UTC, undifferentiated thyroid carcinoma; WIFTC, widely invasive FTC; UNK, uknown; +, present; −, not present; ±, sometimes present.

distinctive gene defects (between brackets) present in the germline of affected patients. Additionally, epidemiologic evidence suggests that follicular cell–derived thyroid cancer may occur in a nonsyndromic familial setting [7]. Although ill defined, linkage studies suggest that the responsible genetic factors associated with this phenomenon reside on the chromosomal loci 1q21, 2q21, 14q32, or 19p13.2 [8]. To date, the most convincing evidence for a pathogenetic cause of thyroid cancer has come from identification of somatic genetic alterations in thyroid cancers [9,10]. Analysis of the genetic pathogenesis of thyroid cancers offers the promise of identifying accurate diagnostic and prognostic markers and targets for novel treatment strategies. Current work focuses on the somatic genetic makeup of follicular cell–derived thyroid cancer and describes the most promising targets for molecular diagnostic, prognostic, and therapeutic improvement.

Follicular thyroid carcinoma

Global genomic profile

The first somatic genetic aberrations described in human thyroid tumors included chromosomal alterations detected by conventional cytogenetic karyotyping and revealed that FTC are characterized by complex karyotypes [11]. The advent of modern cytogenetic screening tools, such as loss of heterozygosity (LOH) analysis and comparative genomic hybridization (CGH), allowed for further refinement of the observed chromosomal alterations (Table 3). Chromosomal aberrations are identified in approximately 60%, 75%, and 75% of FTC when studied by conventional cytogenic karyotyping, CGH, and LOH-based allelotyping, respectively [12–21]. The observed chromosomal changes include balanced chromosomal translocations, unbalanced chromosomal gains and losses, and imbalance in maternally and paternally inherited chromosomal equivalents. Compilation of individual alterations among tumor samples revealed multiple recurrent alterations, suggesting that they are vital for tumor survival. Recurrent alterations include cytogenetic translocation breakpoints located within the chromosomal regions 2q13, 3p13, 3p25, 5q15, 6q16, 7p15, 7q32, 8q24.1, 9q21, 10q11.2, 13q12, 14q11, 17q11, and 22q11. In addition, LOH studies demonstrate allelic imbalance involving 1p, 3p, 7q31.1, 9q, 10q23-24, 11p, 11q13, 13q, 14q, 15q, and 22q. CGH analyses demonstrate genetic deletions of 1p, 13, and 22 and overrepresentations (gains/amplifications) of 1q, 4q, 5q, 7, 12, 17, 18, and X.

Comparison of the molecular constitution of FTC and follicular thyroid adenoma (FTA) supports the concept of disease continuum and has provided insight into the timing of genetic alterations along the progression axis (Fig. 1) [12,22–24]. Consistent with a progressive pathogenetic relationship, FTA and FTC have a significant overlap in genetic aberrations, including chromosomal gains of 3q, 4q, 6q, 9q, 13q, 14q, 5, 7, 12, 17, 19, 20, and 18 and losses of 1p, 2p, 3p, 11p, 11q, 17q, and 19. Some of these changes, including gains of 5, 7, 12, and 17 and loss of chromosome 22q, are identified in a significant number of follicular thyroid hyperplasias, extending the progression concept to preneoplastic processes (see Fig. 1) [22]. Although the overlapping genetic aberrations between these distinct pathologic entities may be unrelated, it is tempting to speculate that they may represent early events in the development of follicular thyroid tumors. In agreement with this concept, FTC contains an increased genomic complexity manifested by a higher absolute number of genetic alterations relative to FTA. Accordingly, early genetic events and later events that are uniquely present in FTC, such as gains of 1q21 and deletions of 13q21-31, may promote malignant transformation.

Individual genetic events

Peroxisome proliferator-activated receptor gamma

Of chromosomal alterations identified in FTA and FTC, 3p25 is the most common, occurring in approximately 30% to 40% of cases [25]. The 3p25 locus typically is involved in balanced translocations, most commonly with 2p13 (t(2;3)(q13; p25)), but it also can be involved in unbalanced translocations, deletions, and overrepresentations [26]. The peroxisome proliferator-activated receptor gamma (PPARγ) gene is identified as a principal target of 3p25 alterations in follicular neoplasms [27]. PPARγ is a member of the nuclear hormone receptor superfamily that includes thyroid hormone, retinoid acid, and androgen and estrogen receptors [28]. When activated by ligand binding, PPARγ functions as a transcription factor that mediates important biologic processes, such as inflammation, tissue remodeling, and atherosclerosis [29,30]. PPARγ is implicated in oncogenesis through its capacity to modulate cell proliferation and apoptosis [30]. Kroll and colleagues [27] reported that the t(2;3)(q13; p25) in thyroid cancer results in fusion of PPARγ to the DNA-binding domain of the PAX8 gene (2q13), a transcription factor essential for thyroid gland development. The PAX8-PPARγ rearrangement can be found in approximately 30% of FTC and an equivalent proportion of FTA (see Table 2) [31–33]. In addition, FTC without t(2;3)(q13;p25) may inactivate PPARγ by other mechanisms, including undefined aberrations that diminish PPARγ expression [34].

The presence of PPARγ alteration in a large proportion of FTA/FTC implicates it as an early and essential event in cancer pathogenesis, which is supported by functional studies. In normal cells, PPARγ signaling imparts a tumor-suppressive effect through several signaling pathways involved in differentiation, senescence, angiogenesis, and apoptosis [30,35]. In vitro and in vivo, PPARγ agonists induce apoptosis in cell lines derived from lung cancer [36–39]. These data are supported by clinical studies showing decreased lung cancer incidence in patients treated with PPARγ agonists, such as the antidiabetic thiazolidinediones [40]. In thyroid cells, in vivo studies also support the role of PPARγ as a tumor suppressor [41,42]. Conditional inactivation of PPARγ in a murine model predisposed to the development of FTC results in increased tumorigenesis, which can be reversed by treatment with PPARγ agonists [43]. Global gene expression analysis comparison of PAX8-PPARγ–positive and –negative FTC demonstrates significantly divergent gene expression profiles, implying involvement of PAX8-PPARγ in multiple oncogenic pathways [44]. Studies by Kroll and colleagues [27] suggest that the key effects of the PAX8-PPARγ fusion protein result from inhibition of wild-type PPARγ activity.

Table 3
Advantages and limitations of commonly used genome-wide screening techniques

Technique	Advantages	Limitations
Conventional cytogenetic karyotyping	Overview of complete karyotype including structural and numeric chromosomal changes	Limited resolution unable to identify origins of marker chromosomes, and double minute chromosomesNeed for tissue culture
Loss of heterozygosity	High-resolution detection of allelic imbalance	No true genome-wide screen Requirement for matched normal reference
	Feasible on archival DNA	Does not identify origins of allelic imbalance (ie, gain, loss, amplification)
Fluorescent in situ hybridization	Highly sensitive and specific gene mapping and detection of numeric and structural changes in metaphase chromosomes and interphase nuclei (ie, feasible on archival tissue)	No true genome-wide screen
		Prior knowledge of aberrations/loci required
Comparative genomic hybridization	Genome-wide detection and mapping of chromosomal gains, loosen, and amplifications	Limited resolution (<5 to 10 Mb)
	Requires only small amount (2 μg) of (archival) DNA	Unable to detect balanced chromosomal changes/ structural aberrations
	No need for tissue culture or matched normal reference DNA	
Spectral karyotyping	High-resolution overview of complete tumor karyotype, including structural and numeric aberrations	Does not detect inversions and subtle deletions
Complementary DNA micrarray	Simultaneous appraisal of expression levels of large number ($>10,000$) of genes in one experiment	Does not detect expression levels of unknown genes or foreign sequences
		Typically needs matched normal reference
Array comparative genomic hybridization	Simultaneous detection of gene copy number of large number of genes without need for culturing, matched-reference DNA or fresh frozen tissue	Does not detect structural aberrations or DNA copy number of unknown genes or foreign sequences (HPV, EBV viral integrations)

Table 3 (*continued*)

Technique	Advantages	Limitations
SAGE	Genome-wide, quantitative evaluation of gene expression, detects expression of all expressed genes within cell	Laborious
Digital karyotyping	High-resolution, quantitative, genome-wide appraisal of DNA copy number Detects foreign sequences (HPV, EBV viral integrations)	Llaborious, small (1000-bp) amplifications or deletions not detected
Quantitative PCR	Highly sensitive, quantitative evaluation of genetic copy number without need for culturing, fresh frozen tissue, or matched-reference DNA	No true genome wide, unbiased evaluation

Abbreviations: EBV, Epstein-Barr virus; HPV, human papilloma virus; SAGE, serial analysis of gene expression.

RAS mutation

The mitogen-activated protein kinase (MAPK) signaling pathway is highly conserved and regulates cellular proliferation, differentiation, and survival in response to a variety of membrane-bound receptor tyrosine kinases (RTKs) (such as epidermal growth factor receptor [EGFR] and ERBB2) and adhesion proteins [45]. MAPK activation results in recruitment and activation of the RAS protein at the cell membrane, which, in turn, binds effector proteins. RAF proteins, including A-RAF, B-RAF, and C-RAF, are key intermediates of the MAPK pathway and important downstream targets of RAS. BRAF is the most potent activator of

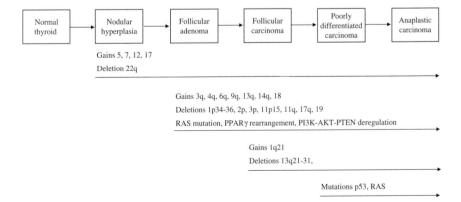

Fig. 1. Tumor progression model for FTC.

downstream intermediates. BRAF activates MEK through phosphorylation. The pathway culminates in activation of the transcription factor ERK. Subsequent translocation of ERK to the nucleus results in transcription of genes involved in differentiation, proliferation, and survival [46].

In normal cells, the MAPK pathway is under stringent control through negative feedback loops and transcriptional repression by multiple senescence and apoptotic signaling pathways. Constitutive activation of its intermediates, however, allows the MAPK pathway to escape regulatory controls in cancer cells. Somatic mutation of RAS is among the most frequent oncogenic alterations in human cancers and results in constitutive activation of the MAPK cascade [47]. In FTC, RAS mutation is present in up to 30% of cases that typically do not harbor the PAX8-PPARγ rearrangement (see Table 2) [48]. Similar to the PPARγ rearrangement, RAS mutation may be an early event in thyroid tumorigenesis, as it is present in a significant number of FTA (see Table 2) [49–51]. A high frequency of RAS mutation also is present in PDTC and ATC but not in PTC (see Table 2) [52,53]. Functional studies also demonstrate the importance of RAS in FTC pathogenesis. Transgenic mice with expressing mutated RAS develop FTC at a high rate [54]. Conversely, analysis of alternative MAPK pathway components, such as the BRAF gene, have not revealed evidence for mutation in FTC [55,56].

AKT activation

In addition to the MAPK pathway, RTKs may activate a second major oncogenic signaling cascade, the phosphoinositide 3-kinase (PI3K)-AKT pathway. In normal cells, PI3K-AKT signaling is activated by ligand binding or receptor homo- or heterodimerization of RTKs, such as EGFR, Her2Neu, and insulin-like growth factor I [57]. This results in the recruitment of PI3K isoforms to the plasma membrane and subsequent generation of 3'-phosphorylated phosphoinositides (PI3,4P; PI3,4,5P). Phosphoinositol triphosphate (PIP3) activates PDK1, which in turn phosphorylates AKT. By phosphorylating key intermediates, AKT affects the function of many downstream targets that mediate cell survival by multiple mechanisms, including cell cycle progression and inactivation of apoptotic pathways. The PTEN, an important antagonist of PI3K-mediated activation of PIP3, induces G1 arrest by decreasing the phosphorylated AKT fraction [58]. The oncogenic properties of the PI3K-AKT cascade are corroborated by its alteration in many human cancers, including melanomas, breast cancer, colorectal cancer, and squamous cell carcinomas [59–63].

The increased rate of thyroid cancer in patients who have Cowden's syndrome, marked by germline mutation in PTEN and resultant increase in AKT activation, supports a role for PI3K-AKT signaling and FTC pathogenesis [64]. Similarly, an increase in follicular thyroid tumor development is noted in heterozygous PTEN negative mice, and crossbreeding of these mice with AKT1 null mice results in reversal of the thyroid tumor predisposition

[65,66]. PTEN silencing through promoter methylation, inactivating point mutation, and LOH is observed in 20% to 30% of FTC (see Table 2) [67–71]. In addition, oncogenic mutation of PI3K and PIK3CA amplification is reported in 10% and 29% of FTC, respectively (see Table 2) [68,72]. PTEN and PI3K-mediated AKT activation mechanisms are mutually exclusive events in FTC [68,72]. Moreover, increased AKT activity is observed relative to normal thyroid tissue in the majority of sporadic human FTC without PTEN or PI3K aberrations, suggesting alternate activation mechanisms may be involved and implicating it as a central process in FTC pathogenesis [73,74].

Papillary thyroid carcinoma

Global genomic profile

Consistent with their divergence in clinicopathologic characteristics and clinical behavior, genetic analysis reveals that PTC and FTC differ significantly in their genotype. The overall chromosomal composition of PTC seems less complex than that of FTC, with detectable chromosomal alterations present in approximately 40% to 50% of PTC when analyzed by conventional karyotyping, CGH, and allelotyping analyses [20,75–79]. In addition to the frequency, the chromosomal aberrations in PTC differ from that occurring in FTC. PTC contains recurrent breakpoints at 1p32-33, 1p12-13, 3p11, 3p25, 3q21, 4p14-15, 5p15, 6q21, 7q33-36, 9q13-21, 10q11.2, 10q21.1, 11q13, 11q23, 12p11, 12q11-13, 13q31, 15q24, 16p12-13, 16q12-13, and 19q13. Also, CGH and LOH studies demonstrate several nonoverlapping chromosomal gains, losses, and LOH events in PTC relative to FTC. Although the overall genomic profile of PTC is highly homogeneous with multiple recurrent alterations, individual cases vary significantly in their complement of chromosomal alterations. For example, several studies show that PTC in patients exposed to the Chernobyl accident contain unique breakpoints detectable on the chromosomal arms 4q, 5q, 6p, 10q, 12q, 13q, and 14q [80,81]. The global genomic analysis of PTC suggests a genetic explanation for its heterogeneous clinicopathologic profile and divergent clinicopathologic profile from FTC. Refinement of some of the involved chromosomal alterations, including cytogenetic breakpoints at 1q21, 10q11, and 7q, has delivered a functional explanation for their recurrent presence in PTC and sheds light on mechanisms involved in the association with prior radiation exposure [75].

Individual genetic events

RET rearrangement

Structural rearrangement of the chromosomal 10q11.2 locus is the most common chromosomal alteration in PTC, occurring in more than 30% of cases [18,82,83]. Cytogenetic analyses show the presence of balanced rear-rangements, including paracentric intrachromosomal inversions and inter-chromosomal translocations [83,84]. In 1987, the RTK, RET, was identified as the target of chromosomal 10q11.2 rearrangements in PTC [85]. The RET proto-oncogene codes for a transmembrane receptor that is essential for neuronal cell survival and differentiation [86]. Accordingly, it is expressed primarily in neural tissue and is crucial for normal neural development.

The RET protein contains three functional domains, including an extra-cellular ligand binding, a hydrophobic transmembrane, and an intracellular tyrosine kinase domain [86]. In normal cells, RET is activated by binding of one of four currently known ligands (glial-derived neurotrophic factor, neu-rturin, persephin, and artemin) to its extracellular portion [50]. On ligand binding, receptor dimerization results in tyrosine autophosphorylation of the intracellular receptor domain and activation of downstream signaling pathways through interaction with specific coreceptors.

In PTC with 10q11.2 rearrangement, RET is activated through fusion of its intracellular tyrosine kinase portion to a heterologous gene sequence containing dimerization motifs and an active promoter [87]. As a result, high levels of the chimeric protein, which is constitutively active through continuous dimerization and consequent autophosphorylation, are ex-pressed. Several different fusion partners are involved in the RET rearrange-ment, giving rise to approximately 11 different chimeric RET/PTC proteins (Table 4). Among these, RET/PTC1, RET/PTC2, and RET/PTC3 are the most common variants, accounting for 20% to 60% of cases [88]. Although the exact function of most RET-containing chimeric proteins is not known, some translocated genes have oncogenic activity. These include PRKAR1A (RET/PTC2), which is responsible for the thyroid tumor predisposing syn-drom Carney compleyx, and the H4 gene (RET/PTC1), which is fused to the

Table 4
Most common tyrosine kinase fusion genes in papillary thyroid cancer

Tyrosine kinase	Activating gene	Oncogene	Chromosomal location
RET	H4	RET/PTC1	10q21
	PRKAR1A	RET/PTC2	17q23-24
	ELE1	RET/PTC3; RET/PTC4	10q11.2
	RFG5	RET/PTC5	14q
	HTIF1	RET/PTC6	7q32-34
	RFG7	RET/PTC7	1p13
	Kinetin	RET/PTC8	14q22.1
	RFG8	RET/PTC9	18q21-22
NTRK1	TPM3	TRK	1q22
	TPR	TRK/T1, TRK/T2, TRK/T4	1q25
	TFG	TRK/T3	3q11-12
BRAF	AKAP9	BRAF-AKAP9	7q

tyrosine kinase gene platelet-derived growth factor receptor beta in atypical chronic myeloid leukemia with t(5;10)(q33;q22) [89,90].

Overall, the prevalence of RET/PTC rearrangement varies considerably due to geographic variation, genetic heterogeneity of PTC, and variation in detection methods [87,91–95]. Independent of these factors, RET/PTC frequency seems higher in patients who have a history of external beam radiation. For example, RET/PTC is detectable in nearly 80% of children exposed to the fallout from the Chernobyl disaster, especially those who had short latency periods for tumor occurrence after the exposure [96,97]. The high rate of RET/PTC formation and resultant thyroid tumorigenesis in patients who have radiation exposure has been attributed to the follicular cell–specific proximity of RET and its fusion genes in the nucleus facilitating aberrant end joining after simultaneous breakage of RET and a potential fusion partner [98]. These data are supported by the finding that ionizing radiation can cause RET/PTC formation in cultured thyroid tumor cells and transplanted human thyroid tissues in mice [99,100]. The large difference in RET/PTC between sporadic PTC and radiation-induced PTC, however, cannot be attributed entirely to this phenomenon, because RET/PTC also is detected at a higher rate in young PTC patients who do not have a history of radiation exposure relative to sporadic PTC in older patients (40%:70%) [95,101]. One potential explanation is that RET/PTC-positive PTC presents at an earlier age.

RET/PTC rearrangements may be considered an early event in thyroid carcinogenesis based on their high frequency in papillary thyroid microcarcinomas [102]. Several investigators also have identified the presence of RET/PTC rearrangement in Hashimoto's thyroiditis, suggesting that it may be an initiating event in carcinogenesis [103–105]. In vivo experiments support an initiating role for RET/PTC in PTC development, as ectopic expression of RET/PTC fusion constructs transform cultured NIH3T3 and thyroid cells with high efficiency [106–108]. Introduction of RET/PTC constructs in cultured cells leads to thyroid cell dedifferentiation with down-regulation of follicular cell–specific genes, such as those coding for thyroglobulin and sodium iodide symporter [109,110]. Moreover, transgenic mice carrying RET/PTC constructs develop PTC at a high rate [110]. RET/PTC rearrangement is not identified in FTA or FTC, supporting their divergent pathogenetic evolution. The finding that RET signaling is mediated through activation of oncogenic MAPK and PI3K cascades explains the transforming potential of constitutively active RET/PTC constructs [109,111–113]. The data show abrogation of RET/PTC-induced transformation in cells with inactivated intermediates of downstream signaling cascades. Expression studies show significant difference in expression profiles between RET/PTC-positive and -negative PTC, including genes involved in inflammatory and immune responses, cell proliferation, cell adhesion, and apoptosis, suggesting that the global functional effects of RET/PTC remain to be defined [114–117].

NTRK1 rearrangement

The second most common cytogenetic abnormality in PTC is 1q21 rearrangements, occurring in approximately 10% of cases [75]. The gene target of this aberration also is a RTK, including the NTRK1 gene [18]. NTRK1 is a transmembrane receptor for nerve growth factor, which regulates growth, differentiation, and apoptosis in the peripheral and central nerve system [118]. In normal cells, binding of nerve growth factor is required for receptor dimerization and consequent autophosphorylation of tyrosine residues and activation of downstream signaling pathways [118]. NTRK1 is constitutively activated in a manner highly reminiscent of RET activation, resulting from fusion of the intracellular NTRK1 tyrosine domain to dimerization motifs and active promotor-containing heterologous partner genes by balanced translocation and intrachromosomal inversions. Several different fusion genes are described, including TRK (TPM3 fusion), TRK-T1 (TPR fusion), TRK-T2 (TPR-variant fusion), and TRK-T3 (TFG fusion) (see Table 4) [18,119–121]. The capability of these genes to activate tyrosine kinase genes is not restricted to NTRK1. TPM3 and TFG are reported to fuse to ALK in anaplastic large cell lymphoma [121]. Also, TFG recently was identified as a novel fusion partner of NOR1 in extraskeletal myxoid chondrosarcoma [122]. Analogous to RET activation, ligand independent activity of the resultant chimeric NTRK1 protein is ensured by autophosphorylation of the TK domain on dimerization [18]. As the physiologic downstream pathways involved in mediation of NTRK1 signaling include the MAPK and PI3K pathways, constitutive activity observed in PTC has significant oncogenic potential [123]. This is confirmed by in vivo experiments demonstrating that transgenic mice containing the TRK-T1 gene develop PTC at a high rate [124].

BRAF mutation

As discussed previously, constitutive activation of the MAPK pathway is an important downstream target of RTK rearrangement in PTC. Evidence for the importance of MAPK activation in PTC is extended by the identification of activating point mutations in the BRAF gene in PTC, which occur in cases without tyrosine kinase rearrangements [125,126]. Point mutations in the BRAF gene at nucleotide 1799 resulting in a thymidine to adenine transversion is the predominant abnormality in PTC [127]. This results in a substitution of a valine to glutamate at residue 600 of the kinase domain of the BRAF protein (BRAF^{V600E}). The substitution disrupts autoinhibitory hydrophobic interactions between the ATP-binding site and the activating loop that maintain the dephosphorylated BRAF protein in an inactive conformation [127]. The resultant conformational change allows for novel interactions that keep the protein in a catalytically active conformation. The result is a constitutively active BRAF kinase and subsequent ERK activation. In the case of differentiated thyroid nodules, BRAF^{V600E} mutations occur exclusively in PTC [128]. BRAF^{V600E} mutations are the genetic alteration most common in PTC, present in approximately 45% of cases (see Table 2) [129]. In contrast to RET/PTC rearrangements and consistent with the mutual exclusivity of both aberrations, BRAF^{V600E} mutation seems to be restricted to adult PTC, with a low prevalence detected in childhood [130,131]. Also, radiation-induced PTC has a low prevalence of BRAF^{V600E} mutations [132–134]. Recent evidence suggests an alternative mechanism may activate BRAF in radiation-induced PTC involving a paracentric inversion of chromosome 7 that creates a fusion of BRAF kinase domain to the A-kinase anchor protein 9 (AKAP9) (see Table 4) [135]. The AKAP9-BRAF fusion is present in 11% of radiation-induced PTC but not in sporadic PTC. The AKAP9-BRAF fusion represents the third variant of intrachromosomal inversion that commonly is seen in radiation-induced PTC, in addition to RET/PTCs and TRKs. The predilection of paracentric inversions for radiation-induced thyroid carcinogenesis is not understood clearly. Balanced chromosomal rearrangements and resultant fusion oncogenes are rare in solid tumors except for those in tissues frequently subject to radiation-induced carcinogenesis, including the thyroid, salivary glands, and mesenchymal tissue [136,137]. Spatial proximity of the involved genes has been held responsible for the high rate of balanced rearrangements in thyroid gland malignancy and may prove relevant in the pathogenesis of sarcomas and salivary gland neoplasms [98,138,139].

BRAF^{V600E} mutations also are found in other tumor types, such as melanomas, colorectal cancers, and ovarian carcinomas, confirming its important role in oncogenesis [140–142]. Evidence suggests that BRAF activation is an early event in oncogenesis, with a prevalence of 85% in premalignant melanocytic nevi and 17% in thyroid microcarcinomas [142,143]. The importance of constitutive BRAF activation in oncogenesis is supported further by in vitro and in vivo work. BRAF^{V600E} and AKAP9-BRAF fusion constructs transform NIH3T3 cells in culture, and introduction of BRAF^{V600E}-positive cell lines into nude mice causes tumor formation [135,144]. Moreover, transgenic mice with thyroid-specific expression of BRAF^{V600E} develop PTC at high frequency [145].

Poorly differentiated and anaplastic carcinomas

Global genomic profile

Clinicopathologic evidence suggests that follicular cell–derived thyroid cancer represents a biologic continuum, progressing from highly curable well-differentiated thyroid cancer (WDTC) to the universally fatal ATC [2,146]. This is supported by the presence of a gradual loss of papillary and follicular growth patterns and simultaneous increase in the presence of mitoses, necroses, and nuclear pleomorphism, with progression from WDTC to PDTC and ATC (see Table 2). Moreover, residual foci of differentiated PTC/FTC are present in the majority of PDTC and ATC. In addition, histopathologic progression can be observed in successive recurrences of WDTC.

PDTC and ATC have a more complex genotype than WDTC, with chromosomal aberration present in 85% to 100% of cases, including multiple structural and numeric aberrations, marker chromosomes, double minute chromosomes, and homogeneously staining regions [18,75,147–150]. Comparative analysis demonstrates a stepwise increase, suggesting that several chromosomal alterations, including 5p, 5q, 8q, 19p, and 19q, and losses of 8 p and 22q are common to WDTC, PDTC, and ATC [151,152], suggesting they may be early events in carcinogenesis. As gains of 1p34–36, 6p21, 9q34, 17q25, and 20q and deletions of 1p11-31, 2q32-33, 4q11-13, 6q21, 11q, and 13q21-31 are uniquely present in PDTC and ATC [151,152], they may represent malignant progression and impart an aggressive phenotype. Consistent with their intermediate position, tall cell variant of PTC (TCV) contain many of the abnormalities present in PDTC and ATC [153]. Congruently, TCV have a higher rate of anaplastic transformation relative to WDTC (Ghossein RA, personal communication). Finally, several chromosomal alterations, including gain of 3p13-14 and 11q13 and loss of 5q11-31, are uniquely identifiable in ATC and may be markers of anaplastic transformation [151,152]. Although functional analysis to support the impact of the chromosomal observations is limited, one study validates their importance, showing that restoration of chromosome 11 deletions by microcell transfer inhibits ATC tumorigenicity in vitro [154]. The collected data suggest that increasing chromosomal instability is an underlying factor of thyroid cancer progression [151,152]. Factors promoting chromosomal instability remain ill defined but may be related to increase in alterations of genes involved in DNA repair and maintenance of genetic stability, including p53, β-catenin, and RAS (discussed later).

Individual genetic events

p53 pathway

Cells contain several pathways that limit cell proliferation and induce programmed cell death (apoptosis) in response to activation of oncogenic signals. The p53 gene codes for a nuclear transcription factor that plays a pivotal role in cellular protection against malignant transformation through its abilities to regulate the cell cycle and safeguard genomic integrity [155]. In case of endogenic or exogenic cellular or oncogenic stress, the p53 protein may induce cell cycle arrest to allow DNA repair or induce apoptosis through a cascade of downstream factors [156]. The critical role of p53 in oncogenesis is evident from the fact that it is mutated in approximately 40% to 50% of human malignancies [9]. When mutated, p53 cannot bind to its cognate DNA sequence, thereby disrupting transcription and expression of multiple downstream targets. Abrogation of p53 function also may be present in cells without p53 mutation. For example, a significant percentage of human tumors overexpress mouse double minute protein 2 (MDM2), a p53-binding protein that promotes ubiquitination-based degradation [157]. Another mechanism for p53 dysfunction involves the inactivation of p14^{ARF} gene within the CDKN2A locus at 9p21, which occurs through homozygous deletion, somatic mutation, or epigenetic silencing. As p14^{ARF} binds to MDM2 and promotes the rapid degradation of MDM2, its inactivation results in accumulation of MDM2 and decreased p53 activity [158,159].

Although p53 mutation rarely, if ever, is detected in WDTC, it is present in approximately 50% and 80% of PDTC and ATC, respectively [160]. Moreover, decrease in MDM2 expression along the progression axis is consistent with the inability of mutated p53 to induce MDM2 expression, as is present in normal cells [161]. In cases of ATC where immunohistochemical analysis detects evidence of p53 mutation, it is not present in the WDTC components of the same tumor [53,162]. The strongest evidence for the role of p53 in anaplastic progression of thyroid cancer comes from murine studies. Mice with thyroid-targeted expression of RET/PTC oncogene develop minimally invasive papillary carcinomas that do not metastasize. Crossbreeding of these mice into a p53$^{-/-}$ background leads to the development of rapidly growing poorly differentiated and anaplastic thyroid tumors [163].

β-catenin

β-catenin, a member of the *Wnt* signaling pathway, is a multifunctional protein involved in a variety of cellular functions, including cell adhesion and signal transduction [164]. In normal cells, *β-catenin* resides at the cytoplasmic surface of the cell membrane [165]. Under normal conditions, *β-catenin* levels are low in the cytosol because of the activity of a multiprotein destruction complex, including APC protein and Axin [166]. When Wnt protein binds to Frizzled receptors on the cell membrane, cytosolic *β-catenin* levels are increased and diverted to the nucleus, where it induces transcription of target genes involved in cell proliferation [166]. The importance of the *Wnt* signaling pathway in oncogenesis is evident by its targeted aberration in a large fraction of human tumors [166]. For example, in 80% of colorectal adenomas and carcinomas, aberrant *Wnt* signaling is mediated through APC mutations, resulting in high cytosolic *β-catenin* [167]. In the remainder of colorectal cancers and several other human tumor types, activating mutations in the *β-catenin* gene (CTNNB1) result in cytosolic stabilization of β-catenin protein and constitutive activation of downstream signaling [168]. The involvement of the *Wnt* signaling pathway in thyroid cancer is evident from the 100-fold increase in papillary thyroid carcinoma in patients who have Gardner's syndrome (germline APC mutations) [3]. Analysis of sporadic thyroid cancer shows a minority of PTC and ATC with APC or *axin* mutations [169]. Comparative analysis, however, shows a progressive increase in *CTNNB1* mutations and associated nuclear localization of *β-catenin* from WDTC (0%) to PDTC (25%/21%) and, finally, to ATC (66%/48%) [170,171]. These data suggests a role for *β-catenin* regulation in thyroid tumor progression.

Signaling pathways

Studies suggest that deregulation of MAPK and PI3K/AKT signaling pathways are involved in thyroid cancer progression. This is supported by an increasing rate of RAS mutations from WDTC (8%) to PDTC (55%) and, finally, to ATC (51%) [52]. Morphologic correlation indicates that BRAF mutations are found at a higher rate in TCV (> 90%) relative to classical PTC (40%) [126,128]. BRAF mutations also are present in PDTC (15%) and ATC (15%), although at lower frequency [129]. The lower frequency of BRAF mutations in these aggressive thyroid tumors may be explained by dilution of FTC-derived PDTC and ATC but this remains to be shown [172]. Mice with targeted expression of BRAF develop PTC that transforms rapidly into PDTC, representing the most convincing evidence of a role for MAPK deregulation in thyroid tumor progression [145]. Activation of the *PI3K-AKT* signaling pathway also increases along the progression axis with the highest rate of *PIK3CA* mutation, *PTEN* silencing, and *AKT* activation in ATC [68,173–176]. In contrast, *RET/PTC* and *NTRK1* mutations do not seem to predispose to anaplastic transformation, as they are present in low frequency in PDTC and ATC [18,53,177,178]. The combined data on molecular analysis suggest a thyroid cancer progression model (Fig. 2; see Fig. 1 and Table 2).

Other factors

The cancer genome is complex, with multiple factors contributing to cancer behavior. Epigenetic alterations play a fundamental role in the

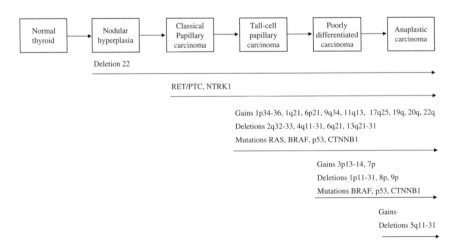

Fig. 2. Tumor progression model for PTC.

regulating gene expression [179]. Two key epigenetic mechanisms that are dysregulated progressively in thyroid cancers are DNA methylation and histone modifications [180,181]. DNA methylation results from a methyl group added to the cytosine residue in a CpG dinucleotide. Gene promoter methylation, particularly near a transcription start site, usually results in silencing of the gene [181]. Several important genes are subject to inactivation by methylation in thyroid cancers, including PTEN, *RASSF1A*, tissue inhibitor of metalloproteinase 3 (*TIMP3*), *SLC5A8*, death-associated protein kinase (*DAPK*), and retinoic acid receptor β2 (*RARβ2*), and are more common with aggressive histopathologic variants [182]. Similarly, other general oncogenic pathways effecting processes, such as angiogenesis, cell division, invasion, and metastasis, are increasingly active in PDTC and ATC, serving as putative progression markers and therapeutic targets [10,183–185].

Clinical value of genetic aberrations in thyroid cancer

Molecular diagnostics

Traditional cancer detection is based on histopathologic analysis and is limited by several factors, including tissue sampling and the subjective histologic definition of neoplasia with resultant interobserver variability, even between highly qualified pathologists. The identification of specific somatic molecular alterations in cancers and their earliest neoplastic precursors coupled with the development of highly sensitive molecular analytic techniques, such as the polymerase chain reaction (PCR), allow for highly accurate cancer diagnosis. In recent years, the emerging value of molecular markers is exemplified by routine use of molecular diagnostics to identify and stage hematologic malignancies and sarcomas [137,186,187]. Although lagging in solid tumors, several examples validate the use of molecular diagnostics. Screening for APC tumor suppressor gene mutations is an example, which can be identified in the stools of 60% of patients who have low-stage colon carcinoma, 50% of patients who have colorectal adenomas, and 0% of control patients who do not have colonic neoplasia [188]. Routine use of immunohistochemistry is another example applicable to thyroid cancers. Expression of thyroglobulin or calcitonin in questionable lesions is nearly pathonomic for the thyroid origin of a given cancer.

In the case of follicular cell–derived thyroid malignancy, fine needle aspiration cytology (FNAC) remains the gold standard for preoperative evaluation [189,190]. FNAC, however, yields an indeterminate specimen in 10% to 30% of cases and an inadequate result in another 5% to 10% of cases, resulting in potentially unnecessary thyroidectomy [190]. The surgical specimens in these cases harbor clinically relevant thyroid cancer in only a minority of cases [190]. In addition, a small rate of false-positive and -negative results adds to the insufficiency of FNAC as a selector for surgery. The specificity of genetic aberrations for thyroid malignancy promises to improve the morbidity and economic burden of inadequate diagnostic hemithyroidectomies significantly. In this context, the high sensitivity of PCR-based BRAF mutation analysis and its 100% specificity for PTC may improve the diagnostic accuracy of FNAC. Several retrospective studies looking at BRAF mutation detection of thyroid cancer in FNAB samples demonstrate a 100% specificity and sensitivity in cases of PTC carrying BRAF mutation [191–193]. Consistent with 50% of PTC having BRAF mutation, nearly half of patients who have PTC can be diagnosed preoperatively based on BRAF mutation analysis [127]. The data has been validated in prospective studies showing that FNAC-guided BRAF mutation detection is feasible economically and technically [127]. Analysis of BRAF mutation is likely to classify approximately 8% of indeterminate FNAB samples that represent PTC [127]. In addition, less-invasive BRAF detection in blood samples is under investigation with promising results [127].

Most significant improvement in the accuracy of FNAC is contingent on identification of reliable markers differentiating malignant from benign follicular thyroid tumors. Several studies have compared global gene expression signatures of follicular adenomas and follicular carcinomas using microarrays, showing significant differences [194–197]. Molecular classifiers were identified that distinguish FTC from follicular adenomas with a high specificity and sensitivity based on analysis of as few as 3 genes. Assessment of the identified molecular classifiers in FNAC specimens promises to improve diagnostic accuracy but remains to be validated.

Recent studies suggest that molecular analysis also may aid in the diagnosis of the follicular-variant PTC (FVPTC), which is contingent on the identification of classical nuclear features of PTC (optically clear nuclei and nuclear grooves/pseudoinclusions) in tumors with an entirely follicular growth pattern [55,198]. Traditionally, all thyroid tumors with an entirely follicular growth pattern were considered follicular adenomas or follicular carcinomas based on the presence or absence of capsular/vascular invasion, respectively [198]. The identification of PTC-type nuclear features in a subset of these tumors and analysis of their clinical behavior in short-term follow-up studies, however, justified their World Health Organization (WHO) reclassification as a PTC follicular variant in the early 1980s. Recently, molecular comparison of classical PTC, FVPTC, and follicular thyroid tumors demonstrated that FVPTC are characterized by a molecular composition equivalent to follicular thyroid tumors [17,199–202]. The genetic profile is characterized by a similar number and type of chromosomal alterations. Moreover, the common presence of RAS mutation and PPARγ rearrangement and absence of BRAF^{V600E} and RET/PTC mutations has generated calls for reclassification of FVPTC [17]. Recently, meticulous clinicomorphologic examination of a large cohort of FVPTC demonstrated that 20% are diffuse/infiltrative unencapsulated tumors and 80% of FVPTC are encapsulated tumors (70% of which were noninvasive) [198]. Encapsulated FVPTC developed lymph node metastasis in 5% of cases (equivalent to follicular carcinoma) compared with 65% in unencapsulated FVPTC (equivalent to classical PTC). Lymph node metastasis was not detected in encapsulated FVPTC without capsular/vascular invasion. Also, no recurrence was identified in patients who had noninvasive encapsulated FVPTC (versus one recurrence in a case of invasive encapsulated FVPTC). The genetic and clinicopathologic data suggest that encapsulated FVPTC belongs to the family of follicular thyroid tumors. The reclassification of FVPTC to FTC would have significant impact, as tumors without capsular/vascular invasion that currently are considered malignant would be reclassified as benign follicular adenomas, consistent with their clinical behavior.

Molecular staging

Variables that predict outcome of thyroid cancers include age greater than 45 years, histopathologic subtype, tumor size greater than 4 cm, extrathyroidal extension, and presence of distant metastases at presentation (Tables 5 and 6) [203,204]. Based on these clinicopathologic factors, individual cases of differentiated thyroid cancer may be assigned to low (99% survival), intermediate (85% survival), or high (42% survival) risk groups. WDTC, however, can manifest highly heterogeneous clinical behavior that is not predicted by the established clinicopathologic criteria. For example, several morphologic variants of WDTC are reported that are more aggressive clinically. TCV and Hürthle cell carcinomas are subtypes of PTC and FTC, respectively, that are associated with a poorer clinical outcome [205,206]. Although combining the morphologic analysis with clinicopathologic prognostic factors improves the overall categorization of patients who have thyroid cancer, it is accepted that overall staging can be improved by the addition of molecular markers.

To date, no markers are identified that meet the level of proof required for inclusion in the risk-group stratification of thyroid cancers but several markers show promise. The complement of chromosomal aberrations in thyroid cancer may have prognostic usefulness. As discussed previously, global genomic analysis of thyroid cancer has revealed several chromosomal alterations associated with PDTC and ATC. Data from Kitamura and

Table 5
Thyroid cancer staging at Memorial Sloan-Kettering Cancer Center

	Low risk	Intermediate risk		High risk
Patient age	<45 y	<45 y	>45 y	>45 y
Tumor size	<4.0 cm	>4.0 cm	<4.0 cm	>4.0 cm
Extrathyroidal extension	Absent	Present	Absent	Present
Distant metastases	Absent	Present	Absent	Present
High tumor grade	Absent	Present	Absent	Present

High tumor grade: poor tumor differentiation, Hürthle cell histology, tall cell histology.

Table 6
Prognostic factors used in different staging systems for differentiated thyroid cancer

	TNM	AGES	AMES	MACIS	MSKCC	EORTC
Patient age	+	+	+	+	+	+
Tumor size	+	+	+	+	+	+
Extrathyroidal extension	+	+	+	+	+	+
Distant metastasis	+	−	+	+	+	+
Tumor grade	−	+	−	−	+	+
Completeness of resection	−	−	−	+	−	−
Gender	−	−	−	−	−	−

Abbreviations: AGES, age, grade, extension, size; AMES, age, metastasis, extension, size; EORTC, European Organisation for Research and Treatment of Cancer; MACIS, metastasis, age, completeness of resection, invasion, size; MSKCC, Memorial Sloan-Kettering Cancer Center; TNM, tumor, node, metastasis; +, present; −, not present.

colleagues [207] suggest that these alterations can be present in WDTC and, when present, predict a poor prognostic outcome. The investigators compared the chromosomal profiles of 24 deceased patients who had PTC and 45 age- and gender-matched surviving controls (>10 years' follow-up). Clinical stage was not significantly different between the groups. Allelic instability at the chromosomal regions 1q, 4p, 7q, 9p, 9q, and 16q was associated with postoperative death due to PTC. Poor prognostic significance of 1q gain and 9q loss was confirmed by CGH analysis by Kjellman and colleagues [78]. The candidacy of 1q as a prognostic marker is strengthened by the identification of MUC1 as a putative amplification target [153]. A comparison of histopathologic subtypes of PTC revealed amplification and up-regulation of MUC1 is associated independently with outcome and is more frequent in TCV. Moreover, analysis of a clinicopathologically matched group of classical PTC with poor and favorable outcome showed that overexpression of *MUC1* predicts survival in PTC. Preclinical studies support the role of MUC1 in promoting an aggressive phenotype of PTC [208,209]. Current efforts include defining the usefulness of MUC1 as a therapeutic target.

In addition to chromosomal alterations, the prognostic usefulness of individual gene alterations associated with thyroid tumor progression is demonstrated, including *β-catenin*, BRAF, RAS, and p53 mutations. Garcia-Rostan and colleagues [52,170] found that *β-catenin* and RAS mutations are predictors of outcome in thyroid cancers, independent of all clinicopathologically predictors except histologic differentiation. Several studies have demonstrated that BRAF mutation also is an independent predictor of disease recurrence. Xing [127] found a cancer recurrence rate of 9% in BRAF-negative cases in contrast to 25% of BRAF-mutated cases. BRAF-mutated cancers also were associated with significantly lower rates of radioactive iodine avidity, likely resulting in the loss of expression of thyroid-specific genes, such as the iodine symporter gene [127,145]. Mutations in p53 are much more common in PDTC and ATC. As such, p53 mutations also predict overall outcome in thyroid cancers [53,55,210].

Molecular therapeutics

Traditional treatment of differentiated thyroid cancers includes surgery and postoperative radioactive iodine treatment. Approximately 90% of new cases are cured with this approach [203]. Surgery and radioactive iodine treatment also are effective in the treatment of local or distant recurrence, with a disease control rate of approximately 90% and 70%, respectively [211–213]. The response to these treatment modalities is significantly lower in the high-risk group thyroid cancer or histologically aggressive thyroid cancers (poorly differentiated, TCV, or Hürthle cell carcinomas), which often are associated with a decreased radioactive iodine uptake [205,206,214]. Although the application of external beam radiation therapy or chemotherapy may confer a survival benefit in some cases, a majority of patients succumb to the disease [215,216]. In addition, ATC are resistant to all forms of treatment and nearly universally fatal [216]. The development of novel therapeutic strategies is an important focus of thyroid cancer research. The identification of somatic molecular alterations specifically present in cancer cells holds a theoretic opportunity for targeted thyroid cancer treatment. Recently, hopes for identification of molecular treatment targets have been fueled by the high sensitivity of chronic leukemia and gastrointestinal stromal tumors with the tyrosine kinase gene alterations for the tyrosine kinase inhibitor, imatinib mesylate [217]. Also, a mutated tyrosine kinase gene EGFR recently was shown to confer sensitivity of non–small cell lung cancers to treatment with EGFR inhibitors, including agents such as gefinitib and erlotinib [218–220].

The common presence of constitutively active tyrosine kinase genes in thyroid cancer makes them logical candidates for targeted treatment. Recently, it was shown that the vandetanib (ZD6474, AstraZeneca), a tyrosine kinase inhibitor, blocks the enzymatic activity of RET-derived oncoproteins and inhibits tumor growth of RET/PTC-transformed NIH3T3 cells in nude mice [221,222]. In addition to RET inhibition, ZD6474 is an orally bioavailable inhibitor of EGFR and VEGF signaling pathways, both of which may be involved in many thyroid cancers [223]. Preclinical studies of ZD6474 have demonstrated antitumor efficacy against multiple human cancer xenograft models [224]. Phase I clinical trials demonstrate that ZD6474 is well tolerated with adverse events, including rash, diarrhea, and asymptomatic QTc prolongation [225,226]. Phase II clinical studies using vandetanib as monotherapy and in combination with docetaxel show promising results in non–small cell lung cancer [226,227]. A phase II trial has completed accrual looking at the efficacy of ZD6474 in unresectable familial modularly thyroid cancer, demonstrating clinical activity as reported by the American Society of Clinical Oncology in 2007 [228]. An international, randomized, placebo-controlled phase II trial of ZD6474 in medullary thyroid cancer is accruing patients. Given the high rates of activation of RET in papillary thyroid cancers, phase II trials using ZD6474 are planned [229]. Moreover, alternative RET inhibitors are under investigation, including pyrazolo-pyrimidine agents, PP1 and PP2 [230,231].

Downstream of RET, the association of MAPK signaling members, including RAS and BRAF, with aggressive thyroid cancer subtypes, includ-ing TCV, PDTC, and ATC, along with their independent prognostic value, makes them ideal subjects for targeted treatment. In vitro and in vivo stud-ies show that inhibition of oncogenic RAS and BRAF leads to tumor shrinkage in several human tumor types [232]. The multikinase inhibitor, BAY 43-9006 (Sorafenib, Bayer), is an effective inhibitor of BRAF and has been assessed in thyroid cancer. The agent inhibited thyroid cancer cell lines with BRAF mutation, including ATC xenografts in nude mice [184]. Sorafenib also inhibited growth of BRAF-negative–RET/PTC-positive thyroid cancer cell lines, likely a consequence of effects on MAPK signaling [127,233]. Cytostatic suppression of MEK signaling, fur-ther downstream along the MAPK cascade, was demonstrated with the agent CI-1040, resulting in tumor growth inhibition of BRAF-mutant xeno-grafts derived from various tumor types [233–235]. Inhibition of oncogenic RAS using farnesyl transferase inhibitors are effective against a variety of RAS-positive tumor types and are undergoing clinical trial in advanced thy-roid cancers [235–237]. RAS and BRAF inhibition results in redifferentia-tion with resultant re-expression of thyroid-specific genes, including the sodium-iodide symporter gene [238,239]. MAPK inhibition not only may inhibit tumor growth but also may restore radioactive iodine avidity in a sig-nificant proportion of dedifferentiated/advanced thyroid cancers.

In addition to MAPK signaling, studies have assessed the feasibility of PI3K-AKT inhibition and p53 targeting in thyroid cancer. Furuya and col-leagues [240] have demonstrated that treatment with LY294002, a potent PI3K inhibitor, inhibited thyroid tumor growth, reduced tumor cell prolif-eration, and decreased cell motility to block metastatic spread of thyroid tumors in a mouse model of FTC. In addition, treatment of thyroid cancer cells with the AKT inhibitor, KP372-1, suppressed AKT activity and cell proliferation and induced apoptosis in thyroid cancer cells [241].

The virtually exclusive presence of p53 mutation in aggressive thyroid cancer is a logical target for molecular therapy. In contrast to blocking the products of proto-oncogenes, re-establishment of tumor suppressor genes in all targeted cancer cells is a challenging undertaking. Thus far, re-establishment of p53 protein expression in thyroid cancer cells has been attempted using genetically modified viral vectors. One of these, agent ONYX-15, is an E1B-deleted adenovirus that replicates exclusively in p53-mutated cells [242]. ONYX-15 kills ATC cells in vitro and in vivo [243,244]. The data underscore the importance of the p53 pathway for sur-vival of aggressive thyroid cancers, but the agent is unlikely to make it to

Box 1. Ongoing clinical trials on molecular targetting of thyroid cancer at the National Cancer Institute

Phase II/III study of Combretastatin and Paclitaxel/Carboplatin in the Treatment of Anaplastic Thyroid Cancer OXC4T4-302

Phase I/II study of Vandetanib in Treating Young Patients With Medullary Thyroid Cancer NCI-07-C-0189

Phase II study of FR901228 in Treating Patients With Recurrent and/or Metastatic Thyroid Cancer That Has Not Responded to Radioactive Iodine MSKCC-04059

Phase II study of Rosiglitazone in Treating Patients With Locoregionally Extensive or Metastatic Thyroid Cancer UCSF-03201

Phase II study of Irinotecan in Patients With Metastatic or Inoperable Locoregional Medullary Thyroid Cancer JHOC-J0459

Phase II study of Bortezomib in Treating Patients With Metastatic Thyroid Cancer That Did Not Respond to Radioactive Iodine Therapy MDA-2004-0059

Phase II study of Sorafenib in Treating Patients With Advanced Anaplastic Thyroid Cancer CASE-5304

Phase II Trial Evaluating Gleevec in Patients With Anaplastic Thyroid Carcinoma UMCC 2003-044

Phase II study of Lenalidomide in Treating Patients With Metastatic Thyroid Cancer That Has Not Responded to Radioactive Iodine and Cannot Be Removed By Surgery UKMC-05-0701-F3R

Phase II study of Sunitinib Malate in Patients With Iodine I 131-Refractory, Unresectable Well-Differentiated Thyroid Cancer or Medullary Thyroid Cancer UCCRC-NCI-7735

Phase II study of Sorafenib in Treating Patients With Metastatic, Locally Advanced, or Recurrent Medullary Thyroid Cancer OSU-06054

Phase II study Of AG-013736 In Patients With Doxorubicin-Refractory Or Intolerant Thyroid Cancer A4061027

An efficacy phase II Study Comparing ZD6474 to Placebo in Medullary Thyroid Cancer D4200C00058

Phase II study of Sunitinib and Imaging Procedures in Treating Patients With Thyroid Cancer FHCRC-6494

Phase I study of NGR-TNF in Treating Patients With Advanced Solid Tumors EORTC-16041

Available at: www.cancer.gov/clinicaltrials/search.

clinical use because of issues of biologic availability. Clinical trials are underway to assess the viability of clinical practice strategies (described previously) (Box 1). In addition, continuous development of novel agents is anticipated to result in significant improvement of aggressive thyroid cancer treatment.

Summary

The common thread that links WDTC to PDTC and ATC is genetic composition. The progressive accumulation of genetic abnormalities serves as the nidus for progression and, once identified, may identify the Achilles heal of thyroid cancers. The completion of the Human Genome Project combined with the advent of novel genetic analytic tools has helped unravel the fibers that compose thyroid carcinogenesis [245]. Beyond basic biology, many of these identified genetic abnormalities have prognostic and therapeutic implications. As understanding continues to expand, there will be an increasing impact of genetics on diagnosis, prognostication, therapy, and, ultimately, patient outcome.

References

[1] Jemal A, Siegel R, Ward E, et al. Cancer statistics, 2007. CA Cancer J Clin 2007;57:43–66.
[2] Rosai J, Saxen EA, Woolner L. Undifferentiated and poorly differentiated carcinoma. Semin Diagn Pathol 1985;2:123–36.
[3] Perrier ND, van Heerden JA, Goellner JR, et al. Thyroid cancer in patients with familial adenomatous polyposis. World J Surg 1998;22:738–42 [discussion: 743].
[4] Eng C. PTEN: one gene, many syndromes. Hum Mutat 2003;22:183–98.
[5] Boikos SA, Stratakis CA. Carney complex: pathology and molecular genetics. Neuroendocrinology 2006;83:189–99.
[6] Ishikawa Y, Sugano H, Matsumoto T, et al. Unusual features of thyroid carcinomas in Japanese patients with Werner syndrome and possible genotype-phenotype relations to cell type and race. Cancer 1999;85:1345–52.
[7] Sippel RS, Caron NR, Clark OH. An evidence-based approach to familial nonmedullary thyroid cancer: screening, clinical management, and follow-up. World J Surg 2007;31: 924–33.
[8] Sturgeon C, Clark OH. Familial nonmedullary thyroid cancer. Thyroid 2005;15:588–93.
[9] Vogelstein B, Kinzler KW. Cancer genes and the pathways they control. Nat Med 2004;10: 789–99.
[10] Kondo T, Ezzat S, Asa SL. Pathogenetic mechanisms in thyroid follicular-cell neoplasia. Nat Rev Cancer 2006;6:292–306.
[11] Rodrigues R, Roque L, Espadinha C, et al. Comparative genomic hybridization, BRAF, RAS, RET, and oligo-array analysis in aneuploid papillary thyroid carcinomas. Oncol Rep 2007;18:917–26.
[12] Roque L, Rodrigues R, Pinto A, et al. Chromosome imbalances in thyroid follicular neoplasms: a comparison between follicular adenomas and carcinomas. Genes Chromosomes Cancer 2003;36:292–302.
[13] Tung WS, Shevlin DW, Kaleem Z, et al. Allelotype of follicular thyroid carcinomas reveals genetic instability consistent with frequent nondisjunctional chromosomal loss. Genes Chromosomes Cancer 1997;19:43–51.

[14] Kitamura Y, Shimizu K, Ito K, et al. Allelotyping of follicular thyroid carcinoma: frequent allelic losses in chromosome arms 7q, 11p, and 22q. J Clin Endocrinol Metab 2001;86: 4268–72.

[15] Zedenius J, Wallin G, Svensson A, et al. Allelotyping of follicular thyroid tumors. Hum Genet 1995;96:27–32.

[16] Castro P, Eknaes M, Teixeir MR, et al. Adenomas and follicular carcinomas of the thyroid display two major patterns of chromosomal changes. J Pathol 2005;206:305–11.

[17] Wreesmann VB, Ghossein RA, Hezel M, et al. Follicular variant of papillary thyroid carcinoma: genome-wide appraisal of a controversial entity. Genes Chromosomes Cancer 2004;40:355–64.

[18] Pierotti MA, Bongarzone I, Borello MG, et al. Cytogenetics and molecular genetics of carcinomas arising from thyroid epithelial follicular cells. Genes Chromosomes Cancer 1996;16:1–14.

[19] Herrmann M. Standard and molecular cytogenetics of endocrine tumors. Am J Clin Pathol 2003;119(Suppl):S17–38.

[20] Hemmer S, Wasenius VM, Knuutila S, et al. DNA copy number changes in thyroid carcinoma. Am J Pathol 1999;154:1539–47.

[21] Roque L, Clode A, Belge G, et al. Follicular thyroid carcinoma: chromosome analysis of 19 cases. Genes Chromosomes Cancer 1998;21:250–5.

[22] Belge G, Roque L, Soares J, et al. Cytogenetic investigations of 340 thyroid hyperplasias and adenomas revealing correlations between cytogenetic findings and histology. Cancer Genet Cytogenet 1998;101:42–8.

[23] Belge G, Roque L, Thode B, et al. [Cytogenetic changes in benign thyroid gland hyperplasias and adenomas correlated with histology]. Verh Dtsch Ges Pathol 1997;81:151–6.

[24] Roque L, Castedo S, Gomes P, et al. Cytogenetic findings in 18 follicular thyroid adenomas. Cancer Genet Cytogenet 1993;67:1–6.

[25] French CA, Alexander EK, Cibas ES, et al. Genetic and biological subgroups of low-stage follicular thyroid cancer. Am J Pathol 2003;162:1053–60.

[26] Kroll TG. Molecular events in follicular thyroid tumors. Cancer Treat Res 2004;122: 85–105.

[27] Kroll TG, Sarraf P, Pecciarini L, et al. PAX8-PPARgamma1 fusion oncogene in human thyroid carcinoma [corrected]. Science 2000;289:1357–60.

[28] Gurnell M, Chatterjee VK. Nuclear receptors in disease: thyroid receptor beta, peroxisome-proliferator-activated receptor gamma and orphan receptors. Essays Biochem 2004;40: 169–89.

[29] Vanden Heuvel JP. The PPAR resource page. Biochim Biophys Acta 2007;1771:1108–12.

[30] Hihi AK, Michalik L, Wahli W. PPARs: transcriptional effectors of fatty acids and their derivatives. Cell Mol Life Sci 2002;59:790–8.

[31] Marques AR, Espadinha C, Catarino AL, et al. Expression of PAX8-PPAR gamma 1 rearrangements in both follicular thyroid carcinomas and adenomas. J Clin Endocrinol Metab 2002;87:3947–52.

[32] Dwight T, Thoppe SR, Foukakis T, et al. Involvement of the PAX8/peroxisome proliferator-activated receptor gamma rearrangement in follicular thyroid tumors. J Clin Endocrinol Metab 2003;88:4440–5.

[33] Cheung L, Messina M, Gill A, et al. Detection of the PAX8-PPAR gamma fusion oncogene in both follicular thyroid carcinomas and adenomas. J Clin Endocrinol Metab 2003;88: 354–7.

[34] Marques AR, Espadinha C, Frias MJ, et al. Underexpression of peroxisome proliferator-activated receptor (PPAR)gamma in PAX8/PPARgamma-negative thyroid tumours. Br J Cancer 2004;91:732–8.

[35] Ehrmann J Jr, Vavrusova N, Collan Y, et al. Peroxisome proliferator-activated receptors (PPARs) in health and disease. Biomed Pap Med Fac Univ Palacky Olomouc Czech Repub 2002;146:11–4.

[36] Kim KY, Ahn JH, Cheon HG. Apoptotic action of peroxisome proliferator-activated receptor-gamma activation in human non small-cell lung cancer is mediated via proline oxidase-induced reactive oxygen species formation. Mol Pharmacol 2007;72:674–85.

[37] Han S, Roman J. Rosiglitazone suppresses human lung carcinoma cell growth through PPARgamma-dependent and PPARgamma-independent signal pathways. Mol Cancer Ther 2006;5:430–7.

[38] Li M, Lee TW, Yim AP, et al. Apoptosis induced by troglitazone is both peroxisome pro-liferator-activated receptor-gamma- and ERK-dependent in human non-small lung cancer cells. J Cell Physiol 2006;209:428–38.

[39] Keshamouni VG, Reddy RC, Arenberg DA, et al. Peroxisome proliferator-activated recep-tor-gamma activation inhibits tumor progression in non-small-cell lung cancer. Oncogene 2004;23:100–8.

[40] Govindarajan R, Ratnasinghe L, Simmons DL, et al. Thiazolidinediones and the risk of lung, prostate, and colon cancer in patients with diabetes. J Clin Oncol 2007;25:1476–81.

[41] Martelli ML, Iuliano R, Le Pera I, et al. Inhibitory effects of peroxisome poliferator-activated receptor gamma on thyroid carcinoma cell growth. J Clin Endocrinol Metab 2002;87:4728–35.

[42] Lui WO, Foukakis T, Liden J, et al. Expression profiling reveals a distinct transcription signature in follicular thyroid carcinomas with a PAX8-PPAR(gamma) fusion oncogene. Oncogene 2005;24:1467–76.

[43] Kato Y, Ying H, Zhao L, et al. PPARgamma insufficiency promotes follicular thyroid carcinogenesis via activation of the nuclear factor-kappaB signaling pathway. Oncogene 2006;25:2736–47.

[44] Giordano TJ, Au AY, Kuick R, et al. Delineation, functional validation, and bioinformatic evaluation of gene expression in thyroid follicular carcinomas with the PAX8-PPARG translocation. Clin Cancer Res 2006;12:1983–93.

[45] Roberts PJ, Der CJ. Targeting the Raf-MEK-ERK mitogen-activated protein kinase cascade for the treatment of cancer. Oncogene 2007;26:3291–310.

[46] Porter AC, Vaillancourt RR. Tyrosine kinase receptor-activated signal transduction path-ways which lead to oncogenesis. Oncogene 1998;17:1343–52.

[47] Giehl K. Oncogenic ras in tumour progression and metastasis. Biol Chem 2005;386:193–205.

[48] Nikiforova MN, Lynch RA, Biddinger PW, et al. RAS point mutations and PAX8-PPAR gamma rearrangement in thyroid tumors: evidence for distinct molecular pathways in thyroid follicular carcinoma. J Clin Endocrinol Metab 2003;88:2318–26.

[49] Nikiforov YE, Nikiforova MN, Gnepp DR, et al. Prevalence of mutations of ras and p53 in benign and malignant thyroid tumors from children exposed to radiation after the Chernobyl nuclear accident. Oncogene 1996;13:687–93.

[50] Suarez HG. Molecular basis of epithelial thyroid tumorigenesis. C R Acad Sci III 2000;323:519–28.

[51] Esapa CT, Johnson SJ, Kendall-Taylor P, et al. Prevalence of Ras mutations in thyroid neo-plasia. Clin Endocrinol (Oxf) 1999;50:529–35.

[52] Garcia-Rostan G, Zhao H, Camp RL, et al. ras mutations are associated with aggressive tumor phenotypes and poor prognosis in thyroid cancer. J Clin Oncol 2003;21:3226–35.

[53] Nikiforov YE. Genetic alterations involved in the transition from well-differentiated to poorly differentiated and anaplastic thyroid carcinomas. Endocr Pathol 2004;15:319–27.

[54] Vitagliano D, Portella G, Troncone G, et al. Thyroid targeting of the N-ras(Gln61Lys) oncogene in transgenic mice results in follicular tumors that progress to poorly differenti-ated carcinomas. Oncogene 2006;25:5467–74.

[55] DeLellis RA. Pathology and genetics of thyroid carcinoma. J Surg Oncol 2006;94:662–9.

[56] Puxeddu E, Moretti S, Elisei R, et al. BRAF(V599E) mutation is the leading genetic event in adult sporadic papillary thyroid carcinomas. J Clin Endocrinol Metab 2004;89:2414–20.

[57] Sansal I, Sellers WR. The biology and clinical relevance of the PTEN tumor suppressor pathway. J Clin Oncol 2004;22:2954–63.

[58] Waite KA, Eng C. Protean PTEN: form and function. Am J Hum Genet 2002;70:829–44.

[59] Singh B, Reddy PG, Goberdhan A, et al. p53 regulates cell survival by inhibiting PIK3CA in squamous cell carcinomas. Genes Dev 2002;16:984–93.

[60] Robertson GP. Functional and therapeutic significance of Akt deregulation in malignant melanoma. Cancer Metastasis Rev 2005;24:273–85.

[61] Kada F, Saji M, Ringel MD. Akt: a potential target for thyroid cancer therapy. Curr Drug Targets Immune Endocr Metabol Disord 2004;4:181–5.

[62] Ollikainen M, Gylling A, Puputti M, et al. Patterns of PIK3CA alterations in familial colorectal and endometrial carcinoma. Int J Cancer 2007;121:915–20.

[63] Chen Q, Wang C, Jiang C, et al. Exogenous PTEN gene induces apoptosis in breast carcinoma cell line MDA468. J Huazhong Univ Sci Technolog Med Sci 2007;27:61–4.

[64] Liaw D, Marsh DJ, Li J, et al. Germline mutations of the PTEN gene in Cowden disease, an inherited breast and thyroid cancer syndrome. Nat Genet 1997;16:64–7.

[65] Yeager N, Klein-Szanto A, Kimura S, et al. Pten loss in the mouse thyroid causes goiter and follicular adenomas: insights into thyroid function and Cowden disease pathogenesis- Cancer Res 2007;67:959–66.

[66] Chen ML, Xu PZ, Peng XD, et al. The deficiency of Akt1 is sufficient to suppress tumor development in Pten+/− mice. Genes Dev 2006;20:1569–74.

[67] Alvarez-Nunez F, Bussaglia E, Mauricio D, et al. PTEN promoter methylation in sporadic thyroid carcinomas. Thyroid 2006;16:17–23.

[68] Hou P, Liu D, Shan Y, et al. Genetic alterations and their relationship in the phosphatidy-linositol 3-kinase/Akt pathway in thyroid cancer. Clin Cancer Res 2007;13:1161–70.

[69] Gimm O, Perren A, Weng LP, et al. Differential nuclear and cytoplasmic expression of PTEN in normal thyroid tissue, and benign and malignant epithelial thyroid tumors. Am J Pathol 2000;156:1693–700.

[70] Eng C. The role of PTEN, a phosphatase gene, in inherited and sporadic nonmedullary thyroid tumors. Recent Prog Horm Res 1999;54:441–52 [discussion: 453].

[71] Halachmi N, Halachmi S, Evron E, et al. Somatic mutations of the PTEN tumor suppressor gene in sporadic follicular thyroid tumors. Genes Chromosomes Cancer 1998;23:239–43.

[72] Wang Y, Hou P, Yu H, et al. High prevalence and mutual exclusivity of genetic alterations in the phosphatidylinositol-3-kinase/akt pathway in thyroid tumors. J Clin Endocrinol Metab 2007;92:2387–90.

[73] Ringel MD, Hayre N, Saito J, et al. Overexpression and overactivation of Akt in thyroid carcinoma. Cancer Res 2001;61:6105–11.

[74] Vasko V, Saji M, Hardy E, et al. Akt activation and localisation correlate with tumour invasion and oncogene expression in thyroid cancer. J Med Genet 2004;41:161–70.

[75] Roque L, Nunes VM, Ribeiro C, et al. Karyotypic characterization of papillary thyroid carcinomas. Cancer 2001;92:2529–38.

[76] Roque L, Clode AL, Gomes P, et al. Cytogenetic findings in 31 papillary thyroid carcinomas. Genes Chromosomes Cancer 1995;13:157–62.

[77] Singh B, Lim D, Cigudosa JC, et al. Screening for genetic aberrations in papillary thyroid cancer by using comparative genomic hybridization. Surgery 2000;128:888–93 [discussion: 884–93].

[78] Kjellman P, Lagercrantz S, Hoog A, et al. Gain of 1q and loss of 9q21.3-q32 are associated with a less favorable prognosis in papillary thyroid carcinoma. Genes Chromosomes Cancer 2001;32:43–9.

[79] Califano JA, Johns MM 3rd, Westra WH, et al. An allelotype of papillary thyroid cancer. Int J Cancer 1996;69:442–4.

[80] Richter H, Braselmann H, Hieber L, et al. Chromosomal imbalances in post-chernobyl thyroid tumors. Thyroid 2004;14:1061–4.

[81] Zitzelsberger H, Lehmann L, Hieber L, et al. Cytogenetic changes in radiation-induced tumors of the thyroid. Cancer Res 1999;59:135–40.

[82] Pierotti MA. Chromosomal rearrangements in thyroid carcinomas: a recombination or death dilemma. Cancer Lett 2001;166:1–7.

[83] Pierotti MA, Santoro M, Jenkins RB, et al. Characterization of an inversion on the long arm of chromosome 10 juxtaposing D10S170 and RET and creating the oncogenic sequence RET/PTC. Proc Natl Acad Sci U S A 1992;89:1616–20.

[84] Sozzi G, Bongarzone I, Miozzo M, et al. A t(10;17) translocation creates the RET/PTC2 chimeric transforming sequence in papillary thyroid carcinoma. Genes Chromosomes Cancer 1994;9:244–50.

[85] Fusco A, Grieco M, Santoro M, et al. A new oncogene in human thyroid papillary carcinomas and their lymph-nodal metastases. Nature 1987;328:170–2.

[86] Arighi E, Borrello MG, Sariola H. RET tyrosine kinase signaling in development and cancer. Cytokine Growth Factor Rev 2005;16:441–67.

[87] Nikiforov YE. RET/PTC rearrangement in thyroid tumors. Endocr Pathol 2002;13: 3–16.

[88] Santoro M, Dathan NA, Berlingieri MT, et al. Molecular characterization of RET/PTC3; a novel rearranged version of the RETproto-oncogene in a human thyroid papillary carcinoma. Oncogene 1994;9:509–16.

[89] Boikos SA, Stratakis CA. Carney complex: the first 20 years. Curr Opin Oncol 2007;19: 24–9.

[90] Schwaller J, Anastasiadou E, Cain D, et al. D.G. H4(D10S170), a gene frequently rearranged in papillary thyroid carcinoma, is fused to the platelet-derived growth factor receptor beta gene in atypical chronic myeloid leukemia with t(5;10)(q33;q22). Blood 2001;97: 3910–8.

[91] Zhu Z, Ciampi R, Nikiforova MN, et al. Prevalence of RET/PTC rearrangements in thyroid papillary carcinomas: effects of the detection methods and genetic heterogeneity. J Clin Endocrinol Metab 2006;91:3603–10.

[92] Chung JH, Hahm JR, Min YK, et al. Detection of RET/PTC oncogene rearrangements in Korean papillary thyroid carcinomas. Thyroid 1999;9:1237–43.

[93] Delvincourt C, Patey M, Flament JB, et al. Ret and trk proto-oncogene activation in thyroid papillary carcinomas in French patients from the Champagne-Ardenne region. Clin Biochem 1996;29:267–71.

[94] Motomura T, Nikiforov YE, Namba H, et al. ret rearrangements in Japanese pediatric and adult papillary thyroid cancers. Thyroid 1998;8:485–9.

[95] Bongarzone I, Fugazzola L, Vigneri P, et al. Age-related activation of the tyrosine kinase receptor protooncogenes RET and NTRK1 in papillary thyroid carcinoma. J Clin Endocrinol Metab 1996;81:2006–9.

[96] Nikiforov YE. Radiation-induced thyroid cancer: what we have learned from chernobyl. Endocr Pathol 2006;17:307–17.

[97] Thomas GA, Bunnell H, Cook HA, et al. High prevalence of RET/PTC rearrangements in Ukrainian and Belarussian post-Chernobyl thyroid papillary carcinomas: a strong correlation between RET/PTC3 and the solid-follicular variant. J Clin Endocrinol Metab 1999;84: 4232–8.

[98] Nikiforova MN, Stringer JR, Blough R, et al. Proximity of chromosomal loci that participate in radiation-induced rearrangements in human cells. Science 2000;290: 138–41.

[99] Mizuno T, Iwamoto KS, Kyoizumi S, et al. Preferential induction of RET/PTC1 rearrangement by X-ray irradiation. Oncogene 2000;19:438–43.

[100] Caudill CM, Zhu Z, Ciampi R, et al. Dose-dependent generation of RET/PTC in human thyroid cells after in vitro exposure to gamma-radiation: a model of carcinogenic chromosomal rearrangement induced by ionizing radiation. J Clin Endocrinol Metab 2005;90: 2364–9.

[101] Fenton CL, Lukes Y, Nicholson D, et al. The ret/PTC mutations are common in sporadic papillary thyroid carcinoma of children and young adults. J Clin Endocrinol Metab 2000; 85:1170–5.

[102] Viglietto G, Chiappetta G, Martinez-Tello FJ, et al. RET/PTC oncogene activation is an early event in thyroid carcinogenesis. Oncogene 1995;11:1207–10.

[103] Nikiforov YE. RET/PTC Rearrangement—a link between Hashimoto's thyroiditis and thyroid cancer.or not. J Clin Endocrinol Metab 2006;91:2040–2.

[104] Nikiforova MN, Caudill CM, Biddinger P, et al. Prevalence of RET/PTC rearrangements in Hashimoto's thyroiditis and papillary thyroid carcinomas. Int J Surg Pathol 2002;10: 15–22.

[105] Arif S, Blanes A, Diaz-Cano SJ. Hashimoto's thyroiditis shares features with early papillary thyroid carcinoma. Histopathology 2002;41:357–62.

[106] Lanzi C, Cassinelli G, Pensa T, et al. Inhibition of transforming activity of the ret/ptc1 oncoprotein by a 2-indolinone derivative. Int J Cancer 2000;85:384–90.

[107] Borrello MG, Alberti L, Arighi E, et al. The full oncogenic activity of Ret/ptc2 depends on tyrosine 539, a docking site for phospholipase Cgamma. Mol Cell Biol 1996;16:2151–63.

[108] Durick K, Yao VJ, Borrello MG, et al. Tyrosines outside the kinase core and dimerization are required for the mitogenic activity of RET/ptc2. J Biol Chem 1995;270:24642–5.

[109] Knauf JA, Kuroda H, Basu S, et al. RET/PTC-induced dedifferentiation of thyroid cells is mediated through Y1062 signaling through SHC-RAS-MAP kinase. Oncogene 2003;22: 4406–12.

[110] Jhiang SM, Cho JY, Furminger TL, et al. Thyroid carcinomas in RET/PTC transgenic mice. Recent Results Cancer Res 1998;154:265–70.

[111] Miyagi E, Braga-Basaria M, Hardy E, et al. Chronic expression of RET/PTC 3 enhances basal and insulin-stimulated PI3 kinase/AKT signaling and increases IRS-2 expression in FRTL-5 thyroid cells. Mol Carcinog 2004;41:98–107.

[112] Ouyang B, Knauf JA, Smith EP, et al. Inhibitors of Raf kinase activity block growth of thyroid cancer cells with RET/PTC or BRAF mutations in vitro and in vivo. Clin Cancer Res 2006;12:1785–93.

[113] Mitsutake N, Miyagishi M, Mitsutake S, et al. BRAF mediates RET/PTC-induced mitogen-activated protein kinase activation in thyroid cells: functional support for requirement of the RET/PTC-RAS-BRAF pathway in papillary thyroid carcinogenesis. Endocrinology 2006;147:1014–9.

[114] Borrello MG, Alberti L, Fischer A, et al. Induction of a proinflammatory program in normal human thyrocytes by the RET/PTC1 oncogene. Proc Natl Acad Sci U S A 2005; 102:14825–30.

[115] Cahill S, Smyth P, Finn SP, et al. Effect of ret/PTC 1 rearrangement on transcription and post-transcriptional regulation in a papillary thyroid carcinoma model. Mol Cancer 2006;5:70.

[116] Puxeddu E, Knauf JA, Sartor MA, et al. RET/PTC-induced gene expression in thyroid PCCL3 cells reveals early activation of genes involved in regulation of the immune response. Endocr Relat Cancer 2005;12:319–34.

[117] Giordano TJ, Kuick R, Thomas DG, et al. Molecular classification of papillary thyroid carcinoma: distinct BRAF, RAS, and RET/PTC mutation-specific gene expression profiles discovered by DNA microarray analysis. Oncogene 2005;24:6646–56.

[118] Lamballe F, Klein R, Barbacid M. The trk family of oncogenes and neurotrophin receptors. Princess Takamatsu Symp 1991;22:153–70.

[119] Greco A, Miranda C, Pagliardini S, et al. Chromosome 1 rearrangements involving the genes TPR and NTRK1 produce structurally different thyroid-specific TRK oncogenes. Genes Chromosomes Cancer 1997;19:112–23.

[120] Mencinger M, Panagopoulos I, Andreasson P, et al. Characterization and chromosomal mapping of the human TFG gene involved in thyroid carcinoma. Genomics 1997;41: 327–31.

[121] Lamant L, Dastugue N, Pulford K, et al. A new fusion gene TPM3-ALK in anaplastic large cell lymphoma created by a (1;2)(q25;p23) translocation. Blood 1999;93:3088–95.

[122] Hisaoka M, Ishida T, Imamura T, et al. TFG is a novel fusion partner of NOR1 in extra-skeletal myxoid chondrosarcoma. Genes Chromosomes Cancer 2004;40:325–8.

[123] Alberti L, Carniti C, Miranda C, et al. RET and NTRK1 proto-oncogenes in human diseases. J Cell Physiol 2003;195:168–86.

[124] Russell JP, Powell DJ, Cunnane M, et al. The TRK-T1 fusion protein induces neoplastic transformation of thyroid epithelium. Oncogene 2000;19:5729–35.

[125] Soares P, Trovisco V, Rocha AS, et al. BRAF mutations and RET/PTC rearrangements are alternative events in the etiopathogenesis of PTC. Oncogene 2003;22:4578–80.

[126] Kimura ET, Nikiforova MN, Zhu Z, et al. High prevalence of BRAF mutations in thyroid cancer: genetic evidence for constitutive activation of the RET/PTC-RAS-BRAF signaling pathway in papillary thyroid carcinoma. Cancer Res 2003;63:1454–7.

[127] Xing M. BRAF mutation in thyroid cancer. Endocr Relat Cancer 2005;12:245–62.

[128] Nikiforova MN, Kimura ET, Gandhi M, et al. BRAF mutations in thyroid tumors are restricted to papillary carcinomas and anaplastic or poorly differentiated carcinomas arising from papillary carcinomas. J Clin Endocrinol Metab 2003;88:5399–404.

[129] Ciampi R, Nikiforov YE. Alterations of the BRAF gene in thyroid tumors. Endocr Pathol 2005;16:163–72.

[130] Penko K, Livezey J, Fenton C, et al. BRAF mutations are uncommon in papillary thyroid cancer of young patients. Thyroid 2005;15:320–5.

[131] Kumagai A, Namba H, Saenko VA, et al. Low frequency of BRAFT1796A mutations in childhood thyroid carcinomas. J Clin Endocrinol Metab 2004;89:4280–4.

[132] Nikiforova MN, Ciampi R, Salvatore G, et al. Low prevalence of BRAF mutations in radiation-induced thyroid tumors in contrast to sporadic papillary carcinomas. Cancer Lett 2004;209:1–6.

[133] Lima J, Trovisco V, Soares P, et al. BRAF mutations are not a major event in post-Chernobyl childhood thyroid carcinomas. J Clin Endocrinol Metab 2004;89:4267–71.

[134] Collins BJ, Schneider AB, Prinz RA, et al. Low frequency of BRAF mutations in adult patients with papillary thyroid cancers following childhood radiation exposure. Thyroid 2006;16:61–6.

[135] Ciampi R, Knauf JA, Kerler R, et al. Oncogenic AKAP9-BRAF fusion is a novel mechanism of MAPK pathway activation in thyroid cancer. J Clin Invest 2005;115:94–101.

[136] Teixeira MR. Recurrent fusion oncogenes in carcinomas. Crit Rev Oncog 2006;12:257–71.

[137] Aman P. Fusion genes in solid tumors. Semin Cancer Biol 1999;9:303–18.

[138] Roccato E, Bressan P, Sabatella G, et al. Proximity of TPR and NTRK1 rearranging loci in human thyrocytes. Cancer Res 2005;65:2572–6.

[139] Nikiforov YE. Spatial positioning of RET and H4 following radiation exposure leads to tumor development. ScientificWorldJournal 2001;1:186–7.

[140] Yuen ST, Davies H, Chan TL, et al. Similarity of the phenotypic patterns associated with BRAF and KRAS mutations in colorectal neoplasia. Cancer Res 2002;62:6451–5.

[141] Sieben NL, Macropoulos P, Roemen GM, et al. In ovarian neoplasms, BRAF, but not KRAS, mutations are restricted to low-grade serous tumours. J Pathol 2004;202:336–40.

[142] Fecher LA, Cummings SD, Keefe MJ, et al. Toward a molecular classification of melanoma. J Clin Oncol 2007;25:1606–20.

[143] Ugolini C, Giannini R, Lupi C, et al. Presence of BRAF V600E in very early stages of papillary thyroid carcinoma. Thyroid 2007;17:381–8.

[144] Liu D, Liu Z, Condouris S, et al. BRAF V600E maintains proliferation, transformation, and tumorigenicity of BRAF-mutant papillary thyroid cancer cells. J Clin Endocrinol Metab 2007;92:2264–71.

[145] Knauf JA, Ma X, Smith EP, et al. Targeted expression of BRAFV600E in thyroid cells of transgenic mice results in papillary thyroid cancers that undergo dedifferentiation. Cancer Res 2005;65:4238–45.

[146] Volante M, Collini P, Nikiforov YE, et al. Poorly differentiated thyroid carcinoma: the Turin proposal for the use of uniform diagnostic criteria and an algorithmic diagnostic approach. Am J Surg Pathol 2007;31:1256–64.

[147] Roque L, Soares J, Castedo S. Cytogenetic and fluorescence in situ hybridization studies in a case of anaplastic thyroid carcinoma. Cancer Genet Cytogenet 1998;103:7–10.

[148] Mark J, Ekedahl C, Dahlenfors R, et al. Cytogenetical observations in five human anaplastic thyroid carcinomas. Hereditas 1987;107:163–74.

[149] Jenkins RB, Hay ID, Herath JF, et al. Frequent occurrence of cytogenetic abnormalities in sporadic nonmedullary thyroid carcinoma. Cancer 1990;66:1213–20.

[150] Rodrigues RF, Roque L, Krug T, et al. Poorly differentiated and anaplastic thyroid carcinomas: chromosomal and oligo-array profile of five new cell lines. Br J Cancer 2007;96: 1237–45.

[151] Wreesmann VB, Ghossein RA, Patel SG, et al. Genome-wide appraisal of thyroid cancer progression. Am J Pathol 2002;161:1549–56.

[152] Rodrigues RF, Roque L, Rosa-Santos J, et al. Chromosomal imbalances associated with anaplastic transformation of follicular thyroid carcinomas. Br J Cancer 2004;90:492–6.

[153] Wreesmann VB, Sieczka EM, Socci ND, et al. Genome-wide profiling of papillary thyroid cancer identifies MUC1 as an independent prognostic marker. Cancer Res 2004; 64:3780–9.

[154] Yoshida A, Asaga T, Masuzawa C, et al. Alteration of tumorigenicity in undifferentiated thyroid carcinoma cells by introduction of normal chromosome 11. J Surg Oncol 1994; 55:170–4.

[155] Hollstein M, Sidransky D, Vogelstein B, et al. p53 mutations in human cancers. Science 1991;253:49–53.

[156] Vogelstein B, Kinzler KW. p53 function and dysfunction. Cell 1992;70:523–6.

[157] Freedman DA, Wu L, Levine AJ. Functions of the MDM2 oncoprotein. Cell Mol Life Sci 1999;55:96–107.

[158] Jin S, Levine AJ. The p53 functional circuit. J Cell Sci 2001;114:4139–40.

[159] Tao W, Levine AJ. P19(ARF) stabilizes p53 by blocking nucleo-cytoplasmic shuttling of Mdm2. Proc Natl Acad Sci U S A 1999;96:6937–41.

[160] Donghi R, Longoni A, Pilotti S, et al. Gene p53 mutations are restricted to poorly differentiated and undifferentiated carcinomas of the thyroid gland. J Clin Invest 1993;91:1753–60.

[161] Saltman B, Singh B, Hedvat CV, et al. Patterns of expression of cell cycle/apoptosis genes along the spectrum of thyroid carcinoma progression. Surgery 2006;140:899–905 [discussion: 896–905].

[162] Matias-Guiu X, Villanueva A, Cuatrecasas M, et al. p53 in a thyroid follicular carcinoma with foci of poorly differentiated and anaplastic carcinoma. Pathol Res Pract 1996;192: 1242–9 [discussion: 1241–50].

[163] La Perle KM, Jhiang SM, Capen CC. Loss of p53 promotes anaplasia and local invasion in ret/PTC1-induced thyroid carcinomas. Am J Pathol 2000;157:671–7.

[164] Mulholland DJ, Dedhar S, Coetzee GA, et al. Interaction of nuclear receptors with the Wnt/beta-catenin/Tcf signaling axis: Wnt you like to know? Endocr Rev 2005;26:898–915.

[165] Van Aken E, De Wever O, Correia da Rocha AS, et al. Defective E-cadherin/catenin complexes in human cancer. Virchows Arch 2001;439:725–51.

[166] Bullions LC, Levine AJ. The role of beta-catenin in cell adhesion, signal transduction, and cancer. Curr Opin Oncol 1998;10:81–7.

[167] Sparks AB, Morin PJ, Vogelstein B, et al. Mutational analysis of the APC/beta-catenin/Tcf pathway in colorectal cancer. Cancer Res 1998;58:1130–4.

[168] Morin PJ, Sparks AB, Korinek V, et al. Activation of beta-catenin-Tcf signaling in colon cancer by mutations in beta-catenin or APC. Science 1997;275:1787–90.

[169] Kurihara T, Ikeda S, Ishizaki Y, et al. Immunohistochemical and sequencing analyses of the Wnt signaling components in Japanese anaplastic thyroid cancers. Thyroid 2004;14: 1020–9.

[170] Garcia-Rostan G, Camp RL, Herrero A, et al. Beta-catenin dysregulation in thyroid neoplasms: down-regulation, aberrant nuclear expression, and CTNNB1 exon 3 mutations are markers for aggressive tumor phenotypes and poor prognosis. Am J Pathol 2001;158: 987–96.

[171] Garcia-Rostan G, Tallini G, Herrero A, et al. Frequent mutation and nuclear localization of beta-catenin in anaplastic thyroid carcinoma. Cancer Res 1999;59:1811–5.

[172] Wang HM, Huang YW, Huang JS, et al. Anaplastic carcinoma of the thyroid arising more often from follicular carcinoma than papillary carcinoma. Ann Surg Oncol 2007;14:3011–8.

[173] Garcia-Rostan G, Costa AM, Pereira-Castro I, et al. Mutation of the PIK3CA gene in anaplastic thyroid cancer. Cancer Res 2005;65:10199–207.

[174] Wu G, Mambo E, Guo Z, et al. Uncommon mutation, but common amplifications, of the PIK3CA gene in thyroid tumors. J Clin Endocrinol Metab 2005;90:4688–93.

[175] Frisk T, Foukakis T, Dwight T, et al. Silencing of the PTEN tumor-suppressor gene in anaplastic thyroid cancer. Genes Chromosomes Cancer 2002;35:74–80.

[176] Dahia PL, Marsh DJ, Zheng Z, et al. Somatic deletions and mutations in the Cowden disease gene, PTEN, in sporadic thyroid tumors. Cancer Res 1997;57:4710–3.

[177] Bongarzone I, Vigneri P, Mariani L, et al. RET/NTRK1 rearrangements in thyroid gland tumors of the papillary carcinoma family: correlation with clinicopathological features. Clin Cancer Res 1998;4:223–8.

[178] Tallini G, Santoro M, Helie M, et al. RET/PTC oncogene activation defines a subset of papillary thyroid carcinomas lacking evidence of progression to poorly differentiated or undifferentiated tumor phenotypes. Clin Cancer Res 1998;4:287–94.

[179] Xing M. Gene methylation in thyroid tumorigenesis. Endocrinology 2007;148:948–53.

[180] Greenberg VL, Williams JM, Cogswell JP, et al. Histone deacetylase inhibitors promote apoptosis and differential cell cycle arrest in anaplastic thyroid cancer cells. Thyroid 2001;11:315–25.

[181] Yoo CB, Jones PA. Epigenetic therapy of cancer: past, present and future. Nat Rev Drug Discov 2006;5:37–50.

[182] Hoque MO, Rosenbaum E, Westra WH, et al. Quantitative assessment of promoter methylation profiles in thyroid neoplasms. J Clin Endocrinol Metab 2005;90:4011–8.

[183] Bunone G, Vigneri P, Mariani L, et al. Expression of angiogenesis stimulators and inhibitors in human thyroid tumors and correlation with clinical pathological features. Am J Pathol 1999;155:1967–76.

[184] Kim S, Yazici YD, Calzada G, et al. Sorafenib inhibits the angiogenesis and growth of orthotopic anaplastic thyroid carcinoma xenografts in nude mice. Mol Cancer Ther 2007;6:1785–92.

[185] Wang Z, Chakravarty G, Kim S, et al. Growth-inhibitory effects of human anti-insulin-like growth factor-I receptor antibody (A12) in an orthotopic nude mouse model of anaplastic thyroid carcinoma. Clin Cancer Res 2006;12:4755–65.

[186] Gray JW, Kallioniemi A, Kallioniemi O, et al. Molecular cytogenetics: diagnosis and prognostic assessment. Curr Opin Biotechnol 1992;3:623–31.

[187] Tkachuk DC, Westbrook CA, Andreeff M, et al. Detection of bcr-abl fusion in chronic myelogeneous leukemia by in situ hybridization. Science 1990;250:559–62.

[188] Traverso G, Shuber A, Levin B, et al. Detection of APC mutations in fecal DNA from patients with colorectal tumors. N Engl J Med 2002;346:311–20.

[189] Shaha AR, DiMaio T, Webber C, et al. Intraoperative decision making during thyroid surgery based on the results of preoperative needle biopsy and frozen section. Surgery 1990; 108:964–7 [discussion: 961–70].

[190] Shaha AR. Controversies in the management of thyroid nodule. Laryngoscope 2000;110: 183–93.

[191] Cohen Y, Rosenbaum E, Clark DP, et al. Mutational analysis of BRAF in fine needle aspiration biopsies of the thyroid: a potential application for the preoperative assessment of thyroid nodules. Clin Cancer Res 2004;10:2761–5.

[192] Kumagai A, Namba H, Akanov Z, et al. Clinical implications of pre-operative rapid BRAF analysis for papillary thyroid cancer. Endocr J 2007;54:399–405.

[193] Chung KW, Yang SK, Lee GK, et al. Detection of BRAFV600E mutation on fine needle aspiration specimens of thyroid nodule refines cyto-pathology diagnosis, especially in BRAF600E mutation-prevalent area. Clin Endocrinol (Oxf) 2006;65:660–6.

[194] Finley DJ, Zhu B, Barden CB, et al. 3rd Discrimination of benign and malignant thyroid nodules by molecular profiling. Ann Surg 2004;240:425–36 [discussion: 427–36].

[195] Weber F, Shen L, Aldred MA, et al. Genetic classification of benign and malignant thyroid follicular neoplasia based on a three-gene combination. J Clin Endocrinol Metab 2005;90: 2512–21.

[196] Fryknas M, Wickenberg-Bolin U, Goransson H, et al. Molecular markers for discrimination of benign and malignant follicular thyroid tumors. Tumour Biol 2006;27:211–20.

[197] Lubitz CC, Gallagher LA, Finley DJ, et al. 3rd Molecular analysis of minimally invasive follicular carcinomas by gene profiling. Surgery 2005;138:1042–8 [discussion: 1048–49].

[198] Liu J, Singh B, Tallini G, et al. Follicular variant of papillary thyroid carcinoma: a clinico-pathologic study of a problematic entity. Cancer 2006;107:1255–64.

[199] Di Cristofaro J, Marcy M, Vasko V, et al. Molecular genetic study comparing follicular variant versus classic papillary thyroid carcinomas: association of N-ras mutation in codon 61 with follicular variant. Hum Pathol 2006;37:824–30.

[200] Zhu Z, Gandhi M, Nikiforova MN, et al. Molecular profile and clinical-pathologic features of the follicular variant of papillary thyroid carcinoma. An unusually high prevalence of ras mutations. Am J Clin Pathol 2003;120:71–7.

[201] Castro P, Rebocho AP, Soares RJ, et al. PAX8-PPARgamma rearrangement is frequently detected in the follicular variant of papillary thyroid carcinoma. J Clin Endocrinol Metab 2006;91:213–20.

[202] Castro P, Roque L, Magalhaes J, et al. A subset of the follicular variant of papillary thyroid carcinoma harbors the PAX8-PPARgamma translocation. Int J Surg Pathol 2005;13: 235–8.

[203] Shaha A. Treatment of thyroid cancer based on risk groups. J Surg Oncol 2006;94:683–91.

[204] Shaha AR, Shah JP, Loree TR. Risk group stratification and prognostic factors in papillary carcinoma of thyroid. Ann Surg Oncol 1996;3:534–8.

[205] Ghossein RA, Leboeuf R, Patel KN, et al. Tall cell variant of papillary thyroid carcinoma without extrathyroid extension: biologic behavior and clinical implications. Thyroid 2007; 17:655–61.

[206] Stojadinovic A, Hoos A, Ghossein RA, et al. Hurthle cell carcinoma: a 60-year experience. Ann Surg Oncol 2002;9:197–203.

[207] Kitamura Y, Shimizu K, Tanaka S, et al. Association of allelic loss on 1q, 4p, 7q, 9p, 9q, and 16q with postoperative death in papillary thyroid carcinoma. Clin Cancer Res 2000;6: 1819–25.

[208] Siragusa M, Zerilli M, Iovino F, et al. MUC1 oncoprotein promotes refractoriness to chemotherapy in thyroid cancer cells. Cancer Res 2007;67:5522–30.

[209] Patel KN, Maghami E, Wreesmann VB, et al. MUC1 plays a role in tumor maintenance in aggressive thyroid carcinomas. Surgery 2005;138:994–1001 [discussion: 1001–2].

[210] Farid NR. P53 mutations in thyroid carcinoma: tidings from an old foe. J Endocrinol Invest 2001;24:536–45.

[211] Shoup M, Stojadinovic A, Nissan A, et al. Prognostic indicators of outcomes in patients with distant metastases from differentiated thyroid carcinoma. J Am Coll Surg 2003;197: 191–7.

[212] Shaha AR, Ferlito A, Rinaldo A. Distant metastases from thyroid and parathyroid cancer. ORL J Otorhinolaryngol Relat Spec 2001;63:243–9.

[213] Stojadinovic A, Shoup M, Nissan A, et al. Recurrent differentiated thyroid carcinoma: biological implications of age, method of detection, and site and extent of recurrence. Ann Surg Oncol 2002;9:789–98.

[214] Hiltzik D, Carlson DL, Tuttle RM, et al. Poorly differentiated thyroid carcinomas defined on the basis of mitosis and necrosis: a clinicopathologic study of 58 patients. Cancer 2006; 106:1286–95.

[215] Patel KN, Shaha AR. Locally advanced thyroid cancer. Curr Opin Otolaryngol Head Neck Surg 2005;13:112–6.

[216] Patel KN, Shaha AR. Poorly differentiated and anaplastic thyroid cancer. Cancer Control 2006;13:119–28.

[217] Jones RL, Judson IR. The development and application of imatinib. Expert Opin Drug Saf 2005;4:183–91.

[218] Riely GJ, Politi KA, Miller VA, et al. Update on epidermal growth factor receptor mutations in non-small cell lung cancer. Clin Cancer Res 2006;12:7232–41.

[219] Pao W. Defining clinically relevant molecular subsets of lung cancer. Cancer Chemother Pharmacol 2006;58(Suppl 1):s11–5.

[220] Manegold C. Gefitinib (Iressa, ZD 1839) for non-small cell lung cancer (NSCLC): recents results and further strategies. Adv Exp Med Biol 2003;532:247–52.

[221] Vidal M, Wells S, Ryan A, et al. ZD6474 suppresses oncogenic RET isoforms in a Drosophila model for type 2 multiple endocrine neoplasia syndromes and papillary thyroid carcinoma. Cancer Res 2005;65:3538–41.

[222] Carlomagno F, Vitagliano D, Guida T, et al. ZD6474, an orally available inhibitor of KDR tyrosine kinase activity, efficiently blocks oncogenic RET kinases. Cancer Res 2002;62: 7284–90.

[223] Hoffmann S, Glaser S, Wunderlich A, et al. Targeting the EGF/VEGF-R system by tyrosine-kinase inhibitors–a novel antiproliferative/antiangiogenic strategy in thyroid cancer. Langenbecks Arch Surg 2006;391:589–96.

[224] Herbst RS, Heymach JV, O'Reilly MS, et al. Vandetanib (ZD6474): an orally available receptor tyrosine kinase inhibitor that selectively targets pathways critical for tumor growth and angiogenesis. Expert Opin Investig Drugs 2007;16:239–49.

[225] Tamura T, Minami H, Yamada Y, et al. A phase I dose-escalation study of ZD6474 in Japanese patients with solid, malignant tumors. J Thorac Oncol 2006;1:1002–9.

[226] Heymach JV. ZD6474–clinical experience to date. Br J Cancer 2005;92(Suppl 1):S14–20.

[227] Lee D. Phase II data with ZD6474, a small-molecule kinase inhibitor of epidermal growth factor receptor and vascular endothelial growth factor receptor, in previously treated advanced non-small-cell lung cancer. Clin Lung Cancer 2005;7:89–91.

[228] Wells S. A phase II trial of ZD6474 in patients with hereditary metastatic medullary thyroid cancer [abstract 5533]. Proceedings of the American Society of Clinical Oncology; 2006.

[229] ZD6474 headed for phase III trials in the fall. Oncology (Williston Park) 2005;19:1140–2.

[230] Carlomagno F, Santoro M. Identification of RET kinase inhibitors as potential new treatment for sporadic and inherited thyroid cancer. J Chemother 2004;16(Suppl 4):49–51.

[231] Carlomagno F, Guida T, Anaganti S, et al. Disease associated mutations at valine 804 in the RET receptor tyrosine kinase confer resistance to selective kinase inhibitors. Oncogene 2004;23:6056–63.

[232] Gollob JA, Wilhelm S, Carter C, et al. Role of Raf kinase in cancer: therapeutic potential of targeting the Raf/MEK/ERK signal transduction pathway. Semin Oncol 2006;33:392–406.

[233] Ji H, Wang Z, Perera SA, et al. Mutations in BRAF and KRAS converge on activation of the mitogen-activated protein kinase pathway in lung cancer mouse models. Cancer Res 2007;67:4933–9.

[234] Pohl G, Ho CL, Kurman RJ, et al. Inactivation of the mitogen-activated protein kinase pathway as a potential target-based therapy in ovarian serous tumors with KRAS or BRAF mutations. Cancer Res 2005;65:1994–2000.

[235] Xiong HQ. Molecular targeting therapy for pancreatic cancer. Cancer Chemother Pharmacol 2004;54(Suppl 1):S69–77.

[236] Johnson BE, Heymach JV. Farnesyl transferase inhibitors for patients with lung cancer. Clin Cancer Res 2004;10:4254s–7s.

[237] Braga-Basaria M, Ringel MD. Clinical review 158: Beyond radioiodine: a review of potential new therapeutic approaches for thyroid cancer. J Clin Endocrinol Metab 2003;88: 1947–60.

[238] Durante C, Puxeddu E, Ferretti E, et al. BRAF mutations in papillary thyroid carcinomas inhibit genes involved in iodine metabolism. J Clin Endocrinol Metab 2007;92:2840–3.

[239] Riesco-Eizaguirre G, Gutierrez-Martinez P, Garcia-Cabezas MA, et al. The oncogene BRAF V600E is associated with a high risk of recurrence and less differentiated papillary thyroid carcinoma due to the impairment of Na+/I- targeting to the membrane. Endocr Relat Cancer 2006;13:257–69.

[240] Furuya F, Lu C, Willingham MC, et al. Inhibition of phosphatidylinositol 3' kinase delays tumor progression and blocks metastatic spread in a mouse model of thyroid cancer. Carcinogenesis 2007.

[241] Mandal M, Kim S, Younes MN, et al. The Akt inhibitor KP372-1 suppresses Akt activity and cell proliferation and induces apoptosis in thyroid cancer cells. Br J Cancer 2005;92: 1899–905.

[242] Nemunaitis J, Ganly I, Khuri F, et al. Selective replication and oncolysis in p53 mutant tumors with ONYX-015, an E1B-55kD gene-deleted adenovirus, in patients with advanced head and neck cancer: a phase II trial. Cancer Res 2000;60:6359–66.

[243] Portella G, Pacelli R, Libertini S, et al. ONYX-015 enhances radiation-induced death of human anaplastic thyroid carcinoma cells. J Clin Endocrinol Metab 2003;88:5027–32.

[244] Portella G, Scala S, Vitagliano D, et al. ONYX-015, an E1B gene-defective adenovirus, induces cell death in human anaplastic thyroid carcinoma cell lines. J Clin Endocrinol Metab 2002;87:2525–31.

[245] Lander ES, Weinberg RA. Genomics: journey to the center of biology. Science 2000;287: 1777–82.

ELSEVIER
SAUNDERS

Surg Oncol Clin N Am
17 (2008) 37–56

SURGICAL
ONCOLOGY CLINICS
OF NORTH AMERICA

Evaluation and Imaging of a Thyroid Nodule

Marc D. Coltrera, MD

Department of Otolaryngology-Head and Neck Surgery, University of Washington,
1959 NE Pacific Street, Seattle, WA 98195, USA

The approach to the thyroid nodule has been incrementally modified over the past decade. The widespread adoption of fine needle aspiration (FNA) in the 1980s, coupled with increased use of serial ultrasound monitoring, arguably led to the biggest changes in recommendations for surgical intervention during the past 50 years. For the office-based practitioner, thyroid nodule presentation patterns are changing with discoveries of more thyroid "incidentalomas" and with new risk-assessment challenges associated with small (<1 cm) nodules. At the same time, improved primary evaluation techniques, most notably the increasing use of small, portable ultrasound imaging units, are making many clinicians more comfortable in recommending less-invasive follow-up.

This article reviews the current thinking regarding the *de novo* thyroid nodule workup. The article is not intended to be an exhaustive review, but rather a focused, practical manual for the workup of the thyroid nodule in the office. The main focus in evaluating a newly discovered thyroid nodule is to weigh the risk of malignancy. The general algorithm is outlined in Fig. 1. During this process, other issues pertaining to thyroid disease status are evaluated and a more benign, but no less important, diagnosis may be made. However, the most common benign diagnoses, such as Hashimoto's thyroiditis and multinodular goiter, do not exclude malignancy, so the clinician's primary focus remains on the task of ruling out malignancy.

For the initial evaluation of the thyroid nodule, many experts rely largely on minimal laboratory tests, ultrasound evaluation, and FNA. The author shares this view and believes that the widespread adoption of routine ultrasound evaluation of the neck in the office setting will solidify this approach in the next decade. The algorithm outlined in Fig. 1 relies on use of ultrasound early in the process. Statistics and incidence figures are presented in

E-mail address: coltrera@u.washington.edu

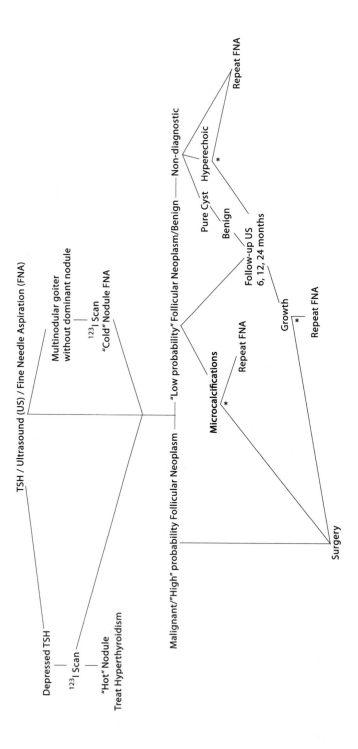

Fig. 1. Algorithm for the initial workup of the thyroid nodule incorporating early use of office-based ultrasound. [123]I, iodine 123; TSH, thyroid stimulating hormone.

this article mainly to support the current recommendations. While there have been some changes, many of the recommendations remain similar to those already published in the North American Clinics series and in other publications. Suggested readings for additional information are provided.

General considerations, including risk factors

Thyroid nodules are commonly found in the general population. Based on long-term, large-cohort health studies, such as the Framingham, Massachusetts, series, it is estimated that 4% to 8% of the general population have palpable thyroid nodules [1,2]. While it is expected that palpation is routinely capable of detecting nodules down to 1 cm, the most common palpable thyroid nodules are first noted when they are 1.5 cm or larger [2]. Over the years, the incidence of thyroid malignancies has been widely quoted as approximately 5% of all thyroid nodules [2,3]. However, this number has typically been derived from palpation-based studies where the bias has been for larger nodules and for growing nodules. Ultrasound studies have been able to demonstrate the presence of smaller nodules down to 0.4 cm in up to 46% of those surveyed [1,4,5]. If all persons with thyroid nodules of any size or history are considered, the overall risk of clinically significant malignancy is probably less. When deciding how aggressively to work up newly discovered thyroid nodules, the clinician must consider the risk factors.

Historical risk factors are a starting point in evaluating a new patient, although the majority of thyroid cancer patients lack a known historical risk factor. The most commonly cited historical risk factors for thyroid malignancies are listed in Box 1. A complete patient history should include questions designed to cover these issues. Radiation exposure is the greatest single risk factor. Studies of children in the United States exposed to external beam radiation for acne and adenoidal reduction have found increased rates of thyroid cancer five to eight times those of the general population [6]. Children exposed in the Ukraine following the Chernobyl nuclear reactor explosion have rates approaching 30 times those of the general population [7]. Most of the nonfamilial, nonsyndromic risk factors have a low correlation with malignant progression and some, such as low-iodine diet, are almost unheard of in the United States [3].

The role of age as a risk factor for thyroid cancer can be confusing. Age features prominently in the staging system for well-differentiated papillary or follicular thyroid cancers (Box 2). The break point in the staging system is placed at 45 years of age. That is, older patients with well-differentiated thyroid cancers have a greater risk of aggressive cancers, with higher risks of recurrence and significant impacts on survival. However, all other risk factors being equal, the older patient with a thyroid nodule does not appear to have a significantly increased risk of having a thyroid cancer until over the age of 70 [3,8]. This is consistent with autopsy data demonstrating

---

Box 1. Risk factors for thyroid malignancies

Historical risk factors
    Low-iodine diet
    Radiation exposure
    Family history
        Multiple endocrine neoplasia
        Gardner syndrome
        Familial polyposis
        Cowden disease
    Recent history of rapid growth
    Age <20 or >70 years old
Physical examination risk factors
    Fixation to skin, surrounding musculature
    Very firm or hard nodules
    Associated neck nodes
    Large nodules (>4 cm)
    True vocal cord fixation
    Persistent diarrhea (medullary carcinoma)
Incidental MRI/CT scan examination risk factors
    Extracapsular spread
    Unilateral lymph node enlargement
    Calcification within a lymph node

---

a high rate of incidental microscopic papillary carcinomas that increases with age at time of death [9]. While thyroid cancer does not always shorten a person's life span, the likelihood of having thyroid cancer increases with age.

Physical findings associated with increased risk of malignancy are limited to signs of gross extracapsular spread and metastases (see Box 1), findings that thankfully are infrequent in *de novo* thyroid nodule evaluations. The so-called "classic" red flag physical finding is true vocal cord paralysis. However, this finding by itself can be of limited help in assessing malignant potential [10,11]. The three main causes of unilateral vocal cord paralysis can be broadly categorized as iatrogenic, malignant, and idiopathic. Reviews of unilateral vocal cord paralysis quote figures for malignancy ranging from 7% to 52% with the vast majority due to lung cancer [10,11]. If lung cancer is excluded, all other malignancies, including thyroid cancer, represent well under 10% of unilateral vocal cord paralysis. In contrast, idiopathic causes account for 30% to 40% of vocal cord paralysis cases. Considering the 46% chance of finding a thyroid nodule on an ultrasound examination in the general population, it is two to three times more likely that the demonstrated nodule will be incidental to the vocal cord paralysis

Box 2. American Joint Committee on Cancer staging system for well-differentiated papillary or follicular thyroid cancer, 6th edition, 2002

Younger than 45 years
    Stage I
        Any T, any N, M0
    Stage II
        Any T, any N, M1
Age 45 years and older
    Stage I
        T1, N0, M0
    Stage II
        T2, N0, M0
    Stage III
        T3, N0, M0
        T1, N1a, M0
        T2, N1a, M0
        T3, N1a, M0
    Stage IVA
        T4a, N0, M0
        T4a, N1a, M0
        T1, N1b, M0
        T2, N1b, M0
        T3, N1b, M0
        T4a, N1b, M0
    Stage IVB
        T4b, any N, M0
    Stage IVC
        Any T, any N, M1

Values: MX, presence of distant metastasis (spread) cannot be assessed; M0, no distant metastasis; M1, distant metastasis is present, involving nonregional lymph nodes, internal organs, bones, etc; NX: regional (nearby) lymph nodes cannot be assessed; N0, no regional lymph node spread; N1, spread to lymph nodes; N1a, spread to lymph nodes in the neck (cervical lymph nodes); N1b, spread to lymph nodes in the upper chest (upper mediastinal lymph nodes); TX, Primary tumor cannot be assessed; T0, no evidence of primary tumor; T1, tumor is 2 cm or smaller; T2, tumor is between 2 cm and 4 cm; T3, tumor is larger than 4 cm or has begun to grow into nearby tissues outside the thyroid; T4a, tumor of any size and has grown extensively beyond the thyroid gland into nearby tissues of the neck; T4b, tumor has grown either back toward the spine or into nearby large blood vessels.

Data from American Joint Committee on Cancer. AJCC cancer staging manual, 6th edition. New York: Springer; 2002. p. 78.

[4,5]. Imaging is very important for demonstrating the proximity of the nodule in question to the recurrent laryngeal nerve and for evaluating evidence of extracapsular spread. The greater value of imaging compared with the physical examination is further underscored by the high likelihood that physical examination alone will miss smaller nodules located deep within the neck near the recurrent laryngeal nerve.

Risk factors and the "incidentaloma"

The increasing use of imaging modalities, such as CT, MRI, and positron emission tomography (PET) scans, has resulted in a general increase in the incidental discovery of thyroid nodules [12,13]. So called "life scans," general survey scans in an otherwise well patient, have burgeoned in the past decade. At the same time, use of CT, MRI, and PET scans has increased in the routine follow-up of patients after cancer treatment. A not uncommon scenario is the incidental finding of a thyroid nodule on a chest CT scan obtained during breast cancer follow-up. This is inevitable when routine thyroid ultrasound can detect nodules in up to 50% of the general population [4,5].

PET scanning has been increasingly used in cancer follow-up because of the focal metabolic activity exhibited by recurrent cancers. Though anecdotal reports exist, the finding of a metabolically active thyroid nodule on PET scan does not clearly indicate a malignancy nor does the lack of metabolic activity obviate the need for an ultrasound evaluation. The overlap in the metabolic rates of benign and malignant thyroid nodules is too great. In a recent study of 7347 PET scans, incidental thyroid focality was demonstrated in 79 patients (1.1%) [13]. Of these 79 patients, 48 had long-term follow-up with definitive diagnosis of benign disease in 31 and malignancy in 15. The differences in mean standardized uptake values were not significant. In the benign lesions, the mean standardized uptake value was 5.6 (range 2.5–53), compared with 6.4 (range 3.5–16) in the malignant lesions.

Once the "incidentaloma" nodule is detected, evaluation is no different from other thyroid nodule evaluations. Because many "incidentalomas" are not palpable, ultrasound-guided FNA must be employed from the outset. Studies have shown that the incidence of malignancy in nonpalpable nodules is similar to that for palpable nodules [14,15]. This poses a potential dilemma if the "incidentaloma" is small (<1 cm) or difficult to biopsy. If an ultrasound-guided FNA is not considered indicated or feasible at the time of initial presentation, the nodule should be followed with serial ultrasounds and checked for growth. If it grows, FNA should be performed when possible or surgical excision entertained, depending on risk factors.

Laboratory tests

Standard laboratory tests employed during thyroid workups include those for thyroid stimulating hormone (TSH), triiodothyronine (T_3), thyroxine (T_4), thyroglobulin, calcitonin and the antithyroid antibody tests including thyroid peroxidase antibodies and microsomal antibodies. Tests for elevated thyroglobulin are useful in monitoring for thyroid cancer recurrence. However, elevated thyroglobulin is much more commonly seen in benign inflammatory conditions [16]. Likewise triiodothyronine, thyroxine, and the antithyroid antibody tests are useful in establishing benign diagnoses, such as Hashimoto's and Grave's Disease. But none of these diagnoses definitively rule out malignancy. Conversely, the majority of thyroid cancer patients are euthyroid with no abnormal thyroid tests [2]. Routine ordering of most thyroid tests in the workup of the new thyroid nodule is not well justified.

The single most useful test essential for all thyroid nodule workups is a third-generation TSH test [2,16,17]. The TSH test uncovers existing hypothyroidism and hyperthyroidism. While a diagnosis of hypothyroidism does not rule out malignancy, it does suggest an alternative hypothesis for recent nodule growth. Then additional testing to diagnose several benign thyroid conditions may be obtained. On the other hand, hyperthyroidism due to a hyperfunctional nodule is the only laboratory diagnosis that significantly lowers the risk of malignancy. A suppressed TSH level should be followed up with a nuclear medicine scan to evaluate the functional status of the thyroid nodule (See the section on the changing role of radioisotope imaging).

Aside from the TSH test, the calcitonin test is the only other laboratory test that by itself can be useful in the diagnosis of thyroid malignancy [18]. Calcitonin elevation strongly correlates with the diagnosis of medullary carcinoma and its associated premalignant lesion, C-cell hyperplasia. Routine calcitonin measurement as part of a thyroid nodule workup is not typically recommended because of the relative rarity of medullary carcinoma. It is frequently obtained after a suspicious FNA or when a definitive pathology specimen is examined. Arguments have been made that calcitonin should be routinely obtained because of its specificity, but the clinical effectiveness and cost-effectiveness of this are questionable [19]. The clinician should obtain a calcitonin level in cases with family history of multiple endocrine neoplasia or familial medullary carcinoma as well as for patients who present with a history of diarrhea or have an appropriately suspicious FNA.

Ultrasound and fine needle aspiration

Complete evaluation of the thyroid nodule in the twenty-first century requires the use of both high-resolution ultrasound and FNA [3,12]. Use of ultrasound early in the workup has been found to change the clinical management in up to two thirds of cases [20]. Even so, FNA is still considered the single most useful evaluation method for a thyroid nodule [19]. The widespread use of FNA has resulted in a 50% reduction in the number of thyroidectomies being performed for questions of malignancy while doubling the percentage of cancers found within the surgical specimens [21]. Since most thyroid nodules come to the attention of the clinician because they are palpable, ultrasound evaluation is usually postponed until after the FNA is first attempted. This approach is changing.

General indications for the use of ultrasound-guided FNA are listed in Box 3. While FNA can be performed with significant success on the palpable nodule by tactile methods alone, a number of studies have shown that the routine use of ultrasound-guided FNA decreases the percentage of inadequate specimens while sensitivity and specificity either increase or remain similar (Fig. 2) [22–24]. Takashima and colleagues [22] looked at 210 patients who underwent an ultrasound-guided FNA for 268 nodules. Palpation-guided FNA was performed on a subset of 62 of these nodules. Nondiagnostic specimens were obtained on 3% (10 of 268) of the ultrasound-guided FNAs and 12 of 62 (19%) of the palpation-guided FNAs. Thirty-four of the cases that were surgically excised had been evaluated by both methods. Comparing those cases with adequate specimens, sensitivity was 88% for the palpation group and 96% for the ultrasound group, while specificity was 90% and 91% respectively. In one of the largest series to date, Danese and colleagues [23] included 9683 consecutive patients with 4986 FNAs performed by palpation and 4697 performed with ultrasound guidance using the same cytologist. The percentage of inadequate specimens was 8.7% in the palpation group and 3.5% in the ultrasound-guided group despite an increased number of mixed cystic-solid lesions in the ultrasound-guided group. Other studies looking at smaller palpable nodules (<2 cm) have found significantly improved sensitivity and specificity for the ultrasound-guided specimens, implying an increased misplacement of the needles in the palpation-guided specimens.

An ultrasound-guided FNA adds modestly to the overall cost of the workup and has the potential to decrease the number of repeat procedures while increasing diagnostic yields. With the advent of affordable, portable high-resolution ultrasound units, the standard of care is evolving toward the routine use of ultrasound-guided FNA in the office at the beginning of the workup. The typical portable ultrasound machine useful in an office setting costs between $20,000 and $50,000 in 2007 dollars (Fig. 3). The biggest determinant of price other than the quality of the basic unit is the

---

Box 3. Ultrasound-guided fine needle aspiration indications

Complex nodules (mixed cystic-solid)
Nonpalpable nodules
Ill-defined palpable nodules
Small palpable nodules (<1.5 cm)
Multinodular goiter
Repeat FNA following nondiagnostic specimen
Adjacent vascular structures

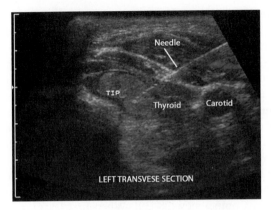

Fig. 2. FNA under ultrasound guidance can decrease the number of nondiagnostic specimens while increasing sensitivity and specificity. Ultrasound guidance can also be useful for avoiding vascular structures.

number and type of transducers included. Several units with adequate resolution are available for less, but lack additional features, such as printers or DVD storage required for clinical documentation if the procedures are to be billed. In addition to manufacturers' claims regarding the affordability of the units, several recent analyses by physicians have demonstrated the cost-effectiveness of incorporating portable ultrasonography into real-world medical practices [25].

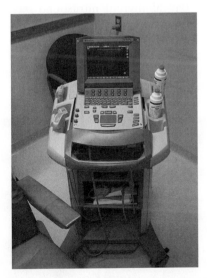

Fig. 3. Example of portable ultrasound unit used in the office setting. Along with the basic unit, one or more transducers and a recording device (eg, printer or DVD recorder) should be included.

In the United States, the main impediment to routine use of office-based ultrasound by nonradiologists has been the lack of formal residency or fellowship training in it. This has already changed most notably for obstetrics gynecology residencies and endocrinology fellowships [26,27]. For endocrine surgeons trained in general surgery or otolaryngology programs, the most common route to obtaining ultrasound competency is through one of the recognized courses offered by the American College of Surgeons, the American Academy of Otolaryngology–Head and Neck Surgery, or the American Association of Clinical Endocrinologists. Having completed the course, a mentorship with an established ultrasonographer needs to be established. Studies of the learning curve for focused examinations, such as the thyroid examination, have generally demonstrated the need for 50 to 75 comparison cases to establish competency [28–30]. When first learning ultrasound, it is instructive to compare portable ultrasound results on patients who are also undergoing high-resolution scans in the radiology suite. Even after gaining ample experience in the use of ultrasound, the author finds it useful to continue to make these comparisons. In the *de novo* evaluation of a thyroid nodule, a radiologist performing a diagnostic ultrasound and an ultrasound-guided FNA procedure will mean billing in two *Current Procedural Terminology* code groups (76536, 76942/10022). Under these circumstances it is cost-neutral and an effective use of a patient's time to perform an ultrasound-guided FNA on the patient's first visit in the office while later obtaining a formal high-resolution scan for complete diagnostic evaluation after the results of the FNA are available. The two scans and their documented images form the basis of an on-going educational process for the clinician.

Performance of a typical thyroid ultrasound includes scanning in the transverse and sagittal planes. By convention, orientation in the transverse plane places the patient's right side on the left side of the image (Fig. 4). This is similar to positioning for traditional plain radiographs, such as chest radiographs, and axial plane CT scans. In the sagittal plane, the rostral

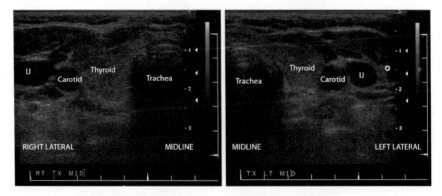

Fig. 4. Transverse ultrasound section. IJ, internal jugular.

direction is to the left and caudal to the right (Fig. 5). For ultrasound of neck structures, the most useful transducer frequencies range from 7 MHz to 13 MHz. The higher frequencies result in greater resolution, which is necessary to detect small structures, such as normal parathyroids [31]. However depth of penetration decreases markedly as the frequency increases, which requires compromise and the use of a lower frequency to adequately evaluate deep structures in a thick neck.

Ultrasound is based on reflectance of sound energy. B-scale ultrasound, the most common type employed in the clinic setting, constructs a two-dimensional image based on the time the reflected wave takes to return to the transducer and the amount of reflected sound energy (see Figs. 4 and 5) [31]. Both of these characteristics are relative measures and must be compared with some standard.

The longer the time required for the sound energy to return, the farther away the object is. To calculate the distance to an object, one needs to know the speed of sound and the time it took for the sound energy to travel through the medium:

$$\text{Distance} = \text{time} \times \text{speed} \div 2$$

The formula includes the factor 2 because the time measured is actually the time it takes for the sound wave to travel to the object and return, twice the actual distance. The speed of sound varies depending on the medium through which it is traveling (Table 1) [31]. To calculate distances, ultrasound machines use an average speed for soft tissues, typically 1540 m/s. The average speed of sound employed is very close to the speed for tissues encountered in the neck, resulting in accurate measurements. Likewise consistent use of this average speed allows for accurate comparisons to be made between serial ultrasound studies.

In B-scale ultrasonography, the greater the reflected energy, the brighter the object appears. The relative amount of reflectance is typically described

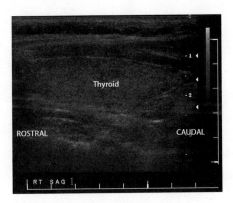

Fig. 5. Sagittal ultrasound section.

Table 1
Speed of sound in commonly encountered media

Medium	Speed (m/s)
Air	330
Fat	1450
Water	1480
Soft tissue average (see text)	1540
Liver	1550
Kidney	1560
Blood	1570
Muscle	1580
Bone	4080

in comparison to another object. The terms used include hypoechoic (less than), isoechoic (equal to) or hyperechoic (greater than). It is standard practice to compare thyroid nodules with adjacent thyroid tissue (Fig. 6). The term anechoic is reserved for objects with no reflectance. The lumens of blood vessels, such as the carotid, are typically anechoic.

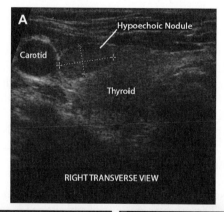

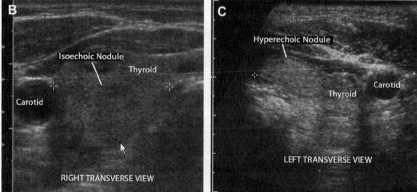

Fig. 6. Examples of hypoechoic (*A*), isoechoic (*B*), and hyperechoic (*C*) thyroid nodules. The nodule echogenecity is expressed relative to the adjacent thyroid tissue.

A standard thyroid ultrasound examination should begin by measuring the length (L), width (W), and depth (D) in centimeters of the individual lobes at their maximal points. The volume or equivalent weight in grams (mass) for each lobe can then be calculated from one of the standard formulas:

$$Mass = 4.9D + 0.07L^2W - 2.3$$

Knowing the volume of the thyroid can be useful when making relative comparisons of nodule growth on subsequent ultrasounds. Individual nodules should be measured in three dimensions and their characteristics noted for future comparison.

While ultrasound findings alone cannot be considered definitive with regard to assessing malignant potential, a number of useful findings are associated with higher or lower risk (Box 4, Fig. 7) [12,14,32,33]. The findings are complementary when coupled with FNA. Three ultrasound findings have significant predictive value by themselves. Purely cystic nodules with thin rims are not associated with malignancy while hyperechoic nodules have only a 2% risk. Conversely, the finding of microcalcifications has a high positive predictive value for malignancy (42%–94%). Microcalcifications are seen on real-time ultrasound as a "starry sky" effect where the small calcified particles wink in and out as the transducer is moved. The effect is usually easy to discern, which increases its diagnostic utility.

CT and MRI scans

Compared with ultrasound, CT and MRI scans are less sensitive for initial detection of thyroid nodules. The most suspicious findings, extracapsular

---

Box 4. Ultrasound findings and correlations with malignancy

Benign associations
  Purely cystic nodules
  Hyperechoic nodules
  Sharp margination
  Coarse calcification
  Halos
  Peripheral vascularity
Malignant associations
  Microcalcifications
  Hypoechoic nodules
  Irregular margins
  Intranodule vascularity
  Extraglandular extension

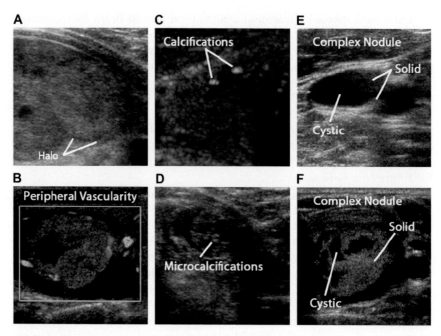

Fig. 7. Typical findings noted on thyroid ultrasound. Halos (*A*) and peripheral vascularity (*B*) are more common in benign nodules. Coarse calcifications (*C*) tend to be associated with benign lesions while microcalcifications (*D*) ("starry sky" effect seen with transducer movements) have a strong association with malignant nodules. Complex cystic and solid nodules (*E* and *F*) come in a wide range of varieties. Placement of the FNA needle within the solid component can be facilitated by ultrasound guidance, decreasing the likelihood of a nondiagnostic specimen.

spread and enlarged lymph nodes with or without calcifications, can be amply demonstrated by high-resolution, real-time ultrasound with one exception. Detection of extracapsular spread deep within a thick neck may be difficult for ultrasound because of the trade-offs between sound penetration and resolution. In the case of mixed cystic and solid structures, ultrasound provides superior resolution and can also be used to ensure proper sampling by FNA (see Figs. 2 and 7 [*E* and *F*]). Calcifications found on CT scan tend to be of the coarse variety more associated with benign than malignant changes (Fig. 8) while microcalcifications, associated with malignancy, are frequently too small to register [32,34]. MRI misses calcifications altogether and their presence needs to be inferred by other findings [34].

Compared with ultrasound, each other modality suffers from other drawbacks, including, in the case of CT scans, increased cost and radiation exposure. A CT scan achieves its best results in evaluating the thyroid and neck nodes using iodinated contrast material. The use of the contrast material carries a relative contraindication in suspected thyroid malignancies. The iodine bolus requires delaying the use of radioactive iodine for treatment or diagnostic scanning for a minimum of 8 to 12 weeks. An MRI scan

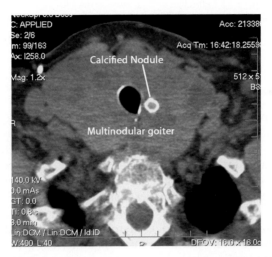

Fig. 8. CT scan of multinodular goiter. Note calcified nodule along with multiple vague, hypo-dense nodules throughout the thyroid.

avoids the use of iodinated contrast material and theoretically can achieve greater resolution than CT scanning, but motion artifact due to breathing, swallowing, and even vascular pulsation degrades the actual resolution.

During the initial evaluation of a thyroid nodule, the main use of CT and MRI scans would be for suspected substernal or retrotracheal thyroid masses (Fig. 9) [35]. While physical examination alone may be sufficient to warrant the use of these scans, the case for first performing an ultrasound is still strong. The ultrasound confirms the continuation of the thyroid into the chest or the retrotracheal area. At the same time, an evaluation of the

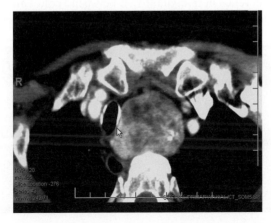

Fig. 9. Substernal goiter. CT scan and MRI are superior to ultrasound for evaluating the extent of substernal goiters and the degree of airway compression. White arrow points to compressed trachea, which is deviated to the patient's right.

accessible thyroid parenchyma helps decide if an FNA will be of any use in the individual case while also demonstrating the fine detail of individual nodules.

The changing role of radioisotope imaging

Radioisotope scans were the mainstay of thyroid imaging beginning in the 1950s [36]. Their utility was always limited, but their use prevailed in the absence of useful alternatives. The need for iodine-restricted diets to optimize results and the attendant radiation exposure presented problems for patients. The scans were not useful in evaluating hypothyroidism or simple goiter or for detecting nodules smaller than 1 cm. Their popularization came from the observation that so-called "cold" nodules, nodules that had less radioisotope uptake than surrounding thyroid tissue, had a higher rate of malignancy compared with "warm" or "hot" nodules. The average malignancy rate in "cold" nodules is commonly stated as around 15% while "warm" nodules are quoted as approximately 8% [37,38]. Neither finding can be considered definitive because the malignancy rates are low for both groups and differ only by a factor of two, resulting in a specificity of 5% and a positive predictive value of 10%. With the advent of widely available high-resolution ultrasound imaging and FNA, the use of radioisotope imaging has significantly declined.

Radioisotope scans are still found useful in three situations encountered in the workup of a new thyroid nodule: when selecting potential FNA targets within multinodular goiters (Fig. 10), when deciding to follow low-grade follicular lesions, and when evaluating a potentially hyperactive nodule [3,39]. In the last instance, the findings can be considered definitive with respect to malignant potential.

While the difference in malignant risk between "cold" and "warm" nodules is not definitive, the relative twofold increase in risk between the two

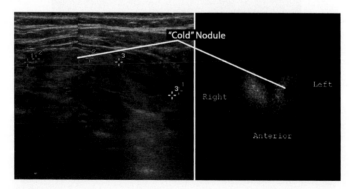

Fig. 10. Multinodular goiter with "cold" nodule. Ultrasound image (*left*) is a composite left sagittal image. Nuclear medicine scan (*right*) demonstrates area of decreased radioisotope uptake consistent with a "cold" nodule. FNA was performed on this nodule.

types is felt to be helpful in guiding the evaluation of multinodular goiters. Because it is impractical to sample all nodules in a multinodular goiter with FNA, the most commonly suggested selection criteria are the dominant nodule or nodules based on size criteria and the presence of known ultrasound risk factors, such as microcalcifications. In the absence of these findings or as an adjunct, radioisotope scanning for "cold" nodules is recommended [39].

When faced with a nondiagnostic FNA, or an FNA result that poses a low risk of follicular neoplasm, the difference between "warm" and "cold" nodules may have some utility in helping decide on continued monitoring versus a surgical procedure for definitive diagnosis [2,21].

In cases of laboratory-documented hyperthyroidism, the demonstration of a "hot" nodule on radioisotope scan is considered very useful because of the low associated risk of malignancy ($<1\%$) [17]. In these cases, the issue quickly shifts from ruling out malignancy to the treatment of the hyperthyroid condition.

The three most commonly used radioisotopes for thyroid imaging are the two radioactive iodine isotopes, iodine 131 (^{131}I) and iodine 123 (^{123}I), and technetium pertechnetate (^{99m}Tc) (Table 2). ^{131}I, the most commonly used agent for both diagnostic imaging and therapy, is a natural byproduct of uranium fission and is produced in significant quantities in nuclear reactors. It has a relatively long half-life (8.02 days), which makes it easy to transport and store for medical purposes. It emits both gamma rays (x-rays) and beta particles (electrons) of relatively high energy (364 KeV). It is this combined high-energy emission that accounts for the superiority of ^{131}I in its therapeutic induction of cell damage and subsequent cell death. The high-energy emission also makes it useful for metastatic workups because of the enhanced tissue penetration of the ^{131}I gamma radiation component. At the same time, the high-energy beta-emission component coupled with the relatively long half-life of ^{131}I makes it less desirable for diagnostic imaging of the *de novo* thyroid nodule. The increased radiation dose is a concern (see Table 2) and, potentially more important for subsequent treatment, the energetic beta emission leads to tissue stunning, which can result in decreased uptake during a subsequent therapeutic dose of ^{131}I [40].

^{123}I is a pure gamma emitter that, compared with ^{131}I, has a lower energy peak (159 KeV) and a significantly shorter half-life (13 hours). When used

Table 2
Most common radioisotopes used for thyroid nodule evaluation

Agent	Half-life	Energy peak	Administered dose	Absorbed radiation dose
^{131}I	8.02 d	364 KeV	100 µCi	75 rad
^{123}I	13 h	159 KeV	100 µCi	0.75 rad
^{99m}Tc	6 h	140 KeV	10 mCi	1.3 rad

for thyroid imaging, the images obtained with ^{123}I are as good or better than those with ^{131}I while resulting in only 1% of the radiation dose (see Table 2). Thus, ^{123}I has become the radioisotope of choice for *de novo* thyroid nodule evaluation and diagnostic imaging. Metastatic workups, particularly when attempting to evaluate bone metastases, may require the greater penetrating power of ^{131}I. Unlike ^{131}I, ^{123}I is not a natural byproduct of other commercial processes and is typically made through cyclotron bombardment of radioxenon. The expense of production and its relatively short half-life can limit its availability.

^{99m}Tc, like ^{123}I, is a pure gamma emitter (140 KeV) with a relatively short half-life (6 hours). Though ^{99m}Tc is taken up by the thyroid, unlike radioactive iodine it is not organified. In the 1970s it was discovered that this difference meant nodules that were "cold" on radioactive iodine scans could be "warm" on ^{99m}Tc scans [41]. For this reason, ^{99m}Tc is generally not used today for the diagnostic workup of the thyroid nodule if radioiodine is available.

Other radioisotopes have been used for thyroid scanning, but few offer any advantages to radioiodine and most suffer from the limitations of ^{99m}Tc. Thallium 201 and ^{99m}Tc methoxyisobutylisonitrile have attracted some interest in the past decade, mostly as an adjunct to radioiodine or ^{99m}Tc scanning [42,43]. Because of their limited applicability and cost considerations, these agents are not routinely used in the initial evaluation of the thyroid nodule.

Summary

The initial evaluation of the thyroid nodule continues to rely chiefly on FNA and ultrasound imaging. The approach to evaluating the thyroid nodule on the first clinical visit has been changing to include earlier and more frequent use of ultrasound both for nodule characterization and as an aid in performing FNA. The use of ultrasound in the initial evaluation has been shown to change the diagnostic plan in a substantial percentage of cases. At the same time, ultrasound-guided FNA in palpable nodules has resulted in significant decreases in insufficient samples. The increased integration of ultrasound in the office setting holds the promise of decreasing uncertainty in diagnosis and improving long-term follow-up while also being cost-effective.

Further readings

Fratas MC, Benson CB, Charboneau JW, et al. Management of thyroid nodules detected by US: Society of Radiologists in Ultrasound consensus statement. Radiology 2005;237:794–800.

Consensus statement on the usefulness of ultrasound for the diagnosis of thyroid neoplasms. Well worth reading for anyone who is interested in using ultrasound to improve their diagnostic acumen.

Baskin HJ, editor. Thyroid ultrasound and ultrasound-guided FNA biopsy. Norwell: Kluwer Academic Publishers; 2000.

Straight forward compendium covering all aspects of thyroid ultrasound. The text can be a bit redundant with overlapping chapters written by different authors, but it is a very accurate representation of the thinking in the endocrine community regarding portable, office-based ultrasound.

Kim N, Lavertu P. Evaluation of a thyroid nodule. Otolaryngol Clin N Am 2003;36:17–33.

This is a concise and complete analysis of the thyroid nodule evaluation. Its salient points remain valid today.

References

[1] Wiest PW, Hartshorne MF, Inskip PD, et al. Thyroid palpation versus high resolution thyroid ultrasonography in the detection of nodules. J Ultrasound Med 1998;17:487–96.

[2] Singer PA, Cooper DS, Daniels GH, et al. Treatment guidelines for patients with thyroid nodules and well-differentiated thyroid cancer. Arch Intern Med 1996;156:2165–72.

[3] Hegedus L. The thyroid nodule. N Engl J Med 2004;351:1764–71.

[4] Carroll BA. Asymptomatic thyroid nodules: incidental sonographic detection. AJR Am J Roentgenol 1982;138:499–501.

[5] Brande A, Viikinkoski P, Nickels J, et al. Thyroid gland: US screening in a random adult population. Radiology 1991;181:683–7.

[6] Schneider AB. Radiation-induced thyroid tumors. Endocrinol Metab Clin North Am 1990; 19:495–508.

[7] Demidchik EP, Mrochek A, Demidchik YU, et al. Thyroid cancer promoted by radiation in young people of Belarus. In: Thomas G, Karaoglou A, Williams ED, editors. Radiation and thyroid cancer. Singapore: World Scientific; 1999. p. 51–60.

[8] Hegedus L, Bonnema SJ, Bennedbaek FN. Management of simple nodular goiter: current status and future perspectives. Endocr Rev 2003;24:102–32.

[9] Mortensen JD, Woolner LB, Bennett WA. Gross and microscopic findings in clinically normal thyroid glands. J Clin Endocrinol Metab 1955;15:1270–80.

[10] Laccourreye O, Papon JF, Kania R, et al. Paralysies laryngees unlaterales: donnees epidemiologiques at evvolution therapeutique. Presse Med 2003;32:781–6.

[11] Loughran S, Alves C, MacGregor FB. Current aetiology of unilateral vocal fold paralysis in a teaching hospital in west Scotland. J Laryngol Otol 2002;116:907–10.

[12] Frates MC, Benson CB, Charboneau JW, et al. Management of thyroid nodules detected by US: Society of Radiologists in Ultrasound consensus statement. Radiology 2005;237:794–800.

[13] Bogsrud TV, Karantanis D, Nathan MA, et al. The value of quantifying 18F-FDG uptake in thyroid nodules found incidentally on whole-body PET-CT. Nucl Med Commun 2007;28:373–81.

[14] Kim EK, Park CS, Chung WY, et al. New sonographic criteria for recommending fine-needle aspiration biopsy of non-palpable solid nodules of the thyroid. AJR Am J Roentgenol 2002;178:687–91.

[15] Hagag P, Strauss S, Weiss M. Role of ultrasound-guided fine-needle aspiration biopsy in evaluation of non-palpable thyroid nodules. Thyroid 1998;8:989–95.

[16] Kane LA, Gharib H. Thyroid testing: a clinical approach. In: Braverman LE, editor. Diseases of the thyroid. 2nd edition. Totawa (NJ): Humana Press; 2003. p. 39–52.

[17] Wong CKM, Wheeler MH. Thyroid nodules: rational management. World J Surg 2000;24: 934–41.

[18] Ozgen AG, Hamulu F, Bayraktar F, et al. Evaluation of routine basal serum calcitonin measurements for early diagnosis of medullary carcinoma in seven hundred seventy-three patients with nodular goiter. Thyroid 1999;9:579–82.

[19] Castro MR, Gharib H. Continuing controversies in the management of thyroid nodules. Ann Intern Med 2005;142:926–31.

[20] Marqusee E, Benson CB, Frates MC, et al. Usefulness of ultrasonography in the management of nodular thyroid disease. Ann Intern Med 2000;133:696–700.

[21] Mazzaferri EL. Management of a thyroid solitary nodule. N Engl J Med 1993;328:553–9.

[22] Takashima S, Fukuda H, Kobayashi T. Thyroid nodules: clinical effect of ultrasound-guided fine needle aspiration biopsy. J Clin Ultrasound 1994;22:535–42.

[23] Danese D, Sciacchitano S, Farsetti A, et al. Diagnostic accuracy of conventional versus sonography-guided fine-needle aspiration biopsy of thyroid nodules. Thyroid 1998;8:15–21.

[24] Carmeci C, Jeffrey RB, McDougall IR, et al. Ultrasound-guided, fine-needle aspiration biopsy of thyroid masses. Thyroid 1998;8:283–9.

[25] Akbar NA, Bodenner DL, Kim LT, et al. Considerations in incorporating office based ultrasound of the head and neck. Otolaryngol Head Neck Surg 2006;135(6):884–8.

[26] Hall R, Ogburn T, Rogers RG. Teaching and evaluating ultrasound skill attainment: competency-based resident ultrasound training for AIUM accreditation. Obstet Gynecol Clin North Am 2006;33(2):305–23.

[27] Zangeneh F, Powell CC, Gharib H. A survey on the use of thyroid ultrasonography in clinical endocrinology training programs. Endocr Pract 2003;9(2):162–3.

[28] Mandavia DP, Aragona J, Chan L, et al. Henderson SO ultrasound training for emergency physicians—a prospective study. Acad Emerg Med 2000;7(9):1008–14.

[29] Rozycki GS. Surgeon-performed ultrasound: its use in clinical practice. Ann Surg 1998;228: 16–28.

[30] McCarter FD, Luchette FA, Molloy M, et al. Institutional and individual learning curves for focused abdominal ultrasound for trauma cumulative sum analysis. Ann Surg 2000;231: 689–700.

[31] Coltrera MD. Essential physics of ultrasound. In: Orloff L, editor. Head and neck ultrasonography. San Diego: Plural Publishing; 2008.

[32] Khoo ML, Asa SL, Witterick IJ, et al. Thyroid calcification and its association with thyroid carcinoma. Head Neck 2002;24:651–5.

[33] Papini E, Guglielmi R, Bianchini A, et al. Risk of malignancy in nonpalpable thyroid nodules: predictive value of ultrasound and color Doppler features. J Clin Endocrinol Metab 2002;87:1941–6.

[34] Fundamentals of diagnostic radiology. Brant WE, Helms CA editors. 3rd edition. Philadelphia: Lippincott, Williams & Wilkins; 2007.

[35] Jennings A. Evaluation of substernal goiters using computed tomography and MR imaging. Endocrinol Metab North Am 2001;30:401–14.

[36] Beierwaltes WH. The history of the use of radioactive iodine. Semin Nucl Med 1979;9:151–5.

[37] Loevner LA. Imaging of the thyroid gland. Semin Ultrasound CT MR 1996;17:539–62.

[38] Yousem DM, Scheff AM. Thyroid and parathyroid. In: Som PM, Curtin HD, editors. Head and neck imaging. 3rd edition. St. Louis (MO): Mosby; 1996. p. 951–72.

[39] Feld S, Garcia M, Baskin HJ, et al. AACE clinical practice guidelines for the diagnosis and management of thyroid nodules. Endocr Pract 1996;2:78–85.

[40] Nordén MM, Larsson F, Tedelind S, et al. Down-regulation of the sodium/iodide symporter explains ^{131}I-induced thyroid stunning. Cancer Res 2007;67(15):7512–7.

[41] Shambaugh GE, Quinn JL, Oyasu R, et al. Disparate thyroid imaging: combined studies with pertechnetate Tc 99m and radioactive iodine. JAMA 1974;228:866–9.

[42] Sinha PS, Beeby DI, Ryan P. An evaluation of thallium imaging for detection of carcinoma in clinically palpable solitary, non-functioning thyroid nodules. Thyroid 2001;11:85–9.

[43] Mezosi E, Bajnok L, Gyory F, et al. The role of technetium-99m methoxyisobutylisonitrile in the differential diagnosis of cold thyroid nodules. Eur J Nucl Med 1999;26:798–803.

ELSEVIER
SAUNDERS

Surg Oncol Clin N Am
17 (2008) 57–70

SURGICAL
ONCOLOGY CLINICS
OF NORTH AMERICA

Pathology and Cytologic Features of Thyroid Neoplasms

Kelly M. Malloy, MD[a], Mary F. Cunnane, MD[b],*

[a]Department of Otolaryngology/Head and Neck Surgery, University of Michigan, 1904
Taubman Health Center, 1500 E. Medical Center Drive, Ann Arbor, MI 48109-0312, USA
[b]Department of Pathology, Anatomy, and Cell Biology, Jefferson Medical College, Suite 283,
Main Building, 132 South 10th Street, Philadelphia, PA 19107, USA

Thyroid cancer is an uncommon neoplasm. The American Cancer Society estimates that thyroid cancer will account for approximately 2% of new cancer cases in 2007 and fewer than 0.5% of cancer deaths [1]. Thyroid cancer is more frequently diagnosed in females. Although it most frequently presents in the fourth and fifth decade, it affects every age group from children to the elderly. Genetic, environmental, and dietary factors all play a role in the pathogenesis of thyroid cancer.

The thyroid is a composite gland, having two distinct cell populations, each producing separate hormones. Neoplasms arise from both cell types; these tumors differ in morphology, epidemiology, and prognosis. Tumors derived from the follicular cells are far more common and comprise 95% of thyroid neoplasms [2]. Most are well differentiated and pursue an indolent course. The few cases of poorly differentiated or anaplastic carcinoma account for most of the deaths attributed to this neoplasm.

Tumors of the C-cells account for approximately 5% of thyroid tumors. Most of these are sporadic, but approximately 20% to 25% occur as part of familial multiple endocrine neoplasia syndromes. C-cell tumors are more aggressive than tumors of follicle cells and account for a substantial fraction of the mortality from thyroid cancer.

The incidence of thyroid carcinoma has increased in recent years, facilitated by two important developments: the widespread use of improved imaging techniques and the popularity of fine-needle aspiration biopsy. Increasingly, new cases of thyroid carcinoma are identified incidentally on imaging performed for indications other than thyroid enlargement.

* Corresponding author.
E-mail address: mary.cunnane@jefferson.edu (M.F. Cunnane).

1055-3207/08/$ - see front matter © 2008 Elsevier Inc. All rights reserved.
doi:10.1016/j.soc.2007.10.012   *surgonc.theclinics.com*

Fine-needle aspiration biopsy has proven to be a safe and reliable procedure to assess thyroid nodules. The sensitivity and specificity of this technique are high, and the overall accuracy is 95%. In most series, 60% to 70% of biopsies are classified as negative. This has resulted in a decline in surgical procedures for benign disease and increased yields of carcinoma in those patients who undergo thyroidectomy [3,4].

This review considers the pathologic features of thyroid neoplasms and highlights those features that contribute to their cytologic diagnosis.

Tumors of follicular cell origin

Most thyroid tumors arise from the follicular cells, and most are well differentiated. Poorly differentiated and undifferentiated tumors are rare. The well-differentiated lesions include papillary and follicular carcinomas and their variants.

Papillary carcinoma

Papillary carcinoma is the most common malignant neoplasm of the thyroid in the United States and in other countries in which dietary iodine is plentiful [5]. It is approximately three times more common in females and occurs in all age groups, including children. The female predominance is not as pronounced in children and in the elderly. There is a definite association with exposure to ionizing radiation in childhood [6,7], as shown by the marked increase in cases in sites near the Chernobyl nuclear accident of 1986 [8]. Some studies have shown a familial association [9,10], and an association with Hashimoto thyroiditis has also been reported [11]. Oncogenes also have an important role in papillary thyroid cancer; rearrangements of the RET oncogene have been found in a substantial proportion of cases [12], including patients who have a history of radiation exposure [13].

Papillary carcinoma typically presents as a gray-white, firm tumor with indistinct borders located in either thyroid lobe or in the isthmus (Fig. 1). Variations of this typical presentation are many: papillary carcinoma may be multifocal, multinodular, encapsulated, or cystic. It may appear as a scar with foci of calcification; rarely, it replaces the entire gland.

Microscopically, architectural and cytologic features are important in the diagnosis of papillary cancer. In classic cases, a papillary architecture is predominant. The papillae are composed of slender fibrovascular stalks, which may be hyalinized. The papillae are complex and branching. They are arranged closely together and appear compressed (Fig. 2). The stalks support a single layer of columnar cells with overlapping nuclei. Psammoma bodies, concentrically laminated calcific concretions, are often present at the tips of the papillae or in the spaces between them. These distinctive structures are believed to represent the ghosts of necrotic tumor cells and are

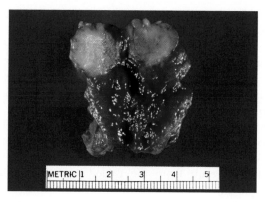

Fig. 1. Papillary carcinoma. Solid, poorly circumscribed tumor distinct from the surrounding thyroid.

present in approximately 50% of cases. Colloid is sparse or absent; when present, it is thick, dense, inspissated, and stains brightly eosinophilic [14].

The most important and diagnostic feature of papillary carcinoma is the distinctive nucleus. Lindsay is credited with drawing attention to the unique nuclear features of papillary cancer [15], and numerous subsequent studies have confirmed that tumors with the nuclear features he described behave clinically like papillary carcinoma. Specifically these neoplasms metastasized to cervical lymph nodes rather than to bone and lung. Further, the metastatic foci exhibited a papillary morphology, with psammoma bodies. In contrast to follicular carcinomas, vascular invasion was infrequent [16,17].

The primacy of nuclear features in the diagnosis of papillary carcinoma is now accepted and is expressed in the World Health Organization's (WHO)

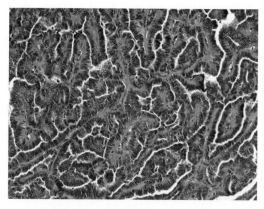

Fig. 2. Typical papillary carcinoma features complex papillae arranged closely together without intervening colloid. Hematoxylin and eosin ×200.

definition of papillary carcinoma: "a malignant epithelial tumor showing evidence of follicular cell differentiation and characterized by distinctive nuclear features" [18]. The distinctive nucleus is enlarged, elongated, oval (rather than round), with finely dispersed chromatin and an inconspicuous small nucleolus, often closely applied to the nuclear membrane. In some cells, the chromatin may be displaced to the periphery of the cell, resulting in the appearance of an optically clear nucleus with a thick nuclear membrane (Orphan Annie nuclei) [17,19]. Ultrastructurally the nuclear membrane is folded and redundant, resulting in the formation of characteristic nuclear grooves. Sharply defined intranuclear inclusions of cytoplasm (nuclear holes) also result from the folded nuclear membrane. Mitotic figures are rarely seen.

Papillary carcinoma has a propensity for lymphatic spread. Intrathyroidal lymphatic dissemination results in multifocal and bilateral foci of tumor in 20% of cases. Metastases to cervical lymph nodes are present in 50% of cases at presentation [20], and often enlarged cervical lymph nodes are the first sign of the disease. Remarkably and in contrast to other neoplasms, cervical lymph node metastases do not seem to affect survival in papillary cancer. Factors that do affect survival include tumor size, extrathyroidal extension, age at diagnosis, and gender. Of these, extrathyroidal extension seems to be the most important. Spread beyond the thyroid and into the soft tissues of the neck occurs in approximately 15% to 25% of patients [21]. Most ominous is posterior extension into the larynx or trachea, which may be associated with uncontrollable neck recurrence. Age is also an important factor—tumors occurring in children have a favorable prognosis regardless of extent [22], but patients older than 60 years of age have a worse prognosis. Large tumors (5 cm or more) and male gender also adversely affect prognosis [23]. Vascular invasion and hematogenous spread are less common in papillary than in follicular carcinoma, although lung metastases may be found in 10% of patients. Pulmonary lesions are often small, may be numerous, and are compatible with prolonged survival. Metastases to bone, liver, and central nervous system are rare.

Patients who have papillary cancer generally have a favorable course and average long-term survival of greater than 95%. Deaths occur in patients who are older than 40 years of age, male, and who have large tumors and distant metastases. In some patients, poor prognosis is the result of progression to poorly differentiated or anaplastic carcinoma [24].

Fine-needle aspiration biopsy is the most useful study in the diagnosis of papillary carcinoma. The sensitivity is 98%, and the positive predictive value of 99% [3]. This excellent success rate is because of the distinctive nuclear features of papillary carcinoma, which are usually found easily in cytologic smears. Aspiration typically yields a cellular specimen with tumor cells arranged in sheets and papillary fronds. The cells display the typical powdery chromatin, nuclear grooves, and intranuclear inclusions of papillary carcinoma (Fig. 3) [25].

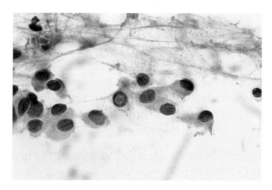

Fig. 3. Cytology of papillary carcinoma. Cells are dispersed with powdery nuclear chromatin and a prominent intranuclear cytoplasmic inclusion. Papanicolaou stain ×1000.

Variants of papillary carcinoma

The WHO recognizes 15 variants of papillary carcinoma, some more common than others [18]. Each of these displays the typical nuclear features of papillary carcinoma but differs in architectural configuration or cytoplasmic details. Some of the variants are noteworthy for their poor prognosis.

Follicular variant. This is the most common variant of papillary carcinoma. In this variant, a follicular architecture predominates and papillae are rare or absent. The lesion closely resembles follicular adenoma or carcinoma. In most cases, the follicles are small (microfollicular) and often contain little or no colloid. They are arranged closely together, giving the appearance of a high cellular nodule. The tumor may or may not be encapsulated. This variant of papillary carcinoma often presents a diagnostic challenge. The characteristic nuclei may be present only focally and may be widely dispersed. In the setting of nodular goiter they are easily overlooked. Encapsulated microfollicular papillary carcinoma may be mistaken for follicular adenoma or an adenomatoid nodule unless the characteristic nuclei are identified. Careful search for the diagnostic nuclear features is required [26]. The macrofollicular variant is rare and displays large follicles distended with colloid, which may have a scalloped border. It may be difficult to separate this lesion from a colloid nodule.

The follicular variant of papillary carcinoma is generally believed to have the same favorable prognosis and long survival as classic papillary carcinoma, although some reports have cited a slightly worse prognosis [27].

Diagnosis of follicular variant papillary carcinoma by fine-needle aspiration is less sensitive than typical papillary carcinoma. Factors that account for a low success rate include architectural features that overlap with follicular lesions (adenoma and carcinoma) and a reduced population of cells with diagnostic nuclear characteristics [28,29].

Tall cell variant. This rare variant was described by Hawk and Hazard [19] in 1976. In this variant, the tumor cells are at least twice as tall as they are wide and display brightly eosinophilic cytoplasm. In contrast to classic papillary carcinoma, mitotic figures are frequently seen and there may be focal necrosis. In most cases the tumor is large, the patient is elderly, and there is evidence of extrathyroidal extension. Recurrences are frequent, and the overall prognosis is worse than for other variants of thyroid carcinoma.

Columnar cell variant. The columnar cell variant of papillary carcinoma is closely related to tall cell papillary carcinoma but is even less common. It, too, has a poor prognosis. The growth pattern is variable, with papillary, follicular, and trabecular areas. The tall columnar cells are distinctive in that they contain subnuclear vacuoles reminiscent of the appearance of early secretory endometrium. The nuclear features of papillary carcinoma are required for the diagnosis; however, these may be difficult to find in some tumors [30].

Diffuse sclerotic variant. This tumor is more common in children and adolescents and typically enlarges the entire thyroid rather than forming a solid mass. Stromal fibrosis and numerous psammoma bodies are conspicuous features. The tumor cells exhibit papillary and follicular patterns of growth with a prominent lymphoid infiltrate and squamous metaplasia. Regional lymph node and lung metastases are often present. Nonetheless, the tumor has a favorable prognosis, possibly because most patients are young [31].

Papillary microcarcinoma

This term refers to a tumor measuring 1 cm or less. The incidence of this tumor is the subject of numerous reports, including autopsy studies and studies involving thyroids removed surgically for benign disease. The frequency depends on the criteria used to define the lesion and the extent of the examination. Figures varying from 25% to 35% have been quoted in the literature. Although this variant has an extremely favorable prognosis, 10% of cases present as metastatic disease in the cervical lymph nodes, and there is no doubt that papillary microcarcinoma is a malignant neoplasm [32].

Encapsulated variant

The encapsulated variant of papillary carcinoma is another lesion with an extremely favorable prognosis and an almost 100% survival rate. The tumor is surrounded by a thick fibrous capsule and has a typical papillary architecture with classic nuclear features. Metastases to regional nodes are present in approximately 25% of cases [33].

Cribriform carcinoma

This unusual tumor is the lesion associated with Gardner syndrome [34]. In this setting, the tumor occurs typically in young women and is bilateral. The architectural pattern is variable and cribriform areas are conspicuous. Some nuclei demonstrate grooves, but others are hyperchromatic. Some authorities regard this as a distinctive tumor rather than a variant of papillary carcinoma.

Follicular carcinoma

Follicular carcinoma is a less common form of differentiated thyroid carcinoma accounting for approximately 5% to 10% of cases. Recent declines in the incidence of follicular carcinoma are attributed to the recognition of the follicular variant of papillary carcinoma and the appropriate classification of follicular patterned lesions with characteristic nuclei of papillary carcinoma. Follicular carcinoma is prevalent in regions in which dietary iodine is deficient, and it is more common in females. It is rare in children and adolescents, and the peak incidence is approximately 1 decade later than that of papillary carcinoma. Follicular carcinoma is divided into minimally invasive and widely invasive types and also includes lesions with oncocytic (Hürthle cell) morphology.

Minimally invasive follicular carcinoma is indistinguishable grossly from follicular adenoma, except for a thick capsule that separates it from the surrounding normal tissue (Fig. 4). Microscopically, too, it is similar to adenoma, composed of small follicles, usually arranged tightly together, and containing scant colloid (Fig. 5). The diagnosis of follicular carcinoma depends entirely on the demonstration of capsular or vascular invasion. The criteria for capsular invasion are somewhat controversial. Some authorities accept any degree of capsular infiltration as evidence of invasion, whereas

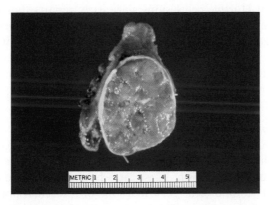

Fig. 4. Follicular carcinoma. A circumscribed tumor with a thick capsule dominates the thyroid lobe.

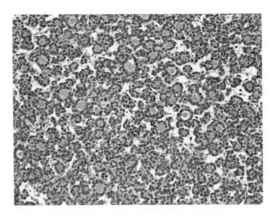

Fig. 5. Follicular carcinoma. Microfollicles contain sparse colloid. Hematoxylin and eosin ×200.

others require full-thickness invasion by a broad front of advancing tumor. Vascular invasion is defined as the presence of tumor in vessels within or outside the capsule. Angioinvasive follicular carcinoma has a greater tendency to metastasize than those lesions that feature capsular invasion only [35].

In contrast to papillary carcinoma, follicular carcinoma infrequently metastasizes to lymph nodes; the most common sites of metastatic disease are lung and bone. In a small number of patients, bone metastases may be the first sign of disease [36].

Hürthle cell follicular carcinoma

A distinctive type of follicular carcinoma is composed of Hürthle cells or oncocytic cells. A Hürthle cell is defined as an altered follicular cell characterized by abundant and distorted cytoplasmic mitochondria. This feature results in an enlarged cell with granular eosinophilic cytoplasm. Controversy has surrounded Hürthle cell lesions since early reports that indicated that Hürthle cell tumors carried a worse prognosis than other thyroid neoplasms [37]. Subsequent studies indicate that Hürthle cell tumors often present at a more advanced stage and with evidence of extrathyroid extension. Most experts agree that the behavior of Hürthle cell tumors is similar to that of other follicular carcinomas of similar stage [38].

Widely disseminated follicular carcinoma

The widely disseminated variant of follicular carcinoma accounts for 5% of cases of follicular cancers. These lesions are not encapsulated and exhibit extensive vascular permeation. Most cases have metastasized at the time of presentation. The tumor cells grow in a solid or trabecular pattern and there is minimal follicle formation. The most conspicuous feature is the extensive vascular invasion. The prognosis for this variant is poor.

Fine-needle aspiration cytology

Fine-needle aspiration cytology is of limited value in follicular carcinoma, because the diagnosis depends on the recognition of invasion. Cytologic smears from patients who have follicular carcinoma are cellular with a predominance of micro-follicles. The cells are arranged in syncytial groups and three dimensional arrays. The diagnosis rendered in most cases is "suspicious." Histologic examination of the excised lesion with careful attention to the capsule is required for definitive diagnosis.

Poorly differentiated carcinoma

This term refers to a group of thyroid carcinomas with a minimal degree of differentiation and a prognosis intermediate between differentiated tumors and anaplastic lesions. Poorly differentiated carcinomas are generally large and are often associated with metastases to lung or bone at the time of presentation. Microscopically the growth pattern may be solid, trabecular, or insular. Mitoses are frequent, and there are foci of necrosis and vascular invasion. The best characterized variant is insular carcinoma, in which the tumor cells grow in sharply circumscribed islands separated by fibrous tissue [39].

Anaplastic carcinoma

This unusual tumor accounts for fewer than 5% of cases of thyroid cancer but more than 50% of thyroid cancer deaths. It affects primarily individuals older than 60 years of age. The female to male ratio is 1.5 to 1. Frequently there is a history of rapid enlargement in a pre-existing goiter. Most cases exhibit signs of regional extension and organ compression, including difficulty breathing and swallowing. The tumor extends locally into the lymph nodes and the skeletal muscle, larynx, and esophagus.

The histomorphology is highly variable. The tumor cells may be spindle-shaped, epithelioid, or giant cells; mixtures of the cell types are frequent. Necrosis and vascular invasion are conspicuous features. Evidence of a pre-existing, well-differentiated thyroid carcinoma, either papillary or follicular, is found in many cases. The prognosis is extremely poor. Even with extremely aggressive therapy, the median survival is less than 6 months [40,41].

Diagnosis by fine-needle aspiration biopsy is generally successful. The smears are cellular and feature a variable population of obviously malignant cells.

Medullary thyroid carcinoma

Medullary thyroid carcinoma (MTC) is a malignant neoplasm derived from the calcitonin-secreting C-cells of the thyroid gland. It is an uncommon malignancy, comprising 3% to 10% of all thyroid cancers and accounting for an estimated 1000 new cases per year in the United States [42]. It is generally accepted that MTC is more aggressive than the well-differentiated thyroid carcinomas; however, recent reports cite survival rates of 80% and 70% at 5 and 10 years, respectively [43]. MTC occurs sporadically in approximately 75% to 80% of cases, with a peak incidence in the fourth decade of life. Hereditary MTC occurs in the context of multiple endocrine neoplasia (MEN) syndromes 2A and 2B and in familial MTC syndrome and comprises 20% to 25% of MTC cases. MEN 2A, or Sipple syndrome, consists of MTC, pheochromocytoma, and parathyroid adenoma. MEN 2B is the constellation of MTC, pheochromocytoma, mucosal neurogangliomas, and marfanoid habitus. Familial MTC syndrome is simply the hereditary form of MTC without other associated endocrine tumors. All three hereditary forms demonstrate autosomal dominant inheritance, early C-cell hyperplasia (often with concomitant elevated serum calcitonin levels) and a pattern of multifocal and bilateral disease. Younger age at presentation of MTC is also a hallmark of the MEN 2 syndromes [44]. Overall, MTC of sporadic and hereditary variants demonstrates a propensity for early cervical lymph node metastases; as many as 80% of patients who have palpable thyroid MTC lesions have lymph node involvement [45]. Distant metastases occur in the lungs, liver, bones, and adrenal glands.

The C-cells of the thyroid gland are embryologically derived from the ultimobranchial bodies and are of neural crest origin. The C-cells exist is highest concentration in the middle to upper posterior aspect of the thyroid lobes; therefore, MTC originates primarily in this region. Grossly, MTC lesions are nonencapsulated solid tumors with well-defined circumscribed borders. The tumors vary from soft to firm to fibrotic in consistency when sectioned, and appear white, tan, or pink in contrast to the surrounding thyroid parenchyma. Large tumors may be more granular in consistency and have areas of calcification. Advanced lesions may replace a thyroid lobe and invade locally into the soft tissues of the strap muscles and trachea.

Microscopically, MTC is characterized by sheets of round, polygonal, or spindle cells that grow in a solid pattern. The nuclei are round, oval, or elongated. The cytoplasm is eosinophilic with fine granules, but may be clear. Mitotic figures are infrequent in most specimens. Necrosis, hemorrhage, and high mitotic rate are uncommon in MTC, particularly in smaller tumors (less than 1.5 cm). The nests of tumor cells of MTC are separated by a stroma that is vascular and contains abundant collagen and amyloid (Fig. 6). The amyloid of MTC stains positively for amyloid with Congo red and demonstrates the classic green birefringence in polarized light.

Although the tumors appear grossly well circumscribed, they do demonstrate microscopic invasion into normal thyroid parenchyma at the margins of the lesions. Advanced tumors may exhibit vascular and lymphatic invasion at their margins also. Specimens from patients who have hereditary

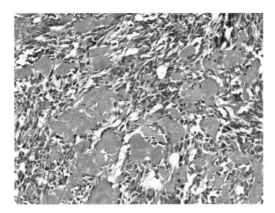

Fig. 6. Medullary carcinoma. Spindle-shaped tumor cells separated by amyloid. Hematoxylin and eosin ×200.

forms of MTC also show areas of C-cell hyperplasia surrounding the primary tumor and in other foci. This is not the case in the sporadic MTC.

Immunohistochemistry is useful in the diagnosis of MTC. Calcitonin staining is present in 80% of MTC cases. Other markers, including calcitonin gene-related peptide, carcinoembryonic antigen (CEA), chromogranin, histaminase, ACTH, and serotonin, are also positive [46]. Patients who have MTC demonstrate elevated serum levels of calcitonin and CEA also, and these markers are used to follow patients postoperatively. A recent study demonstrated that calcitonin doubling-time was the only independent predictor of survival on multivariate analysis [47]. Monitoring of CEA levels can be helpful in patients who have advanced disease, because the tumor may lose the ability to produce calcitonin but continue to secrete CEA.

Fine-needle aspirates of MTC are cellular with a high degree of pleomorphism. Cells may be round, oval, polyhedral, cuboidal, or spindle-shaped, and they are dispersed singly or in loose clusters. Their nuclei are often eccentrically positioned within pale cytoplasm and may exhibit a "salt and pepper" chromatin pattern. Amyloid may be seen in smears, and its presence supports the diagnosis [48].

Overall more than 95% of patients who have hereditary MTC syndromes display germline point mutations of the RET proto-oncogene. Patients who have sporadic MTC demonstrate somatic mutations of the RET gene domain in nearly 70% of cases [49]. Genetic testing for RET proto-oncogene mutation is essential, and testing of close relatives is also important in cases of suspected hereditary MTC.

Thyroid lymphomas

Primary lymphomas represent 5% of thyroid tumors. Most cases occur in patients who have Hashimoto thyroiditis, and there is a distinct female predominance. Recent studies indicate that most thyroid lymphomas are B-cell neoplasms of mucosal associated lymphoid tissue type. A minority are classified as diffuse large B-cell lymphoma. The overall survival is 80% with appropriate therapy. Prognosis depends on the stage of the tumor and the histologic grade [50].

Fine-needle aspiration biopsy is useful in the diagnosis of lymphoma. The correlation of morphology with flow cytometry results in a high degree of accuracy.

Metastatic tumors

Metastases to the thyroid are rare. The most common sites of primary tumor are lung, breast, and kidney.

Summary

Most thyroid neoplasms arise from follicular cells and are well differentiated. Anaplastic and poorly differentiated carcinomas are rare and have a high mortality. Five percent of tumors are of C-cell origin and 20% to 25% of these are hereditary. Thyroid lymphoma is rare and occurs in the setting of Hashimoto thyroiditis. Fine-needle aspiration biopsy is the best diagnostic tool to classify thyroid neoplasms.

References

[1] Jemal A, Siegel R, Ward E, et al. Cancer statistics. CA Cancer J Clin 2007;57:43–66.
[2] Rosai J. Thyroid gland. In: Rosai and Ackerman's surgical pathology. 9th edition. New York: Elsevier; 2004. p. 515–94.
[3] Gharib H, Goellner JR, Johnson DA. Fine-needle aspiration cytology of the thyroid. A 12-year experience with 11,000 biopsies. Clin Lab Med 1993;13(3):699–709.
[4] Gharib H. Fine-needle aspiration biopsy of thyroid nodules: advantages, limitations, and effect. Mayo Clin Proc 1994;69(1):44–9.
[5] Schlumberger MJ. Papillary and follicular thyroid carcinoma. N Engl J Med 1998;338:297–306.
[6] Ron E, Lubin JH, Shore RE, et al. Thyroid cancer after exposure to external radiation: a pooled analysis of seven studies. Radiat Res 1995;141:251–77.
[7] Shore RE. Issues and epidemiological evidence regarding radiation induced thyroid cancer. Radiat Res 1992;131:98–111.
[8] Kazakov VS, Demidchik EP, Astabova LN, et al. Thyroid cancer after Chernobyl. Nature 1992;359:21.
[9] Malchoff CD, Malchoff DM. Familial nonmedullary thyroid carcinoma. Cancer Control 2006;13(2):106–10.
[10] Goldgar DE, Easton DF, Cannon-Albright LA, et al. Systemic population-based assessment of cancer risk in first degree relatives of cancer probands. J Natl Cancer Inst 1994;86:1600–8.
[11] Ott RA, Calandra DB, McCall A, et al. The incidence of thyroid carcinoma in patients with Hashimoto's thyroiditis and solitary cold nodules. Surgery 1985;98:1202–6.
[12] Fenton CL, Lukes Y, Nicholson D, et al. The ret/PTC mutations are common in sporadic papillary thyroid carcinoma of children and young adults. J Clin Endocrinol Metab 2000; 85:1170–5.

[13] Rabes HM, Demidchik EP, Sidorow JD, et al. Pattern of radiation-induced RET and NTRK1 rearrangements in 191 post-Chernobyl papillary thyroid carcinomas: biological, phenotypic, and clinical implications. Clin Cancer Res 2000;6:1093–103.

[14] Carcangiu ML, Zampi G, Pupi A, et al. Papillary carcinoma of the thyroid. A clinicopathologic study of 241 cases treated at the University of Florence, Italy. Cancer 1985;55: 805–28.

[15] Lindsay S. Carcinoma of the thyroid gland. A clinicopathologic study of 293 patients at the University of California Hospital. Springfield (IL): Charles C. Thomas; 1960.

[16] Chen KTK, Rosai J. Follicular variant of thyroid papillary carcinoma: a clinicopathologic study of six cases. Am J Surg Pathol 1977;1:123–30.

[17] Hapke MR, Dehner LP. The optically clear nucleus. A reliable sign of papillary carcinoma of the thyroid. Am J surg Pathol 1979;3:31–8.

[18] DeLellis RA, Lloyd RV, Heitz PU, et al, editors. World Health Organization Classification of Tumours. Pathology and genetics of tumours of endocrine organs. Lyon (France): IARC Press; 2004. p. 57.

[19] Hawk WA, Hazard JB. The many appearances of papillary carcinoma of the thyroid. Cleve Clin Q 1976;43:202–16.

[20] Carcangiu ML, Zampi G, Rosai J. Papillary thyroid carcinoma: a study of its many morphologic expressions and clinical correlates. Path Annu 1985;20(1):1–44.

[21] Morton RP, Ahmad Z. Thyroid cancer invasion of neck structures: epidemiology, evaluation, staging and management. Curr Opin Otolaryngol Head Neck Surg 2007;15: 89–94.

[22] Collini P, Mattavelli F, Pellegrinelli A, et al. Papillary carcinoma of the thyroid gland of childhood and adolescence: morphologic subtypes, biologic behavior and prognosis. A clinicopathologic study of 42 sporadic cases treated at a single institution during a 30 year period. Am J Surg Pathol 2006;30:1420–6.

[23] Rosai J, Carcangiu ML, DeLellis RA. Papillary carcinoma. In: Rosai J, editor. Tumors of the thyroid gland, atlas of tumor pathology [Third Series Fascicle 5]. Washington, DC: Armed Forces Institute of Pathology; 1992. p. 95.

[24] DeGroot LJ, Kaplan EL, McCormick M, et al. Natural history, treatment, and course of papillary thyroid carcinoma. J Clin Endocrinol Metab 1990;71:414–24.

[25] DeMay M. Papillary thyroid carcinoma. In: Practical principles of cytopathology. Chicago: ASCP Press; 1999. p. 215–7.

[26] Suster S. Thyroid tumors with a follicular growth pattern: problems in differential diagnosis. Arch Path Lab Med 2006;130:984–8.

[27] Hagag P, Hod N, Kummer E, et al. Follicular variant of papillary thyroid carcinoma: clinical-pathological characterization and long-term follow-up. Cancer J 2006;12(4): 275–82.

[28] Baloch AW, Gupta PK, Yu GH, et al. Follicular variant of papillary carcinoma. Cytologic and histologic correlation. Am J Clin Pathol 1999;111:216–22.

[29] Lin HS, Komisar A, Opher E, et al. Follicular variant of papillary carcinoma: the diagnostic limitations of preoperative fine-needle aspiration and intraoperative frozen section evaluation. Laryngoscope 2000;110:1431–6.

[30] Evans HL. Columnar cell carcinoma of the thyroid: a report of two cases of an aggressive variant of thyroid carcinoma. Am J Clin Pathol 1986;85:77–80.

[31] Carcangiu ML, Bianchi S. Diffuse sclerosing variant of papillary thyroid carcinoma. Clinicopathologic study of 15 cases. Am J Surg Pathol 1989;13:1041–9.

[32] Baloch ZW, LiVolsi VA. Microcarcinoma of the thyroid. Adv Anat Pathol 2006;13(2): 69–75.

[33] Evans HL. Encapsulated papillary neoplasms of the thyroid. A study of 14 cases followed for a minimum of 10 years. Am J Surg Pathol 1987;11:592–7.

[34] Perrier ND, van Heerden JA, Goellner JR, et al. Thyroid cancer in patients with familial adenomatous polyposis. World J Surg 1998;22:738–42.

[35] Baloch ZW, LiVolsi VA. Our approach to follicular-patterned lesions of the thyroid. J Clin Pathol 2007;60:244–50.

[36] Evans HL. Follicular neoplasms of the thyroid. A study of 44 cases followed for a minimum of 10 years, with emphasis on differential diagnosis. Cancer 1984;54:535–40.

[37] Thompson NW, Dunn EL, Batsakis JG, et al. Hürthle cell lesions of the thyroid gland. Surg Gynecol Obstet 1974;139:555–60.

[38] Carcangiu ML, Bianchi S, Savino D, et al. Follicular Hürthle cell tumors of the thyroid gland. Cancer 1991;68:1944–53.

[39] Volante M, Collini P, Nikiforov YE, et al. Poorly differentiated thyroid carcinoma: the Turin proposal for the use of uniform diagnostic criteria and an algorithmic diagnostic approach. Am J Surg Pathol 2007;31:1256–64.

[40] Haigh PI, Ituarte PHG, Wu HS, et al. Completely resected anaplastic thyroid carcinoma combined with adjuvant chemotherapy and irradiation is associated with prolonged survival. Cancer 2001;91:2335–42.

[41] Cornett WR, Sharma AK, Day TA, et al. Anaplastic thyroid carcinoma: an overview. Curr Oncol Rep 2007;9:152–8.

[42] Hubner RA, Houlston RS. Molecular advances in medullary thyroid cancer diagnostics. Clin Chim Acta 2006;370:2–8.

[43] DeLellis RA. Pathology and genetics of thyroid carcinoma. J Surg Oncol 2006;94:662–9.

[44] Blankenship DR, Chin E, Terris DJ. Contemporary management of thyroid cancer. Am J Otolaryngol 2005;26:249–60.

[45] Fialkowski EA, Moley JF. Current approaches to medullary thyroid carcinoma, sporadic and familial. J Surg Oncol 2006;94:737–47.

[46] Barbet J, Campion L, Kraeber-Bodere F, et al. Prognostic impact of serum calcitonin and carcinoembryonic antigen doubling-times in patients with medullary thyroid carcinoma. J Clin Endocrinol Metab 2005;90:6077–84.

[47] Machens A, Ukkat J, Hauptmann S, et al. Abnormal carcinoembryonic antigen levels and medullary thyroid cancer progression. Arch Surg 2007;142:289–93.

[48] Das DK, Mallik MK, George SS, et al. Secretory activity in medullary thyroid carcinoma: a cytomorphological and immunocytochemical study. Diagn Cytopathol 2007;35:329–37.

[49] Machens A, Dralle H. Multiple endocrine neoplasia type 2 and the RET protooncogene: from bedside to bench to bedside. Mol Cell Endocrinol 2006;247:34–40.

[50] Derringer GA, Thompson LDR, Frommelt RA, et al. Malignant lymphoma of the thyroid gland. A clinicopathologic study of 108 cases. Am J Surg Pathol 2000;24:623–39.

ELSEVIER
SAUNDERS

Surg Oncol Clin N Am
17 (2008) 71–91

SURGICAL
ONCOLOGY CLINICS
OF NORTH AMERICA

Initial Surgical Management
of Thyroid Cancer

Robert L. Witt, MD, FACS[a,b],*

[a]Head and Neck Oncology, Helen F. Graham Cancer Center, Christiana Health Care System,
4701 Ogletown-Stanton Road, Newark, DE 19713-2070, USA
[b]Jefferson Medical College, Department of Otolaryngology-Head and Neck Surgery,
925 Chestnut Street, 6th Floor, Philadelphia, PA 19173-2070, USA

Thyroid cancer, the most common endocrine cancer, represents approximately 1% of all human malignancy. Approximately 5% to 10% of solitary thyroid nodules and 3% of multiple nodules are malignant in the general population. Approximately 30,000 cases of thyroid cancer are diagnosed per year in the United States; 7000 cases are diagnosed in men and approximately 23,000 cases occur in women. This number compares to 150,000 to 160,000 new cases of colon cancer, approximately 210,000 new cases of breast cancer, and just under 200,000 cases of lung cancer. The increase in the incidence of thyroid cancer is approaching 7% a year in the United States, far greater than any other cancer. Fifty percent of the increase is caused by papillary cancers smaller than 1 cm [1]. This dramatic increase in diagnosis likely represents early detection of subclinical disease.

The range of thyroid glands harboring microscopic or occult papillary thyroid cancer (PTC) and follicular thyroid cancer (FTC) ranges from 5% to 10%. Autopsy studies identify PTC in 5% to 36% of cases [2]. The relatively small number of deaths from thyroid cancer, the small number of clinical thyroid cancers, and the huge number of incidental thyroid cancers indicate how little we understand the biology of this disease. Follicular cell-derived thyroid carcinomas (PTC, FTC) are most common. FTC, like PTC, occurs more frequently in women but approximately a decade later. Using a demographic of 53,856 patients, Hundahl and colleagues [3] found that 79% of cases were papillary, 13% were follicular, 3% were Hürthle cell, 3% to 4% were medullary, and 2% were undifferentiated/anaplastic.

* Corresponding author. Helen F. Graham Cancer Center, Christiana Health Care System, 4701 Ogletown-Stanton Road, Newark, DE 19713-2070.
E-mail address: robertlwitt@aol.com

1055-3207/08/$ - see front matter © 2008 Elsevier Inc. All rights reserved.
doi:10.1016/j.soc.2007.10.010   *surgonc.theclinics.com*

Although most patients who have thyroid cancer do well, 5% to 6% succumb to their disease.

PTC presents most commonly between 30 and 50 years of age, with a female/male ratio of 2:1. Nodules are more likely to be malignant in patients younger than 25 years of age or in men, particularly older than age 60 (Fig. 1). The thyroid cancer risk with repeated diagnostic radiographs has not been conclusive. PTC has been associated with therapeutic external gamma radiation for head and neck disease and is the source of 5% to 10% of PTCs. Atomic explosions (the use of atomic weapons in Japan during World War II and among Pacific Islanders during nuclear testing in the 1950s and 1960s) or nuclear facility releases are associated with more aggressive cancers. For example, the maximum risk is 20 years after exposure for therapeutic radiation but only 4 years after exposure from nuclear fallout. The Chernobyl nuclear accident in 1986 led to a nearly fourfold increase in the incidence of PTC in fallout regions, with a higher rate of extrathyroidal spread and distant metastasis at the time of diagnosis [4]. Most children were under age 10 at time of presentation; children under age 4 at time of exposure had the highest risk of thyroid cancer.

PTC is more common in high iodine intake regions (ie, Iceland), and FTC (also anaplastic thyroid carcinoma [ATC]) is more common in iodine-deficient areas. Despite the overall increase in thyroid cancer, FTC is declining in the United States, likely because of the eradication of iodine deficiency. These changes induced by iodine supplementation have been noted in the United States over the last six decades. They parallel the decreased recurrence rates in low-risk younger patients from 16% to 3% and decreased mortality rates from 8% to 0.7%. Anaplastic carcinoma also has declined from 20% to 1% to 2% [5].

Familial nonmedullary thyroid cancer represents approximately 3% to 5% of PTC. It is more aggressive than sporadic cases. Autosomal dominant inheritance with partial penetrance is the mode of inheritance. Familial thyroid cancer is associated with familial adenosis polyposis, Gardner's

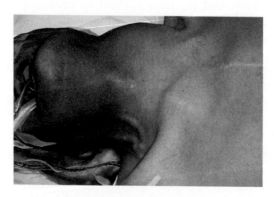

Fig. 1. PTC in a 65-year-old man.

syndrome (colonic polyps, osteomas, epidermal cysts, dermoid tumors, and retinal pigmentation), Cowden's disease (mucocutaneous hamartomas, keratosis, fibrocystic breast disease, and gastrointestinal polyps), and multiple endocrine neoplasia (MEN) type I. Personal or family history of thyroid cancer and previous endocrine malignancy increase the likelihood of thyroid cancer. The receptor tyrosine kinase (ret) proto-oncogene located on chromosome 10qll.2 is the main molecular alteration in papillary carcinoma.

Extent of surgery for differentiated thyroid cancer

Most American surgeons and an even higher number of endocrinologists advocate total thyroidectomy for most cases of DTC. This follows a paradigm shift from treatment of macroscopic disease to the treatment of macroscopic and microscopic disease by increasingly sensitive tests, including serial ultrasound, stimulated thyroglobulin levels, and even the detection of thyroglobulin messenger RNA with polymerase chain reaction. Commonly known multifactorial risk stratification schemes have been developed, although they are frequently not included in decision making for extent of surgery for DTC. A partial list includes AGES (age, grade, extent, and size) [6], AMES (age, metastases [distant] extent, size) [7], MACIS (metastasis, patient age, completeness of resection, local invasion and tumor size) [8], MSKCC (Memorial Sloan-Kettering Cancer Center) [9], and TNM (tumor, nodes, metastasis) (Box 1) [10]. Patients determined to be low risk by various classification systems report 10- to 20-year mortality rates and recurrence rates of 2% to 5% and 10%, respectively, whereas high-risk patients have mortality and recurrence rates of 40% to 50% and 45%, respectively [11].

Important favorable patient factors include age older than 16 and less than 45 and nonfamilial DTC. Mortality rates are higher in men, probably because they are older than women at the time of diagnosis. Two subtypes of DTC that have a particularly excellent prognosis are occult PTC and minimally invasive FTC. For the purpose of this article, a low-risk patient (for recurrence and mortality) is defined by the TNM system (see Box 1) [10] as T1 or T2, N0, M0, younger than 45 years and older than 16 years, with PTC, without aggressive histologic variant (ie, tall cell variant), without family history of DTC, and without bilateral disease or FTC with minimal capsule invasion. High-risk patients in this article are defined as having any TNM stage III and IV, any T3 or any T4 (extrathyroidal spread), any N1 (regional metastasis) or M1 (distant metastasis), any patient older than 45 years and younger than 16 years. Seventy-five percent of patients are in the low-risk group.

Patients at high risk are treated with total thyroidectomy. There is no role for nodulectomy, and the minimum operation is thyroid lobectomy. Low-risk patients are currently treated by thyroid lobectomy or total thyroidectomy, but more commonly the latter procedure is used. A randomized, prospective, double blind trial comparing thyroid lobectomy and total

---

Box 1. TNM staging for papillary and follicular carcinoma

Primary tumor (T)
T1: Tumor ≤2 cm
T2: Tumor >2 cm and <4 cm
T3: Tumor >4 cm, may include minimal extrathyroidal spread
T4a: Tumor of any size with extrathyroidal spread, including
    subcutaneous soft tissues, larynx, trachea, esophagus,
    and recurrent laryngeal nerve
T4b: Tumor invades prevertebral fascia or encases carotid artery
    or mediastinal vessels

Regional lymph nodes (N)
N0: No regional lymph node metastases
N1: Regional lymph node metastases
N1a: Metastasis to level VI (pretracheal, paratracheal,
    and prelaryngeal)
N1b: Metastasis to unilateral, bilateral, or contralateral cervical
    or superior mediastinal lymph nodes

Distant metastasis (M)
M0: No distant metastasis
M1: Distant metastasis

Staging groupings
Younger than age 45
    Stage 1: any T, any N M0
    Stage 2: any T, any N M1
Age 45 and older
    Stage 1: T1 N0 M0
    Stage 2: T2 N0 M0
    Stage 3: T3 N0 M0, T1-T3 N1a M0
    Stage 4a: T4a N0 M0, T4a N1a-b M0, T1-3 N1b M0
    Stage 4b: T4b, any N M0
    Stage 4c: Any T, any N M1

Data from Kebebew E, Clark OH. Differentiated thyroid cancer: "complete" rational approach. World J Surg 2000;24:942–51.

---

thyroidectomy has not been performed. It is unlikely to occur because of the long follow-up (15–25 years) required to differentiate mortality and recurrence given the favorable long-term prognosis for most patients. A comparison of both surgical procedures for the treatment of low-risk DTC continues to be germane.

Arguments for thyroid lobectomy for low-risk papillary thyroid microcarcinoma

Papillary thyroid microcarcinomas (defined as PTC <1 cm) can be treated with thyroid lobectomy. They are often discovered as incidental findings in thyroids removed for other reasons. They almost never result in distant metastasis and only rarely in death.

The National Comprehensive Cancer Network recommends either thyroid lobectomy (the term lobectomy implies thyroid lobectomy and isthmusectomy) or total thyroidectomy for low-risk patients [12]. The argument for thyroid lobectomy for low-risk patients who have PTC centers around the higher morbidity of total thyroidectomy (Box 2). A patient care evaluation study from the United States Thyroid Cancer Study Group reported from a prospective cohort study of 5583 cases of thyroid carcinoma that the rates of hypoparathyroidism and recurrent laryngeal nerve injury were 10% and 1.3%, respectively [3]. Thyroid surgery remains a leading cause of bilateral vocal fold immobility. It is possible that complication rates are even higher than reported. For inexperienced or infrequent thyroid surgeons, the risks of total thyroidectomy are unacceptable. Regardless of surgical expertise, the complication rate rises with the extent of surgery.

The long-term survival rate in the low-risk group exceeds 98%. Shah and colleagues [13] at Memorial Sloan-Kettering Cancer Center studied patients who had DTC in a matched-pair analysis. They showed no statistical difference in the long-term outcome based on the extent of thyroidectomy, arguing the unlikelihood that additional treatment in this group would modify long-term outcome. Hay and colleagues [14] and Mazzaferri [15] reported higher recurrence rates with thyroid lobectomy but not higher mortality rates. Shaha and colleagues [16] and Sanders and Cady [17] found no significant difference in recurrence rates or mortality rates for low-risk patients.

Few experts argue a higher mortality rate for low-risk patients undergoing thyroid lobectomy. The unresolved question is the risk of higher recurrence rates in thyroid lobectomy in low-risk patients. Proponents for thyroid lobectomy for low-risk patients argue that local recurrences can be treated with surgery. Excellent long-term outcome with lobectomy alone occurs in

---

Box 2. Arguments for lobectomy in low-risk patients

1. Total thyroidectomy increases the risk of complication of recurrent laryngeal nerve injury and hypoparathyroidism.
2. There is a low risk of mortality (possible increase in recurrence).
3. Multifocal disease does not adversely affect survival rate.

low-risk patients as predicted by AGES [6], AMES [7], MACIS [8], MSKCC [9], and TNM [10].

Multifocal disease may not adversely affect survival rate. The high incidence of microscopic foci in the opposite lobe does not correlate with the clinical recurrence rate. Recurrence in the opposite lobe arises in less than 5% of patients. Tollefsen and colleagues [18] reported that in PTC the rate of occult cancer in the contralateral lobe was 38%, a rate eight times greater than the incidence of clinically recurrent carcinoma in the opposite lobe after initial lobectomy. Remnant resection of recurrence is infrequent when all macroscopic disease has been removed during initial lobectomy [19]. The presence of microscopic foci in PTC does not mean development of clinically significant cancer.

In the United States, advocates of total thyroidectomy for low-risk patients note a rate of up to 85% of microscopic disease in the contralateral lobe but generally do not argue in favor of concomitant elective lateral neck dissection for clinically negative necks, although up to 90% of patients have positive nodes in the lateral neck on close pathologic inspection and a 10% rate of recurrence in the neck. In contrast, practice patterns in Japan favor thyroid lobectomy and lateral neck dissection for PTC rather than total thyroidectomy [20]. Anaplastic transformation of PTC to a remnant thyroid lobe is rare and is felt by some authors to be a weak argument for total thyroidectomy in low-risk patients [21].

Thyroid lobectomy for low-risk follicular thyroid cancer

The most important factor to consider is the invasiveness of the tumor noted intraoperatively by the surgeon and the findings of the pathologist. Well-differentiated FTC with minimal capsular invasion, no vascular invasion, patient age less than 45, and tumors smaller than 4 cm are associated with 100% survival with thyroid lobectomy [22]. Adjuvant radioactive iodine (RAI), thyroglobulin measurement follow-up, and even thyroid suppressive therapy are questioned in FTC with minimal capsule invasion.

Follicular carcinoma most often cannot be differentiated from follicular adenoma on fine-needle aspiration or frozen section. Lobectomy is generally performed with a diagnosis of follicular neoplasm if the opposite lobe is clinically normal. If the final pathology report reveals minimally invasive carcinoma without vascular invasion in a patient younger than age 45, completion thyroidectomy and RAI are not mandatory if the patient can be followed closely. Deaths from minimally invasive thyroid cancer can occur occasionally, however. If the final pathology report reveals major capsular invasion or vascular invasion, this is not a low-risk patient and completion thyroidectomy should be performed with RAI ablation. Clinical nodal disease in adult FTC is less frequent than PTC (approximately 15%–20%). If no nodes are appreciated, central compartment clearance (zone 6) and elective neck dissection are unnecessary.

Arguments for total thyroidectomy for low-risk papillary thyroid cancer

A historical trend over the last several decades shows more total thyroid-ectomies being performed and fewer thyroid lobectomies for PTC, including low-risk patients who have PTC (Box 3). Analysis of surgical procedures per-formed in more than 1500 US hospitals revealed that among 5584 patients who had thyroid cancer, most (77.4%) underwent total thyroidectomy regardless of tumor histology and stage [23]. The American Thyroid Associ-ation and the American Association of Clinical Endocrinologists advocate total thyroidectomy for low-risk patients who have PTC [24,25]. The expec-tations of endocrinologists have been established by these documents.

The arguments for total thyroidectomy for PTC in low-risk patients include unequivocal superior surveillance with diagnostic RAI scans and thyroglobulin measurements. Either of these tests is difficult to interpret in the presence of large amounts of residual thyroid tissue. RAI can be used to diagnose and treat any residual thyroid carcinoma locally, regionally, and distantly. Adjuvant radioiodine therapy is less effective and has a higher incidence of side effects, such as radiation thyroiditis, if excessive thyroid remnant tissue remains.

Mazzaferri and colleagues [26] noted that an undetectable serum thyro-globulin level measured during thyroid hormone suppression of thyroid-stimulating hormone is often misleading. Twenty-one percent of 784 patients who had no clinical evidence of tumor on baseline serum thyroglob-ulin levels (usually <1 µg/L) during thyroid hormone suppression therapy had a rise in serum thyroglobulin to more than 2 µg/L in response to recombinant human thyroid-stimulating hormone. When this occurred, 36% of the patients were found to have metastases that were identified in 91% by a recombinant human thyroid-stimulating hormone–stimulated thyroglobulin of more than 2 µg/L. Diagnostic whole-body scanning, after

---

Box 3. Arguments for total thyroidectomy in low-risk patients

Superior surveillance with RAI scanning and thyroglobulin
  measurement
Low rate of recurrent laryngeal nerve dysfunction and
  hypoparathyroidism in expert hands
Death and recurrence in a small percentage of low-risk patients
Relief of patient anxiety regarding the possible higher rate of
  recurrence with lobectomy
Elimination of the risk of contralateral lobe recurrence
Elements of classification systems are only available
  postoperatively and can be limited in their ability to direct
  initial surgical therapy

either recombinant human thyroid-stimulating hormone or thyroid hormone withdrawal, identified only 19% of cases of metastasis.

In expert hands, the risk of vocal fold dysfunction and hypoparathyroidism can be kept acceptably low (Fig. 2). Surgeons who performed fewer than ten procedures per year had a fourfold higher complication rate than more active thyroid surgeons [27]. Patients who underwent near total and total thyroidectomy have been compared without an increase in recurrence, even in high-risk patients [28]. Near total thyroidectomy may reduce the risk of permanent hypoparathyroidism.

Total thyroidectomy advocates note that deaths and recurrences that cannot be predicted preoperatively by various classification systems occur and are observed even in patients with low-risk thyroid cancer. Elements of certain prognostic classification systems are only available postoperatively and can be limited in their ability to direct initial surgical treatment. Approximately 5% to 10% of patients who have DTC (mostly high risk) die of their disease. Total thyroidectomy alleviates patient anxiety with respect to recurrence and the need for additional surgery. Kebebew and colleagues [29] used a decision analysis model to compare total thyroidectomy and thyroid lobectomy. Overall, prospective patients viewed thyroid cancer recurrence as less desirable than a thyroidectomy complication; 61.5% of individuals viewed occurrence of thyroid complication as better than a thyroid recurrence. The time and expense of repeated operations in recurrence must be considered.

Up to 85% of patients with clinically unilateral papillary malignancy have microscopic cancer in the opposite lobe. Recurrence develops in the contralateral lobe in 5% of patients. Total thyroidectomy eliminates contralateral lobe disease. Many, but not all, retrospective studies [14,15] with long-term follow-up demonstrate decreased recurrence (although not

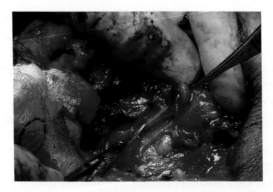

Fig. 2. Recurrent laryngeal nerve bifurcates (hemostat) with superior parathyroid noted (forceps).

mortality) in patients who have total thyroidectomy and RAI ablation compared with lobectomy for low-risk patients.

Asa and colleagues demonstrated that tumors in multicentric PTC carry different *ret/PTC* oncogene rearrangements. This finding suggests that these tumors seem to arise de novo, synchronously or metachronously, from thyroid tissue prone to developing carcinoma, as opposed to the concept that they merely represent intraglandular metastases [30]. To be discovered, genetic and tumor markers may one day accurately predict a tumor's local aggressiveness and metastatic potential.

Multicentric PTC, including bilateral thyroid cancer, occurs in up to 85% of cases, with neck metastasis in 80% to 90% of cases in which the neck is carefully dissected. Central recurrence is associated with substantial mortality. Central compartment neck dissection without grossly involved nodes at the time of total thyroidectomy has been advocated, because re-operation for central compartment recurrence has a significantly higher risk of recurrent laryngeal nerve injury and permanent hypoparathyroidism than does central compartment dissection at the time of initial operation. Others argue that if the paratracheal and tracheoesophageal groove do not have grossly involved nodes, elective central neck dissection is not necessary. Again, failure of long-term prospective studies leaves this an open question.

Massin and colleagues [31] showed that the risk of pulmonary metastasis is reduced as a function of the extent of initial thyroid resection. Pulmonary metastases occurred in 11 of 831 (1.3%) patients who were treated with total thyroidectomy plus iodine-131 and in 91 of 831 (11%) who had thyroid lobectomies.

Total thyroidectomy for high-risk papillary thyroid cancer and invasive follicular thyroid cancer patients

Total thyroidectomy is indicated for patients with tumors larger than 4 cm, extrathyroidal spread (most commonly muscle, followed by recurrent laryngeal nerve, followed by trachea), regional (approximately one third of patients have clinically evident cervical metastasis) or distant metastasis, high histologic grade, and age younger than 16 and older than 45 (Fig. 3). Mortality rates in association with recurrences in high-risk patients approach 40% to 50%. Total thyroidectomy results in less recurrence and mortality over thyroid lobectomy in high-risk patients who have DTC. Two aggressive histologic subtypes of PTC, tall-cell variant and columnar cell variant, warrant strong consideration for total thyroidectomy in otherwise low-risk patients. Multicentricity is not limited to PTC because it occurs in 23% of patients with FTC [32]. The incidence of distant metastasis at presentation is 10% to 15% for FTC. No curable recurrences have been reported in a series with FTC [22].

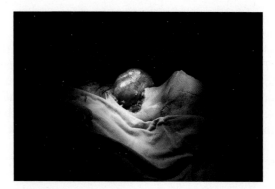

Fig. 3. High-risk PTC: tumor larger than 4 cm, patient age older than 60.

Pediatric differentiated thyroid cancer

Patients younger than age 21 make up 10% of patients who have thyroid cancers. A higher percentage of pediatric thyroid nodules are malignant compared with adults. Pediatric DTC is twice as common in girls, and most cases are PTC (85%–90%). Between 7% and 11% of children treated with radiation develop thyroid cancer; the risk is greatest if radiation was before age 10 [33]. Previous radiotherapy is known to increase the risk of thyroid cancer in children (and adults) but does not influence prognosis in children [34]. Up to 70% of sporadic and radiation-induced PTCs in children carry *ret*/PTC mutations, compared with less than 40% in adults [35].

The argument for total thyroidectomy for pediatric DTC is the higher incidence of distant metastatic dissemination (10% to 15%) versus adults (2%) [36]. In contrast to adult DTC, in which FTC has a higher distant metastatic rate than PTC, in children PTC metastasizes to distant sites at a greater frequency than does FTC. Pulmonary metastases, present in approximately 10% of pediatric cases, are detected more often than in adults. Bone metastases are less common. Multiple foci of disease, incidence of regional lymph node involvement (present in 60%–80%), extrathyroidal tumor infiltration, and distant metastasis are higher particularly in children younger than age 15. Multifocal disease is a predictor of recurrence (but not mortality) after surgical treatment of DTC in the pediatric population [37]. The presence of palpable cervical lymph nodes in children at diagnosis is associated with more invasive forms of malignancy and is a predictive factor of recurrence regardless of the extent of the initial surgery [34]. Diffuse sclerosing variant of papillary carcinoma, which is more frequently observed in children than adults, is associated with aggressive behavior [34]. A higher rate of RAI avidity can be expected compared with adults. Paradoxically, although children who have DTC may present with more advanced disease, they generally have an excellent long-term prognosis, with survival rates more than 90%. Distant metastasis, however, is associated with mortality in half the pediatric patients. DTC recurs in 25% of pediatric patients, sometimes months or years after initial treatment. Long-term monitoring is important. The prevalence of undifferentiated forms is less common.

Uniformity of opinion does not exist for the extent of thyroidectomy with pediatric DTC because of the low mortality rate and high surgical complication rate. Newman and colleagues [38] reported that the recurrence rate after total or subtotal thyroidectomy was identical to the results of lobectomy. La Quaglia and colleagues [39] reported that the risk of a major complication in children younger than age 6 was more than 60%. Others have reported more local recurrences with lobectomy compared with total thyroidectomy [40]. Jarzab and colleagues [41] showed a 97% rate of children in a group treated with Iodine 131 were disease free after 5 years compared with 40% relapse rate without Iodine 131.

Differentiated thyroid cancer during pregnancy

Thyroid nodules in pregnant women are more likely malignant, affecting 1 in 1000. The prognosis of thyroid cancer detected during pregnancy is similar to that for nonpregnant women. Delaying surgery until after delivery prevents maternal complication and fetal death. Human chorionic gonadotropin released during pregnancy accelerates the growth of thyroid carcinoma, and operating during the second trimester allows the tumor to undergo operation at a potentially smaller size. Surgical outcome, with regard to type of operation, operation time, perioperative complications, length of hospital stay, and treatment outcome, did not differ significantly between a group of patients operated during the second trimester when compared with surgery after delivery, despite a slight tumor size increase [42].

Differentiated thyroid cancer in patients younger than age 45

Gemsenjager and colleagues [22] confirmed the impact of age on survival: young patients (<45 years) had a mortality rate of 0% despite stage T4 in 18%, N1 in 35%, and M1 in 7%. Patients younger than age 45 with nodal metastasis do not have a higher mortality rate.

Differentiated thyroid cancer in elderly persons

Ten percent of DTC cases occur in patients older than 65. The risk of recurrence and death increases linearly with age, particularly after age 50. For any 10-year difference in age, there is a near doubling of risk. The death rate for patients over age 70 is more than 50% [43]. Tumors in elderly patients frequently show extrathyroidal spread, with a higher incidence of distant metastases in bones and lungs. The tumors are often not iodine avid. The

prevalent histologic type is papillary, often with features of poor differentiation and a less favorable prognosis compared with younger adults [44].
Nodal metastases in older patients who have DTC are an unfavorable prognostic factor. Total thyroidectomy with postoperative RAI is widely
recommended.

Hürthle cell carcinoma and other aggressive histologic subtypes of differentiated thyroid cancer

Aggressive histologic subtypes of PTC include oxyphilic, tall cell, diffuse
sclerosing, and columnar variants; Hürthle cell carcinoma and insular are
variants for FTC. The incidence of neck metastasis in Hürthle cell carcinoma is approximately 10% (Fig. 4). Hürthle cell carcinoma is associated
with the highest incidence of distant metastases among DTC. Hürthle cell
carcinoma with no or minimal capsular invasion is unlikely to recur and
can be treated adequately with thyroid lobectomy. Total thyroidectomy
with evaluation of the central node compartment is necessary for Hürthle
cell carcinoma with invasion. Hürthle cell carcinoma responds poorly to
RAI treatment; however, ablation of any remaining thyroid tissue is recommended to facilitate the use of serum thyroglobulin levels as a tumor marker
and allow detection of recurrent or metastatic disease that may take up RAI.
Total thyroidectomy with evaluation of the central node compartment is the
treatment for histologically aggressive subtypes of DTC. It should be
strongly considered even in otherwise low-risk patients.

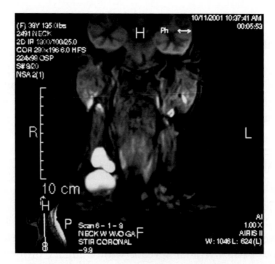

Fig. 4. Hürthle cell thyroid carcinoma metastatic to the neck.

Medullary thyroid cancer

Medullary thyroid carcinoma (MTC) is a neuroendocrine malignancy of the thyroid C cells. It presents as a neck mass in sporadic MTC and index cases of hereditary MTC. Spread of MTC occurs initially to zone 6 nodes and mediastinal lymph nodes (zone 7) and subsequently to lateral cervical nodes. Distant metastasis occurs in 10% of cases on presentation. Diarrhea as a chief complaint is most often associated with metastatic disease with high levels of calcitonin. MTC cells do not concentrate RAI and are not sensitive to hormonal manipulation. Surgery is the mainstay of therapy for primary and recurrent disease.

MTCs produce the polypeptide hormone calcitonin, measurement of which indicates the presence of tumor in at-risk individuals and the effectiveness of therapy in treated patients. The routine use of calcitonin for a thyroid nodule has not been widely practiced in the United States. Basal and stimulated (with calcium gluconate or pentagastrin) serum calcitonin levels are important diagnostic markers. Stimulated tests allow identification of C-cell hyperplasia or early MTC before clinical disease is apparent and are the most sensitive.

Immunostaining for calcitonin can improve the sensitivity of fine-needle aspiration. Preoperative measurement of plasma-free metanephrine and neck ultrasonograpy should always be done if the diagnosis of MTC is known preoperatively. CT of the neck, chest, and abdomen are also important. Sporadic MTC occurs typically in the third decade, manifests as a solid neck tumor (often bilaterally), and accounts for 60% to 70% of patients who have MTC. Hereditary MTC includes MEN type 2 and familial MTC. MTC is present in almost all patients with MEN-2. Hereditary MTC is autosomal dominant with a 90% penetrance. C-cell hyperplasia is a precursor of hereditary MTC, and hereditary MTC is often multicentric and bilateral. C-cell hyperplasia in sporadic cases is of less significance because it can be seen in normal patients and patients who have Grave's disease.

MEN-2 occurs as MEN-2A, also called Sipple's syndrome (MTC, pheochromocytoma, primary hyperparathyroidism, and occasionally lichen amyloidosis and/or Hirschsprung's disease). It represents 90% of patients who have MEN-2. Pheochromocytoma occurs in approximately 50% of patients, may present before or after MTC, and—if present—must be addressed initially. Parathyroidectomy occurs in approximately 30% of patients, and prophylactic parathyroidectomy is not performed without laboratory confirmation of disease. MEN-2B (MTC, pheochromocytoma [occurs in 50%], marfanoid body habitus, thick lips, everted eyelids, mucosal neuromas, and intestinal ganglioneuromatosis) and familial MTC (no other endocrinopathy) are less common. The age of diagnosis in unscreened patients with MEN-2A is 20 to 30 years of age, MEN-2B is younger than 20, and familial MTC is in the fourth decade. MTC makes up approximately 10% of childhood thyroid cancers.

The *ret* gene underlies the oncogenesis of all hereditary and some sporadic MTC. Approximately 60% of patients who have sporadic MTC have somatic *ret* mutations and an associated comparatively more aggressive course. The physiologic function of *ret* includes neural crest cell migration and gastrointestinal and genitourinary development. The *ret* gene encodes a transmembrane tyrosine kinase receptor, *ret* (*rearranged during transfection*). A single *ret* germline mutation results in a proto-oncogene in the pericentriomeric region of chromosome 10 (locus 10q11.2) that consists of 21 exons. Various mutations are noted in different codons, with codon 634 *ret* mutation (exon 11) being the most common and associated with classic MEN-2A. Many known mutated codons result in different phenotypes of the disease and predict the age of onset of MTC. Codons 768 (exon 13) and 891 (exon 15) are more specific for familial MDC [45]. The mutation in MEN-2B is almost always at codon-918 (exon 16) [46]. *Ret* mutations, identified by polymerase chain reaction amplification, are identified in approximately 98% of MEN-2A and 93% of MEN-2B families [47]. All first-degree relatives of persons who have MTC must be screened. *Ret* testing in sporadic MTC is also performed because it may represent the index case of familial MTC in 1% to 7% of cases [47].

The importance of early diagnosis for MEN-2 is important. Normal calcitonin levels are less than 10 pg/mL. If the only evidence of MTC is a minimally increased peripheral plasma calcitonin level (ie, 25–100 pg/mL), the chance of curing a patient is 95%; for calcitonin levels between 1000 and 5000 pg/mL the cure rate is approximately 90%; when the preoperative stimulated plasma calcitonin level exceeds 10,000 pg/mL, the cure rated falls to 40% [48].

Biochemical screening of abnormal pentagastrin-stimulated calcitonin levels has been replaced by genetic screening of all relatives at risk. Almost half the thyroidectomy specimens from *ret*-positive children with positive calcitonin testing have microscopic MTC [49]. Currently, practice standards include genetic testing at birth with total thyroidectomy in children with *ret* mutations; ideally before age 5 in patients who have MEN-2A and familial MTC and in the first 6 months of life for patients who have MEN-2B [50]. Central but not lateral neck dissection is performed unless clinically suspicious lateral nodes are noted intraoperatively. Parathyroid tissue should be autotransplanted to the forearm in patients who have MEN-2A caused by a codon 634 *ret* mutation to facilitate excision if hyperparathyroidism develops. *Ret* testing may have reduced mortality from MEN-2 to less than 5% [47].

For sporadic cases or index hereditary cases, total thyroidectomy and central lymph node dissection are the standard and minimum treatments for MTC. Positive lymph nodes correlate with the size of the primary lesion. Positive lymph nodes are found in 11% of patients who have a tumor smaller than 1 cm. They are found in 60% of tumors larger than 2 cm [51]. Patients with palpable unilateral intrathyroidal tumors have nodal metastases present in 81% of central nodes, 81% of ipsilateral selective (zones II to V) neck dissections, and 44% of contralateral selective (zones II to V) neck dissections [52]. Palpable MTC should be treated with total thyroidectomy, central neck lymph node dissection, and bilateral neck dissection.

The 10-year survival rate for MTC is approximately 80%. Prognosis is unpredictable. Although some patients with metastatic disease live for years, others with a similar stage succumb rapidly. Patients with raised postoperative calcitonin and no clinical or radiographic evidence of disease may not develop overt disease. Sporadic MTC is associated with a 50% to 75% survival rate; however, when matched for age and extent of disease, it is similar to hereditary MTC [53]. Familial MTC has a more indolent course. Favorable prognostic factors are young age, female gender, and tumor confined to the gland.

Postoperative stimulated calcitonin is more sensitive than basal levels. Patients with elevated calcitonin levels (or carcinoembryonic antigen levels) should have imaging by CT scan, MRI, meta-iodobenzylguanidine scan, or fluorodeoxyglucose positron emission tomography to identify sites of recurrence and metastasis. The role of radiation therapy is not well defined. It has been used in the postoperative setting and for bone metastasis. There is currently no effective systemic therapy for MTC.

Activating mutations in a tyrosine kinase receptor gene are present in most MTCs, and experience with tyrosine kinase inhibitors in the setting of clinical trials is critical for the identification of effective systemic treatment. ZD6474 (vandetanib) selectively targets vascular epidermal growth factor receptor, epidermal growth factor receptor, and *ret* tyrosine kinase activity. Therapeutic nuclids (90Yttrium-labeled octreotide), and chemoembolization of liver metastases are currently other promising therapeutic concepts in patients with distant metastases.

Anaplastic thyroid cancer

ATC presents as a rapidly growing neck mass with progressive dysphagia and airway obstruction (Figs. 5 and 6). ATC does not concentrate iodine or express thyroglobulin. Tumors larger than 4 cm, vocal fold immobility, and tracheal invasion are common. Horner's syndrome also may occur. Distant metastasis can occur in multiple organ sites but is most common in the lung. Death within months is the most common outcome. ATC generally occurs in the seventh decade of life, with a female/male ratio of 2:1. Thyrotoxicosis secondary to rapid thyroid tissue destruction from necrosis can be seen. Approximately half the patients have a history of prior DTC or goiter in the resected specimen. ATC may arise from dedifferentiation of a DTC in up to 20% of cases [54]. Fine-needle aspiration is the best initial test. True cut needle biopsy or open biopsy may be required. All ATCs are

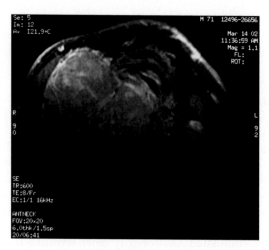

Fig. 5. ATC with airway obstruction.

American Joint Commission on Cancer stage IV. Diminishing incidence is likely related to iodine supplementation.

Airway protection (either tracheotomy or, when not feasible, endotracheal stenting) and nutritional support are initial goals. Radical surgery must be tempered with the knowledge that less than 10% of patients survive, and survival depends on feasibility of resection, complications of resection, and presence of distant metastasis. Long-term survivors who undergo combined surgery and radiation often have had only small foci of ATC in association with DTC [55]. The rare survival with ATC is associated with complete resection and associated with tumors smaller than 5 cm, patients younger than age 70, and no distant metastasis. Because ATC does not

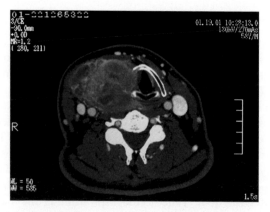

Fig. 6. ATC with erosion of thyroid cartilage.

accumulate iodine, the extent of thyroidectomy is less important as long as negative margins are achieved. Distant metastasis, mostly to the lung, is reported in 50% of patients at time of presentation [56]. Chemotherapy (with 5-fluorouracil and cisplatin) and radiotherapy followed by debulking surgery results in palliation but little hope of long-term survival. Preoperative radiotherapy to 3000 rad with doxorubicin IV, subsequent debulking surgery, and postoperative radiation therapy to 4600 rad led to 4 patients in a series of 33 with no evidence of disease surviving for more than 2 years [57]. Manumycin, a farnesyl protein transferase inhibitor, blocks *ras* oncogene function. ATC may involve mutations in the *ras* proto-oncogene. Enhanced cytotoxic effects and cell apoptosis in ATC have been reported with manumycin [58]. Combretastatin A4 phosphate, a vascular targeting agent, causes a rapid and selective shutdown of tumor blood vessels leading to massive necrosis. Combretastatin A4 phosphate may be efficacious when combined with conventional chemotherapeutic drugs or radiation [59].

Thyroid lymphoma

Thyroid lymphoma occurs most often in the sixth decade of life, with a female predominance (4 to 1). It often can present before age 60. Exposure to radiation does not increase the risk of thyroid lymphoma. Its increased frequency is paralleled with the increase in Hashimoto's thyroiditis, which increases a patient's risk of thyroid lymphoma by 70-fold [60]. The associated large B-cell type lymphoma is often accompanied by chronic lymphocytic thyroiditis. Hodgkin's disease can involve the thyroid gland secondarily, although it is rare. The thyroid contains no native lymphoid tissue.

Like ATC, thyroid lymphoma can present as a rapidly expanding thyroid mass often fixed to surrounding structures. It also can present as a slow-growing solid nodule, often with cervical and mediastinal involvement (stage IIE) (Table 1). Fine-needle aspiration may not be able to distinguish thyroid lymphoma from ATC, and core needle or open biopsy may be required. Advances in immunohistochemistry and flow cytometry will reduce the need for open biopsy or core needle biopsy. Differentiating low-grade mucosa–associated lymphoma and thyroiditis may continue to require

Table 1
Staging of thyroid lymphoma

Stage	Disease extent
IE	Thyroid alone
IIE	Thyroid and regional lymph nodes
IIIE	Thyroid and node involvement above and below diaphragm
IV	Thyroid and diffuse organ involvement

open biopsy. CT of the brain, head and neck, chest, abdomen, and pelvis and bone marrow biopsy is requisite. PET scan can be positive with thyroiditis or malignancy. High standardized uptake values are more likely cancer. Most patients have diffuse large B-cell lymphoma or mixed mucosa-associated lymphoid type (MALT) lymphoma or mixed mucosa-associated lymphoid type (MALT) lymphoma and diffuse large B-cell lymphoma. They are treated with combined radiation therapy and chemotherapy. Lymphomas with mucosa-associated lymphoid type (MALT) lymphoma characteristics present as indolent localized extranodal tumor and at stage IEA can be treated with surgery or radiotherapy alone.

Summary

The disturbing rise in the number of cases of DTC is likely based on earlier surveillance. High-risk patients who have thyroid cancer are treated with total thyroidectomy. In the United States, low-risk patients who have DTC (T1 or T2, N0, M0, <45 years of age and >16 years of age, with PTC, without aggressive histologic variant, without family history of DTC, and without bilateral disease or FTC with minimal capsule invasion) currently are treated predominantly with total thyroidectomy. Persuasive arguments for total thyroidectomy and thyroid lobectomy have been made for low-risk patients who have DTC. Clearly a different biology exists for most patients with low-risk DTC when compared with high-risk DTC. Yet-to-be discovered tumor markers ultimately will lead to a trend of less aggressive thyroid surgery. Activating mutations in a tyrosine kinase receptor gene are present in most MTCs, and experience with tyrosine kinase inhibitors in the setting of clinical trials is critical for the identification of effective systemic treatment.

References

[1] Davies L, Welch HG. Increasing incidence of thyroid cancer in the United States, 1973–2002. JAMA 2006;295(18):2164–7.

[2] Busnardo B, De Vido D. The epidemiology and etiology of differentiated thyroid carcinoma. Biomed Pharmacother 2000;54:322–6.

[3] Hundhal SA, Fleming ID, Fremgen AM, et al. A National Cancer Data Base report on 53,856 cases of thyroid carcinoma treated in the US, 1985–1995. Cancer 1998;83:2638–40.

[4] Geiger JD, Thompson NW. Thyroid tumors in children. Otolaryngol Clin North Am 1996; 29(4):711–9.

[5] Cady B. Hayes Martin Lecture. Our AMES is true: how an old concept still hits the mark; or, risk group assignment points the arrow to rational therapy selection in thyroid cancer. Am J Surg 1997;174(5):462–8.

[6] Hay ID, Grant CS, Taylor WF, et al. Ipsilateral lobectomy versus bilateral lobar resection in papillary thyroid carcinoma: a retrospective analysis of surgical outcome using a novel prognostic scoring system. Surgery 1987;102:1088–95.

[7] Cady B, Rossi R. An expanded view of risk-group definition in differentiated thyroid carcinoma. Surgery 1988;104:947–53.

[8] Hay ID, Bergstralh EJ, Goellner JR, et al. Predicting outcome in papillary thyroid carcinoma: development of a reliable prognostic scoring system in a cohort of 1779 patients surgically treated at one institution during 1940–1989. Surgery 1993;114:1050–8.

[9] Shaha A, Loree TR, Shah JP. Intermediate-risk group for differentiate carcinoma of thyroid. Surgery 1994;116:1036–41.

[10] Greene FL. American Joint Committee on Cancer: updating the strategies in cancer staging. Bull Am Coll Surg 2002;87(7):13–5.

[11] Kebebew E, Clark OH. Differentiated thyroid cancer: "complete" rational approach. World J Surg 2000;24:942–51.

[12] National Comprehensive Cancer Network. Thyroid carcinoma: clinical practice guidelines in oncology, version 2. 2007. Available at: www.nccn.org/professionals/physician_gls/PDF/thyroid.pdf. Accessed November 10, 2007.

[13] Shah JP, Loree T, Dharker D, et al. Prognostic factors in differentiated carcinoma of the thyroid: a matched pair analysis. Am J Surg 1992;166:331–5.

[14] Hay ID, Grant CS, Bergstralh EJ, et al. Unilateral total lobectomy: is it sufficient surgical treatment for patients with AMES low-risk papillary thyroid carcinoma? Surgery 1998; 124:958–64.

[15] Mazzaferri EL. An overview of the management of papillary and follicular thyroid carcinoma. Thyroid 1999;9:421–7.

[16] Shaha AR, Shah JP, Loree TR. Low-risk differentiated thyroid cancer: the need for selective treatment. Ann Surg Oncol 1997;4:328–33.

[17] Sanders LE, Cady B. Differentiated thyroid cancer: reexamination of risk groups and outcome of treatment. Arch Surg 1998;133:419–25.

[18] Tollefsen HR, Shah FP, Huvos AG. Papillary carcinoma of the thyroid: recurrence in the thyroid gland after initial surgical treatment. Am J Surg 1972;124:468–72.

[19] Beahrs OH. Surgical treatment for thyroid cancer. Br J Surg 1984;71:976–9.

[20] Shigematsu N, Takami H, Nobutake I, et al. Nationwide survey on the treatment policy for well-differentiated thyroid cancer: results of a questionnaire distributed at the 37th meeting of the Japanese Society of Thyroid Surgery. Endocr J 2005;52:479–91.

[21] Cohn KH, Backdahl M, Forsslund G, et al. Biologic considerations and operative strategy in papillary thyroid carcinoma: arguments against the routine performance of total thyroidectomy. Surgery 1984;96:957–71.

[22] Gemsenjager E, Heitz PU, Seifert B, et al. Differentiated thyroid carcinoma. Swiss Med Wkly 2001;131:157–63.

[23] Hundahl SA, Cady B, Cunningham MP, et al. Initial results from a prospective cohort study of 5583 cases of thyroid carcinoma treated in the United States during 1996. US and German Thyroid Cancer Study Group. An American College of Surgeons commission on cancer patient care evaluation study. Cancer 2000;89:202–17.

[24] Cooper DS, Doherty GM, Haugen BR, et al. Management guidelines for patients with thyroid nodules and differentiated thyroid cancer. Thyroid 2006;16(2):109–41.

[25] Cobin RH, Gharib H, Bergman DA, et al. AACE/AAES medical/surgical guidelines for clinical practice: management of thyroid carcinoma. Endocr Pract 2001;7(3):202–20.

[26] Mazzaferri EL, Robbins RJ, Spencer CA, et al. A consensus report of the role of serum thyroglobulin as a monitoring method for low-risk patients with papillary throid carcinoma. J Clin Endocrinol Metab 2003;88:1433–41.

[27] Sosa JA, Bowman HM, Tielsch JM, et al. The importance of surgeon experience for clinical and economic outcomes from thyroidectomy. Ann Surg 1998;3:320–30.

[28] Grant CS, Hay ID, Gough IR, et al. Local recurrence in papillary thyroid carcinoma: is extent of surgical resection important? Surgery 1988;104(6):954–62.

[29] Kebebew E, Duh QY, Clark OH. Total thyroidectomy or thyroid lobectomy in patients with low-risk differentiated thyroid cancer: surgical decision analysis of a controversy using a mathematical model. World J Surg 2000;24:1295–302.

[30] Sagg SL, Ezzat S, Rosen IB, et al. Distinct multiple *RET/PTC* gene rearrangements in multifocal papillary thyroid neoplasia. J Clin Endocrinol Metab 1998;83:4116–22.

[31] Massin JP, Savoie JC, Garnier H, et al. Pulmonary metastases in differentiated thyroid carcinoma: study of 58 cases with implications for the primary tumor treatment. Cancer 1984;53:982–92.

[32] Hay ID, McConahey WM, Goellner JR. Managing patients with papillary thyroid carcinoma: insights gained from the Mayo Clinic's experience of treating 2512 consecutive patients during 1940 through 2000. Trans Am Clin Climatol Assoc 2002;113:241–60.

[33] McClellan DR, Francis GL. Thyroid cancer in children, pregnant women, and patients with Grave's disease. Endocrinol Metab Clin North Am 1996;25(1):27–48.

[34] Borson-Chazot F, Causeret S, Lifante JC, et al. Predictive factors for recurrence from a series of 74 children and adolescents with differentiated thyroid cancer. World J Surg 2004;28: 1088–92.

[35] Puxeddu E, Fagin JA. Genetic markers in thyroid neoplasia. Endocrinol Metab Clin North Am 2001;30(2):493–513.

[36] Giuffrida D, Scollo C, Pellegriti G, et al. Differentiated thyroid cancer in children and adolescents. J Endocrinol Invest 2002;25:18–24.

[37] Harness JK, Thompson NW, McLeod MK, et al. Differentiated thyroid carcinoma in children and adolescents. World J Surg 1992;16:547–54.

[38] Newman KD, Black T, Heller G, et al. Differentiated thyroid cancer: determinants of disease progression in patients < 21 years of age at diagnosis. A report from the surgical discipline committee of the children's cancer group. Ann Surg 1988;227:533–41.

[39] La Quaglia MP, Corbally MT, Heller G, et al. Recurrence and morbidity in differentiated thyroid carcinoma in children. Surgery 1988;104:1149–56.

[40] Welch Dinauer CA, Tuttle RM, Robie DK, et al. Extensive surgery improves recurrence-free survival for children and young patients with class I papillary thyroid carcinoma. J Pedeatr Surg 1999;34:1799–804.

[41] Jarzab B, Handkiewicz J, Wloch J, et al. Multivariate analysis of prognostic factors for differentiated thyroid carcinoma in children. Eur J Nucl Med 2000;27:834–41.

[42] Nam K, Yoon JH, Chang H, et al. Optimal timing of surgery in well-differentiated thyroid carcinoma detected during pregnancy. J Surg Oncol 2005;91:199–203.

[43] Cady B. Presidential address. Beyond risk groups: a new look at differentiated thyroid cancer. Surgery 1998;124(6):947–57.

[44] Vini L, Hyer SL, Marshall J, et al. Long-term results in elderly patients with differentiated thyroid carcinoma. Cancer 2003;97:2736–42.

[45] Eng C, Clayton D, Schuffenecker I, et al. The relationship between specific RET proto-oncogene mutations and disease phenotype in multiple endocrine neoplasia type 2: international RET mutation consortium analysis. JAMA 1996;276:1575–9.

[46] Santoro M, Carlomagno F, Romano A, et al. Activation of RET as a dominant transforming gene by germline mutations of MEN2A and MEN2B. Science 1995;267:381–3.

[47] Brandi ML, Gagel RF, Angeli A, et al. Consensus: guidelines for diagnosis for MEN type 1 and type 2. J Endocrinol Metab 2001;86(12):5658–71.

[48] Wells SA Jr, Dilley WG, Farndon JA, et al. Early diagnosis and treatment of medullary thyroid carcinoma. Arch Intern Med 1985;145(7):1248–52.

[49] Cote CJ, Wohllk N, Evans D, et al. RET proto-oncogene mutations in multiple endocrine neoplasia type 2 and medullary thyroid carcinoma. Bailleres Clin Endocrinol Metab 1995; 9(3):609–30.

[50] Pacini F, Romei C, Micolli P, et al. Early treatment of hereditary medullary thyroid carcinoma after attribution of multiple endocrine neoplasia type 2 gene carrier status by screening for ret gene mutations. Surgery 1995;118(6):1031–5.

[51] Duh QY, Sancho JJ, Greenspan FS, et al. Medullary thyroid carcinoma: the need for early diagnosis and total thyroidectomy. Arch Surg 1989;124(10):1206–10.

[52] Moley JF, De Benedetti MK. Patterns of nodal metastases in palpable medullary thyroid carcinoma: recommendations for extent of node dissection. Ann Surg 1999;229(6):887–8.

[53] Samaan NA, Schultz PN, Hickey RC. Medullary thyroid carcinoma: prognosis of familial versus sporadic disease and the role of radiotherapy. J Clin Endocrinol Metab 1988;67: 801–5.

[54] Spires JR, Schwartz MR, Miller RH. Anaplastic thyroid carcinoma: association with differentiated thyroid cancer. Arch Otolaryngol Head Neck Surg 1988;114(1):40–4.

[55] Demeter JG, DeJong SA, Lawrence AM, et al. Anaplastic thyroid carcinoma: risk factors and outcome. Surgery 1991;110(6):956–61.

[56] Pierie JP, Muzikansky A, Gaz RD, et al. The effect of surgery and radiotherapy on outcome of anaplastic thyroid carcinoma. Ann Surg Oncol 2002;9(1):57–64.

[57] Tennvall J, Tallroth E, elHassan A, et al. Anaplastic thyroid carcinoma: doxorubicin, hyperfractionated radiotherapy and surgery. Acta Oncol 1990;29(8):1025–8.

[58] Yeung SC, Xu G, Pan J, et al. Manumycin enhances the cytotoxic effect of paclitaxel on anaplastic thyroid carcinoma cells. Cancer Res 2000;60(3):650–6.

[59] Thorpe PE. Vascular targeting agents as cancer therapeutics. Clin Cancer Res 2004;10(2): 415–27.

[60] Holm LE, Blomgren H, Lowenhagen T. Cancer risks in patients with chronic lymphocytic thyroiditis. N Engl J Med 1985;312(10):601–4.

ELSEVIER
SAUNDERS

Surg Oncol Clin N Am
17 (2008) 93–120

SURGICAL
ONCOLOGY CLINICS
OF NORTH AMERICA

Surgery for Thyroid Cancer

Ziv Gil, MD, PhD, Snehal G. Patel, MD*

*Head and Neck Service, Department of Surgery, Memorial Sloan-Kettering Cancer Center,
1275 York Avenue, New York, NY 10065, USA*

Surgical resection of the thyroid gland is standard treatment for management of carcinomas and is performed by a variety of specialists, including general surgeons, otolaryngologists, endocrine surgeons, and oncologic surgeons. Oncologic thyroid surgery has three main objectives: to assure complete removal of one or both of the thyroid lobes, to preserve the parathyroid (PT) glands and their blood supply, and to prevent injury to the superior and recurrent laryngeal nerves (RLNs). To perform safe and efficient thyroid surgery, surgeons should be familiar not only with the anatomy of the thyroid gland and the vital structures along the course of the gland but also with the anatomic variations in regional anatomy. Although postoperative complications are infrequent in experienced hands, hypocalcemia and vocal cord paralysis can lead to significant morbidity and impaired quality of life. The operation of thyroidectomy has been performed for more than a century [1] and is well described in the literature with the expected variation in the actual technique of the procedure.

This article describes the technique of thyroidectomy in detail as practiced by the authors at Memorial Sloan-Kettering Cancer Center for the surgical treatment of thyroid cancer. A technique that facilitates complete extracapsular resection of the thyroid, preserves the PT glands with their blood supply, the RLNs, and the superior laryngeal nerves, and minimizes postoperative complications is emphasized. Management of certain specific situations, such as retrosternal goiter, locally invasive thyroid cancer, and reoperative surgery for locally recurrent cancer, is discussed but management of the regional lymph nodes is not addressed here.

Standard surgical technique of thyroidectomy

The extent of surgical resection of the thyroid gland for well-differentiated thyroid cancer (WDTC) has been debated extensively and the

* Corresponding author.
  E-mail address: patels@mskcc.org (S.G. Patel).

1055-3207/08/$ - see front matter © 2008 Elsevier Inc. All rights reserved.
doi:10.1016/j.soc.2007.10.014   *surgonc.theclinics.com*

indications and pros and cons of hemi- versus total thyroidectomy are discussed in the article by Witt elsewhere in this issue. The authors practice a policy of risk stratification in deciding the extent of surgery, and the technique of unilateral extirpation of the thyroid lobe is described, as bilateral resection is performed in a similar fashion.

Skin incision planning

Skin incision preferably should be marked with patients awake and sitting up. The skin incision is planned so that it provides optimal surgical exposure for safe conduct of the operation and results in the best cosmetic outcome. A suitable transverse line of relaxed skin tension in the lower neck most commonly fulfills these requirements.

Variability in body habitus and the extent of access required dictate the location and length of the skin incision, and the site and length of the incision never should be based on cosmetic considerations alone. Planning of the incision should take into account the length and width of the patient's neck, the size of the thyroid gland, and presence of previous surgical scars (Fig. 1). Patients who have a long neck may require selection of a higher skin crease to allow full access to the superior poles of the thyroid gland, which are located more cephalad than in patients who have a short neck. If the usual lower skin crease is chosen in patients who have a long neck, a longer incision is required in order to provide sufficient access to the superior poles. Careful planning of the incision in female patients who have large breasts is especially important, because the skin over the manubrium tends to ride up into the neck when the patient is supine on the operating table. A higher skin crease may need to be selected in these patients in order to avoid a wide, hypertrophic scar and poor cosmetic outcome is seen not uncommonly in incisions that come to lie on the skin of the upper chest.

An incision that extends from the anterior border of one sternocleidomastoid muscle to the other generally is adequate for routine thyroidectomy. This incision usually is sufficient to provide access for paratracheal node dissection, but lateral extension along the skin crease to the anterior border of the trapezius muscle is required for access to levels II–V in the lateral neck. Lateral extension of the incision also may be required for delivery of a large goiter.

Positioning and draping

The patient is placed on the operating room table in a supine position. General anesthesia is administered and an oral endotracheal tube inserted by an anesthesiologist. Unless there are specific medical requirements, a 6- to 6.5-mm size endotracheal tube is used routinely in order to minimize trauma to the vocal cords. Lacrilube ophthalmic ointment is applied to both eyes before they are taped shut with Microfoam tape. Venodyne pressure

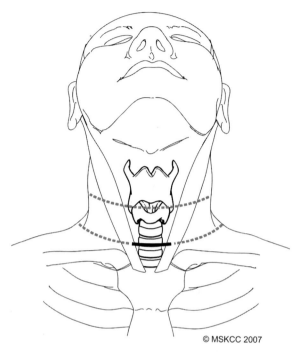

© MSKCC 2007

Fig. 1. A transverse skin crease in the lower neck is chosen most commonly for the skin incision (*bold line*). This incision can be extended laterally if neck dissection is required or, alternatively, a higher skin crease can be selected (*dotted lines*). (*Courtesy of* the Memorial Sloan-Kettering Cancer Center, New York, NY; with permission.)

devices are used routinely, although deep vein thrombosis is uncommon after thyroid surgery. The head is stabilized with a soft donut holder and the operating table is elevated at a 30° angle with the head up (reverse Trendelenburg) and the neck in extension (Fig. 2). Exceptions may need to be made for patients who have restricted mobility of the spine and special care must be taken to avoid injury. Adequate extension of the neck may not be attained in obese patients unless folded sheets are placed under the shoulders to elevate them.

Severe neuropraxia of the brachial plexus is prevented by avoiding stretching of the arms. Injury to the ulnar nerves is avoided by protecting the elbows with adequate padding.

Hypotensive anesthesia is preferable for minimizing bleeding, and communication with the anesthesiologist is crucial in this regard. Prophylactic antibiotics have been shown ineffective in reducing infections after thyroid surgery [2] and the authors do not administer them routinely.

The surgeon should be aware of the possibility that extension of the neck may pull the endotracheal tube out 2 to 4 cm from its original location. Caudal repositioning of the tube may be required, and the position of the tube

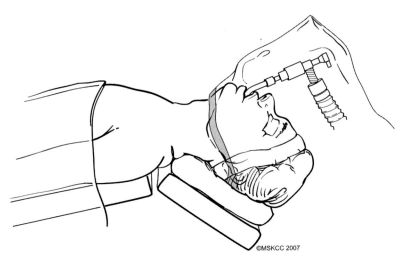

©MSKCC 2007

Fig. 2. The patient is positioned supine on the operating table, which is maintained in a reverse Trendelenburg position with the neck extended. A transparent plastic drape allows continuous monitoring of the endotracheal tube and anesthesia circuit. (*Courtesy of* the Memorial Sloan-Kettering Cancer Center, New York, NY; with permission.)

should always be confirmed before prepping and draping. The patient is prepped and draped in a standard surgical fashion. A transparent plastic drape is used to drape the head (from the level of the jaw line upward) to allow continuous monitoring of the endotracheal tube and anesthesia circuit (see Fig. 2).

Development of cutaneous flaps

The skin is incised with a #15 blade and subsequent dissection is performed with electrocautery at the lowest effective setting. The platysma muscle is incised and cutaneous flaps are developed in the subplatysmal plane (Fig. 3). This plane separates the superficial cervical fascia from the superficial layer of the deep cervical fascia. Care is taken to prevent injury to the anterior jugular veins, which are maintained on the superficial layer of the deep cervical fascia. The superior flap is developed to a point approximately 1 cm cephalad to the thyroid notch and the inferior flap to the level of the superior border of the manubrium sterni. The flaps are retracted and held in place using elastic stay hooks or a Mahorner retractor.

Exposure and management of the strap muscles

The superficial layer of the deep cervical fascia is divided along the avascular midline between the infrahyoid strap muscles. Small veins interconnecting the anterior jugular veins are clamped and divided. The isthmus of the thyroid gland lies immediately deep in the midline and care is taken to

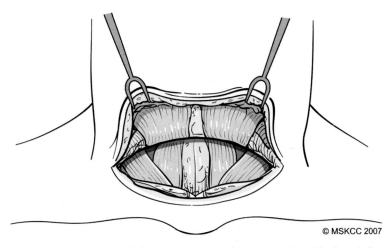

© MSKCC 2007

Fig. 3. The platysma muscle is incised and cutaneous flaps are developed in the subplatysmal plane. (*Courtesy of* the Memorial Sloan-Kettering Cancer Center, New York, NY; with permission.)

avoid injury to the thyroid tissue and vessels during this part of the dissection. After incision of the midline fascia from the level of the cricoid to sternal notch, dissection and appropriate management of the infrahyoid strap muscles is the next step in exposure of the thyroid lobes, especially the superior poles.

A small thyroid gland can be exposed adequately without dividing the sternothyroid muscles (STMs). In this scenario, the strap muscles are retracted laterally and elevated meticulously off the thyroid capsule by dissecting in the avascular areolar tissue that separates the two structures, allowing full exposure of the thyroid lobe. Lateral retraction of the infrahyoid strap muscles almost always provides adequate exposure of the lower pole and body of the thyroid lobe. Adequate exposure of the superior pole and its anatomic relations, however, may be inadequate unless the STM is divided close to its attachment to the thyroid cartilage. Further division of the fascia between the sternohyoid muscle (SHM) and the medial border of the sternocleidomastoid muscle is a useful maneuver that allows wider retraction and better exposure of the superior pole of the thyroid without division of the STM. If lateral retraction of the strap muscles does not provide adequate exposure of the superior pole, the surgeon should have a low threshold for division of the STM. In such instances, the SHM is separated from the STM using the electrocautery. Bipolar electrocautery is used to coagulate blood vessels in the areolar tissue between the two strap muscles. Lateral retraction of the SHM while retracting the thyroid lobe medially allows exposure of the STM and its attachment to the thyroid cartilage. The internal jugular vein can be demonstrated at the lateral border of the STM. The superior attachment of the STM is identified clearly and the electrocautery is used to carefully divide the muscle close to this attachment. Division of the STM close to its superior attachment facilitates exposure of the superior thyroid artery and relevant anatomy and preserves muscle innervation by the ansa hypoglossus.

The divided STM then is retracted laterally for the remainder of the operation and no attempt is made to suture it back it into place. In selected instances, a segment of the STM may need to be resected in continuity with the underlying thyroid gland. Gross extrathyroidal extension (ETE) of tumor that is identified clinically, radiologically, or intraoperatively is an indication for such a maneuver. The STM also may be resected in order to provide an adequate surgical margin if ETE is suspected either pre- or intraoperatively. After division of the STM close to its superior attachment, the muscle is transected inferiorly at the level of the sternal notch so that the segment that abuts the tumor is left in situ on the thyroid lobe.

Although division of the STM is required not infrequently, the SHM only rarely needs to be divided in the absence of gross involvement by tumor. Exposure and delivery of a large goiter, especially with retrosternal extension, may be facilitated, however, by division of both infrahyoid strap muscles.

After exposure of the thyroid gland, both lobes are inspected carefully and palpated before proceeding further. If the contralateral lobe is normal on intraoperative examination and total thyroidectomy is indicated, the authors generally prefer to start with the normal side before dissecting the abnormal lobe. Apart from allowing safe dissection and preservation of the PT glands and RLN in the presence of undistorted normal regional anatomy, this approach provides the surgeon an indication of potential anatomic variations on the contralateral pathologic side.

Exposure of the superior thyroid pole and preservation of the superior laryngeal nerve

Dissection of the thyroid lobe begins by delineating the extent of its superior pole. If the STM is not divided, retraction of the strap muscles with a Richardson retractor laterally and with a right angle retractor cephalad, facilitates exposure of the tip the superior pole. The most important anatomic relation of the superior thyroid pedicle is the external branch of the superior laryngeal nerve (ESLN), but the surgeon also should be aware of the superior PT gland and its vascular supply during this dissection. Division of the superior thyroid vascular pedicle is an important initial step in mobilization of the thyroid lobe.

Mass ligature of the superior pedicle is ill advised for several reasons: (1) the extent of thyroid parenchymal tissue at the superior thyroid pole is variable and its cephalad-most portion easily can be left behind after thyroidectomy, causing superfluous uptake during postsurgical radioactive iodine (RAI) scanning; (2) the ESLN often accompanies the superior thyroid vessels and may be injured during mass ligation of the pedicle; (3) high ligation of the superior thyroid artery may compromise blood supply to the superior PT gland; (4) the superior PT gland occasionally is located posteriorly at the superior pole and inadvertently may be resected with the specimen; and (5) bleeding from a mass ligated superior pedicle may be difficult to control, because the vessels retract cephalad and the ESLN is at risk for injury if blind application of hemostats is attempted. Before ligation of the superior thyroid vessels, the surgeon should be aware of three anatomic variants of the main trunk of ESLN (Fig. 4). In the first variant, the ESLN descends superficial to the inferior constrictor muscle, traveling along the superior thyroid vessels before innervating the cricothyroid muscle. In the second variant, the ESLN pierces the inferior constrictor muscle approximately 1 cm above the cricothyroid membrane. In the third variant, the ESLN runs deep to the inferior constrictor muscle, thereby protecting the nerve from unintended injury [3]. High and mass ligation of the superior thyroid pedicle increases the risk for inadvertent injury to the ESLN in the first two anatomic variants, and the nerve would be safe only in the third variant where it runs deep to the fibers of the inferior constrictor muscle. For the reasons discussed previously, the authors prefer to ligate the individual branches of the superior thyroid artery and veins. These vessels frequently are found anterior to the medial aspect of the superior pole. The technique

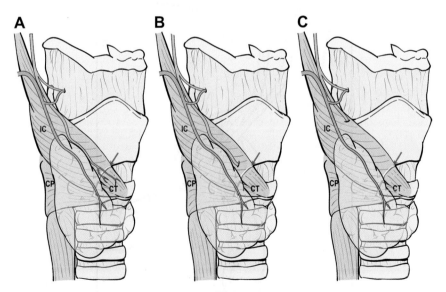

Fig. 4. Variations in the anatomic relationship of the main trunk of the ESLN to the inferior constrictor (IC) muscle and superior thyroid pedicle. (A) The ESLN descends superficial to the IC muscle along the superior thyroid vessels so that it is visible in its entire course before innervating the cricothyroid (CT) muscle. (B) The ESLN pierces the IC muscle approximately 1 cm above the cricothyroid membrane (red arrow) so that only its upper portion is at risk for injury. (C) The ESLN runs deep to the IC muscle and, therefore, is protected from unintended injury during dissection in the vicinity of the superior thyroid pole. The cricopharyngeus muscle is marked CP.

of individual vessel ligation allows the surgeon to delineate the thyroid parenchymal tissue at the superior pole from its surrounding structures
(Fig. 5). Division of the anterior branches releases the tethered pole, expos-
ing its superior and posterior borders. As the dissection continues along the
posterior border of the superior pole, the pole gradually drops down caudally, away from the ESLN, and the remaining small posterior vessels can
be cauterized safely with a fine-tipped bipolar electrocautery (Fig. 6). Separation of the superior pole from its superomedial attachment to the fascia
surrounding the cricothyroid muscles often is required. Within this tissue,
tiny vessels not infrequently interconnect the superior thyroid vessels to
the fascia covering the cricothyroid muscles. These vessels should be cauterized carefully with a bipolar electrocautery close to the gland in order to prevent inadvertent injury to the ESLN.

*Capsular dissection of the thyroid lobe and preservation
of the parathyroid glands*

After mobilization of the superior pole of the thyroid lobe, the next step
is medial rotation of the lobe to provide exposure to its posterolateral

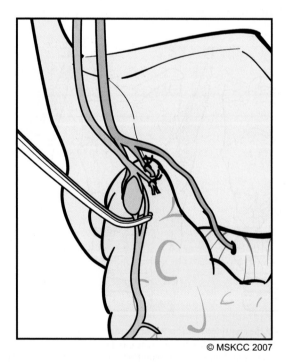

© MSKCC 2007

Fig. 5. The technique of individual vessel ligation allows the surgeon to delineate the thyroid
parenchymal tissue at the superior pole from its surrounding structures, minimizing risk for injury to the ESLN. (*Courtesy of* the Memorial Sloan-Kettering Cancer Center, New York, NY;
with permission.)

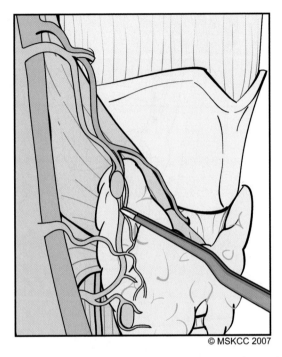

© MSKCC 2007

Fig. 6. As the superior pole tissue drops down away from the ESLN, the remaining small blood vessels, especially those in the vicinity of the superior PT gland, can be cauterized safely with fine-tipped bipolar electrocautery. (*Courtesy of* the Memorial Sloan-Kettering Cancer Center, New York, NY; with permission.)

surface. The middle thyroid vein, if present, is divided and ligated. Hemostatic clamps are applied carefully to the capsule of the thyroid lobe along its lateral edge. Gentle medial retraction of these clamps combined with lateral retraction of the strap muscles provides the surgical exposure required for identification of the PT glands and the RLN. As a general rule, the authors do not attempt to identify the RLN laterally in the paratracheal groove as the initial step. Instead, the focus of the dissection at this stage should be to identify and preserve the PT glands along with their vascular supply.

A technique of capsular dissection is recommended in order to prevent devascularization of the PT glands. The aim of this maneuver is to sweep the posterior capsular fascia off the thyroid parenchyma. This fascia consists of multiple thin layers of connective tissue that encapsulate the thyroid gland and its superficial vasculature. The PT glands frequently are embedded in this capsular tissue and receive their blood supply from branches of the inferior thyroid artery (ITA) and less frequently from the superior thyroid artery (Fig. 7). With the thyroid lobe rotated medially into the surgical wound, the areolar tissue on the posterior surface of the lobe is incised longitudinally and stripped away laterally from the thyroid. Small blood

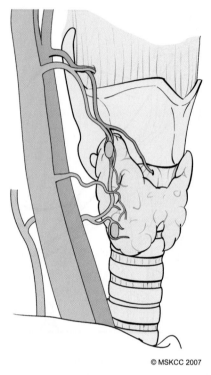

© MSKCC 2007

Fig. 7. The PT glands receive their blood supply from branches of the ITA and, less frequently, from the superior thyroid artery. (*Courtesy of* the Memorial Sloan-Kettering Cancer Center, New York, NY; with permission.)

vessels encountered during this dissection are cauterized carefully with a fine-tipped bipolar forceps or ligated.

During lateral reflection of the visceral fascia, the terminal branches of the ITA are encountered distal to the PT gland after they have supplied these glands. These distal branches are divided carefully and ligated and the adventitial tissue around the thyroid capsule is peeled away along with the PT gland (Fig. 8). As described in the following section, further dissection during preservation of the inferior PT gland inevitably leads to identification of the RLN.

This technique allows identification and preservation of the superior and inferior PT glands along with their blood supply that is contained within the adventitial tissue surrounding the thyroid capsule. The PT glands can be distinguished from the underlying thyroid parenchyma by their yellowish brown color (café ole), fatty consistency, and teardrop shape. On a rare occasion, the surgeon may need to harvest a small sliver of an assumed PT gland for intraoperative pathologic examination to confirm the diagnosis. Devascularization of the PT gland leads to change in the color of the gland from light to dark brown within a few minutes. If a PT gland is detached

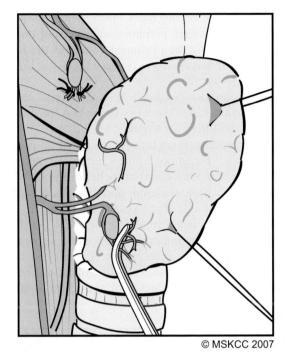

© MSKCC 2007

Fig. 8. The terminal branches of the ITA that are encountered distal to the PT gland after they have supplied these glands are divided and ligated carefully. As the areolar tissue around the thyroid capsule is peeled away along with the PT gland, the RLN comes into view. (*Courtesy of* the Memorial Sloan-Kettering Cancer Center, New York, NY; with permission.)

from its blood supply, the authors recommend reimplantation of the gland after confirming its histology using intraoperative frozen section analysis. PT gland reimplantation is performed by mincing the devascularized gland and placing it into a small pocket created by blunt dissection of the fibers of the sternocleidomastoid muscle. The site of reimplantation is marked with nonabsorbable suture or small titanium clips in case the site needs to be identified at future surgery.

Identification of the recurrent laryngeal nerve and its anatomic variations

The authors' routine practice is to avoid dissection and identification of the RLN laterally in the paratracheal groove as the initial step. As described previously, capsular dissection during preservation of the inferior PT gland normally allows exposure of the RLN as it lies in relationship to the branches of the ITA. The authors prefer this approach rather than lateral dissection in order to avoid several pitfalls. First, lateral dissection for identification of the RLN away from the thyroid capsule increases the risk for devascularization of the PT glands. Second, blind dissection with a clamp along the suspected course of the RLN inadvertently may traumatize the nerve causing temporary or even permanent paralysis of the nerve. Finally, injury to blood vessels along the presumed course of the RLN may cause bleeding and attempts at hemostasis may place the as-yet unidentified nerve at risk for injury.

The alternative technique described here takes into consideration the normal anatomic relationship of the RLN to the ITA, the tuberculum Zuckerkandl, the trachea, and the esophagus.

The technique of capsular dissection is predicated on precise and meticulous surgical technique. Fine-tipped microclamps are used to spread alveolar tissue gently and clamp the distal branches of the ITA before division and ligation. Blind application of clamps and mass ligation of tissue is to be avoided at all costs. Identifiable blood vessels should be divided and ligated individually to prevent accidental injury to the RLN. As dissection of the branches of the ITA distal to the inferior PT gland nears completion, the RLN generally comes into view at this point. A small vasa nervosum vessel that accompanies the nerve can facilitate its identification and differentiation from other structures. The relationship of the RLN to the ITA and its

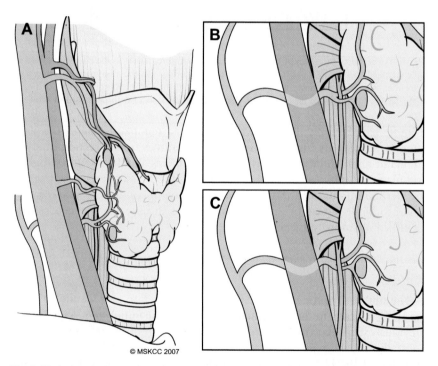

© MSKCC 2007

Fig. 9. Variations in the relationship of the RLN to the ITA and its branches. Most commonly, the RLN courses deep to the inferior thyroid artery and its branches (*A*), but it may lie between the branches (*B*) or anterior (*C*) to the artery. (*Courtesy of* the Memorial Sloan-Kettering Cancer Center, New York, NY.)

branches, however, is variable and bears special attention (Fig. 9). In most individuals, the RLN is located deep to the ITA but it may lie between the branches or anterior to the artery [4]. The RLN generally courses deep to the tuberculum Zuckerkandl and superficial to the lateral border of the trachea. Variations in anatomic relationships of the RLN to the tuberculum Zuckerkandl are not infrequent, however, and the surgeon should be familiar with these in order to avoid injury to the RLN, especially when nodular pathology affects this part of the gland (Fig. 10). The relationship of the RLN to the tracheoesophageal groove also bears notice (Fig. 11). In more than half of cases, the RLN is located along the tracheoesophageal groove and passes deep to Berry's ligament (the posterior suspensory ligament of the thyroid). In the remaining cases, the RLN may pierce Berry's ligament or lie between the ligament and the thyroid parenchyma. The RLN also can ascend along the paraesophageal line posterior to the tracheoesophageal groove. Other variations in the location of the RLN are related to the side of the operated neck. In the left side of the neck, the RLN crosses anterior to the aortic arch, loops under it, and ascends in a relatively constant position along the tracheoesophageal groove (Fig. 12). The course of the right RLN is less predictable, because it crosses anterior to the subclavian artery and ascends posterior to the artery starting a point more lateral than in the left neck.

As the capsular dissection continues, the RLN is exposed laterally or medial to the tuberculum Zuckerkandl. After identification, the RLN is

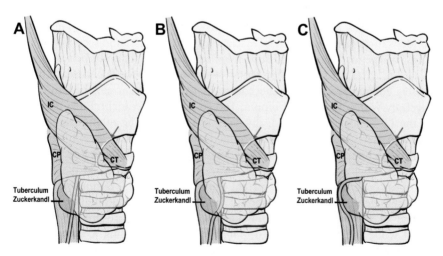

Fig. 10. Variations in anatomic relationships of the RLN to the tuberculum Zuckerkandl. The RLN generally courses deep to the tuberculum Zuckerkandl and superficial to the lateral border of the trachea (*A*) but it may run medial to it (*B*). Nodular enlargement of thyroid tissue in the location of the tuberculum (*C*) may displace the RLN laterally around it, placing the nerve at risk for injury if this variation is not recognized. IC, inferior constrictor muscle; CP, cricopharyngeus muscle; CT, cricothyroid muscle.

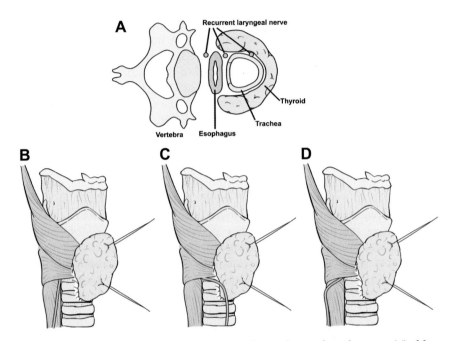

Fig. 11. Anatomic relationship of the RLN to the tracheoesophageal groove (*A*). Most commonly, the RLN courses along the tracheoesophageal groove (*B*) and passes deep to Berry's ligament. Variations include an RLN that ascends anterior to the tracheoesophageal groove (*C*) or along the paraesophageal line posterior to the tracheoesophageal groove (*D*).

dissected gently away from the gland toward Berry's ligament. This dense condensation of the pretracheal fascia overlying the first and second tracheal rings "suspends" the thyroid lobe from the trachea. A fine-tipped hemostat is used to carefully spread the areolar tissue overlying the RLN. Small blood vessels encountered during the course of this dissection can be cauterized carefully with a fine-tipped bipolar forceps, but larger identifiable branches of the ITA must be clamped, divided, and ligated. The relationship of the RLN to Berry's ligament is determined and fine blood vessels in the ligament are clamped carefully with a fine-tipped microclamp before division with a scalpel and ligation. Special care must be exercised in placing this clamp in order to avoid inadvertent injury to the RLN. Similarly, the surgeon's finger or instrument should be oriented longitudinally along the course of the RLN so that the ligature does not exert pressure on the RLN while the knot is secured. The authors prefer using a needle driver to tie knots in this area, as this allows precise control and avoids inadvertent tearing of tissue and blood vessels. Bleeding from a loose or torn ligature on these vessels can be troublesome and it is important to avoid blind attempts at hemostasis with clamps. The safest course of action in this situation is to apply gentle pressure with a swab to achieve temporary hemostasis. This allows identification of the divided vessel and its safe ligation without

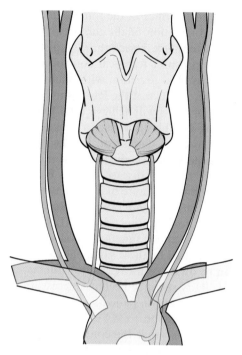

Fig. 12. The left RLN crosses anterior to the aortic arch, loops under it, and ascends in a relatively constant position along the tracheoesophageal groove.

placing the RLN at risk for injury. If the area of Berry's ligament continues to ooze, hemostasis can be achieved by placing a piece of hemostatic Surgicel instead of undue manipulation in attempts to place hemostatic ligatures. As it approaches the larynx, the nerve may run in a single bundle or may divide into 2 to 6 small branches before entering the cricothyroid junction. It is important to recognize this fact so that all branches of the RLN are preserved during dissection.

On rare occasions, a posteriorly located thyroid tumor may adhere to the perineurium of the RLN or may infiltrate deep into the perineural space in the region of Berry's ligament. Isolated invasion of the RLN without involvement of adjacent structures, such as the cricothyroid membrane, cricoid cartilage, tracheal rings, and esophageal musculature, is rare. If the RLN is paralyzed preoperatively and intraoperative exploration shows neural invasion by cancer, the RLN should be sacrificed in order to achieve gross total resection of the tumor. Decision making becomes difficult, however, in cases of minimal neural invasion by WDTC with normal RLN function. The decision to sacrifice a normally functioning RLN in patients who have WDTC is based on several factors, especially because WDTC generally is a RAI avid tumor so that microscopic residual tumor theoretically is amenable to RAI therapy. The primary intraoperative consideration in this decision is whether or not sacrifice of the functioning RLN would make the difference between total resection of the tumor with microscopically negative margins and an incomplete resection. Complete surgical resection of WDTC offers the best prospect for local control and every effort should be made to achieve gross total resection with microscopically negative surgical margins. Therefore, sacrifice of the RLN is indicated in the presence of gross invasion by tumor if this will achieve total tumor resection. Alternatively, the surgeon may be able to dissect a functioning RLN away from the tumor leaving microscopic disease on it. The functional consequences of RLN dysfunction need to be weighed against the likelihood of local recurrence if microscopic residual disease on the RLN fails to respond to RAI therapy. Older patients are more likely to have non–RAI-avid tumors; microscopic residual disease on the RLN is unlikely to respond to adjuvant RAI in this group. Resection of a functioning RLN becomes a valid consideration in these situations; yet, the functional consequences of RLN sacrifice are least likely to be tolerated by these same patients. If a tumor is adherent to the RLN and can be dissected away easily, a functioning RLN generally should be preserved. RLN sacrifice becomes necessary, however, for gross invasion of the nerve, especially in patients who have undifferentiated carcinoma that is unlikely to respond to RAI. Prior to sacrificing a functional nerve, it should be confirmed that the contralateral nerve is free of tumor and can be preserved safely. This is another reason for performing lobectomy on the contralateral side before approaching the diseased lobe or the side of the more prominent pathology.

Division of Berry's ligament frees the thyroid lobe from its attachment to the trachea. The inferior thyroid veins are divided and ligated close to the thyroid gland to complete mobilization of the lower pole of the lobe. In 10% of patients, a thyroid ima artery may be present anterior to the trachea. This artery emerges directly from the arch of the aorta or occasionally from the brachiocephalic trunk to supply the inferior pole of the gland and should be ligated at the level of the thyroid capsule.

Subsequent mobilization of the thyroid lobe off the anterolateral surface of the upper tracheal rings is accomplished with an electrocautery. Attention is given to identification and dissection of the pyramidal "lobe," which is found in more than 50% of individuals [5,6]. The pyramidal lobe can branch off from the left or right thyroid lobes or from the isthmus. The lobe is dissected free from the underlying cricothyroid muscle using electrocautery in a superior-to-inferior direction to maintain it in continuity with the rest of the thyroid gland. If thyroid lobectomy is planned, the thyroid lobe and isthmus are dissected off the trachea and a Kocher clamp is placed vertically across the junction of the isthmus with the contralateral lobe. The thyroid parenchyma then is divided over the clamp with a #15 scalpel to deliver the specimen. The cut edge of the remnant thyroid gland is oversewn with a continuous 3-0 chromic catgut suture. Alternatively, if total thyroidectomy is planned, lobectomy is performed on the contralateral side (as described previously) to deliver the specimen containing both thyroid lobes en bloc. Accurate orientation of the specimen is important and pertinent details of the tumor, such as intraoperative suspicion of ETE, must be communicated to a pathologist in order to ensure meaningful interpretation of histopathologic findings.

Hemostasis, drains, and wound closure

After delivery of the specimen, the wound is irrigated copiously with saline. The lower jugular, paratracheal, pretracheal, and superior mediastinal lymph node basins are inspected and palpated for any suspicious lymphadenopathy. After total thyroidectomy, the surgeon should examine the surgical bed for any remaining thyroid tissue that may be the source of a positive RAI uptake scan and elevated thyroglobulin after surgery. The common sites of residual thyroid tissue after total thyroidectomy are the superior poles, the thyroid tissue around Berry's ligament, and the pyramidal lobe (Fig. 13).

If hypotensive anesthesia is used, the anesthesiologist should return the blood pressure to normal at this stage in order to ensure adequate hemostasis. As described previously, great caution must be exercised around the RLN and indiscriminate use of electrocautery and hemostats should be avoided.

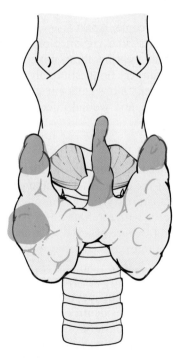

Fig. 13. The common sites of residual thyroid tissue after total thyroidectomy are the superior poles, the thyroid tissue around Berry's ligament, and the pyramidal lobe.

The relevance of placing drains in the thyroid bed is debated and there is evidence to show that draining wounds does not reduce the risk for postoperative hematoma [7,8]. The authors prefer to drain most total thyroidectomy wounds with a Penrose drain, which generally is removed before discharge from hospital the next morning.

The wound then is closed in layers. The fascia overlying the SHMs is sutured loosely in the midline using a few interrupted chromic catgut sutures. Avoidance of a watertight closure of the strap muscles in the midline leaves a conduit between the deep and superficial neck compartments to allow shift of blood in case of expanding hematoma. If a Penrose drain is used, the drain is brought out laterally or in the midline and skin is sutured with 5-0 nylon. The wound is cleaned and smeared with Bacitracin ointment. Loose gauze fluff is used to cover the Penrose drain. After the drain is removed, patients are instructed to shower in 2 days and apply Bacitracin ointment to the suture line, which is kept exposed without dressings.

Postoperative care and management of complications

Postoperative complications are infrequent in experienced hands and best prevented by meticulous surgical technique as described previously. Early recognition and prompt initial management of complications are equally important to successful outcome. Apart from close supervision by the surgeon, this requires awareness and vigilance on the part of all members of the multidisciplinary team treating these patients. The most debilitating complications of thyroid surgery unquestionably are RLN injury and hypocalcemia. Other less frequent but significant complications include hematoma, seroma, ESLN injury, and wound infection.

Hemorrhage and hematoma

Neck hematoma or bleeding after thyroid surgery is rare and reportedly occurs in less than 1% of the cases [9]. The time period for development of postoperative hematoma can vary from 5 minutes to 5 days after surgery, but most hematomas occur within 6 hours after surgery. Patients undergoing thyroid surgery, therefore, are believed to benefit from close monitoring for a minimal period of 6 hours after thyroid lobectomy and overnight after total thyroidectomy [10].

Hematoma is prevented best by appropriate identification and ligation of blood vessels during surgery and by meticulous wound irrigation and hemostasis before wound closure. To identify potential bleeding vessels before wound closure, the anesthesiologist should normalize the patient's blood pressure, because hypotension and vasoconstriction may obscure potential sources of bleeding that may become manifest only after extubation. A simulated Valsalva maneuver can help identify potential venous bleeders when the anesthesiologist raises and maintains the intrapulmonary pressure. Most delayed bleeding is of venous origin and a major source rarely is apparent at wound exploration in hematomas that have occurred slowly over the post-operative course.

Rapidly expanding hematoma, alternatively, occurs most commonly from a bleeding artery. This life-threatening condition should be identified and managed as early as possible. Failure to identify impending hematoma after surgery may occur if the strap muscles are sutured tightly in the midline, allowing the hematoma to cause an increase in the central compartmental pressure with impingement of the airway. The strap muscles, therefore, should be approximated only loosely in the midline, leaving free communication between the deep and superficial neck spaces. Other causes of post-thyroidectomy hematomas include slipping of ligature on major vessels and reopening of cauterized vessels. Factors, such as elevated postoperative blood pressure and use of anticoagulant therapy, may contribute to a higher risk. Increased blood pressure immediately after extubation may be related to Valsalva maneuvers caused by bucking or vomiting and from inappropriate management of hypertensive patients during the early postoperative period. All these situations are preventable by close cooperation with the anesthesiologist.

Although small and stable seroma or hematoma can be monitored closely or evacuated by needle aspiration, significant or expanding hematoma of the neck should be managed surgically because of high risk for airway compromise. Symptoms, such as difficulty breathing, pressure in the neck, and voice changes with an obvious collection in the wound, require surgical intervention without delay. Patients who do not have obvious airway compromise and who have a stable hematoma should be brought to the operating room for re-exploration as early as possible after they are hemodynamically stable. In contrast, patients who have airway symptoms need emergency intervention at the bedside. The hematoma in such patients should be managed by opening the thyroidectomy wound at the bedside and evacuating the clotted blood. Release of central compartment tension by this maneuver usually ameliorates airway symptoms and ends the emergency. In a small percentage of patients, however, airway compromise may persist even after evacuation of the hematoma. Immediate endotracheal intubation should be performed by an experienced clinician, because these patients may develop severe airway obstruction resulting from edema of the larynx as a result of the hematoma. Emergency tracheostomy rarely may become necessary if an endotracheal airway cannot be secured. This is straightforward technically, because the trachea lies exposed in the thyroidectomy wound. All patients should be brought back to the operating room for complete wound exploration after any urgent bedside procedure. After evacuation of the hematoma, the wound should be irrigated copiously and the bleeding vessels identified and ligated. Great care must be taken to avoid injury to the RLN and PT glands, and it is prudent to avoid the use of suction directly in the wound during this phase of the operation. If emergency tracheostomy is performed, closure of the wound becomes challenging, because the tracheotomy now lies within the otherwise clean thyroidectomy wound with the potential for sepsis. The thyroidectomy wound in such instances can be closed over a Penrose drain and the tracheostomy is fashioned in the midline to isolate it from the thyroidectomy wound by suturing the edges of the tracheotomy to the cutaneous edges of the thyroidectomy wound.

The surgeon must be aware of the risk for pneumothorax and postobstructive pulmonary edema that can develop after acute airway obstruction. A chest radiograph, therefore, should be performed after exploration of hematoma in the neck to identify and treat these conditions. Patients who require re-exploration for neck hematoma should be monitored closely for at least 48 hours, because they have an increased risk for airway compromise from laryngeal edema or RLN palsy.

Recurrent laryngeal nerve injury

Temporary nerve palsy may occur in up to 5% of cases [11], whereas permanent RLN injury and vocal cord paralysis occurs in less than 2% to 3% of patients. The causes of transient nerve palsy include significant manipulation and dissection along the RLN, thermal injury, and traction injury. Alternatively, most permanent RLN injuries occur because of transaction of the nerve during surgery. Bilateral RLN injury is rare and was reported in 1 of 1000 thyroid surgeries [11]. This is an especially debilitating situation, as it creates the need for permanent tracheostomy. The surgeon should be aware of a higher risk for bilateral RLN palsy when unilateral RLN paralysis is diagnosed preoperatively, if RLN is sacrificed during the operation, or in patients undergoing reoperative thyroid surgery.

If bilateral RLN injury goes unrecognized intraoperatively, patients generally require reintubation immediately after the operation. Rarely, bilateral injury may not present for up to several hours after extubation. Recurrent failure to extubate patients clearly suggests the possibility of bilateral vocal cord paralysis. If the surgeon is confident that the RLNs are preserved during the operation, it is acceptable to treat the patient with systemic steroids and assisted endotracheal ventilation for several days. The patient then can be weaned off the ventilator gradually and an attempted extubation performed in the operating room. If flexible fiberoptic evaluation of the larynx clearly demonstrates an adequate airway with functioning vocal cords, no further intervention is required [12]. If, however, patients fail extubation or laryngoscopy reveals bilaterally paralyzed vocal cords with or without airway compromise, tracheostomy is indicated. Most of these patients who require tracheostomy generally have temporary RLN palsy of at least one nerve. In such cases, patients can be weaned from the tracheostomy 3 to 9 months after the operation, which is the time required for the RLNs to recover. Laryngeal electromyography may be used to assess the likelihood of future decannulation.

Patients who have unilateral RLN palsy often suffer from hoarseness, although normal voice is not infrequent in this population. Symptomatic patients who have RLN injury also may suffer from dysphagia and aspiration. As discussed previously, recovery of a nerve that is paralyzed temporarily can take several months. Symptomatic patients and those who have permanent paralysis should be considered for vocal cord medialization to improve the quality of their voice and for prevention of aspiration.

Hypocalcemia and hypoparathyroidism

Hypocalcemia secondary to iatrogenic injury to the PT glands occurs in 5% to 25% of patients after thyroid surgery [12,13]. Transient hypocalcemia is more common than permanent hypocalcemia and is believed caused by impaired vascularity of the PT glands after surgery. Permanent hypocalcemia, alternatively, usually occurs because of unintentional compromise of all PT glands. A recent study from the authors' institution found that the incidence of inadvertent excision of a PT gland is approximately 8%; however, removal of three or more PT glands is rare [14]. The risk for hypocalcemia increases in reoperative thyroid surgery or after paratracheal neck dissection. The postoperative measured serum calcium level also may be reported low because of surgical stress caused by inappropriate antidiuretic hormone secretion, low serum albumin level, or laboratory error. In these cases, the free or ionized calcium remains unchanged and this condition does not need correction with calcium supplementation.

Most patients who have transient hypocalcemia usually are asymptomatic. Symptomatic patients usually complain of perioral numbness, tingling, abdominal cramps, paraesthesias, or muscle spasm, especially in their upper extremities. Bedside evaluation of symptomatic patients may include tapping on the facial nerve trunk at the preauricular area, producing muscle twitches (Chvostek's sign), or occlusion of the brachial artery for 3 minutes, producing carpopedal spasm (Trousseau's sign). Failure to recognize and treat severe hypocalcemia may lead to cardiac arrhythmia and seizures.

Calcium levels are drawn routinely between 8 and 12 hours after the operation and then at 20 to 22 hours, immediately before discharge from hospital. Subsequent management is based not only on actual serum levels but also on the trend in the levels over time. Patients who have low calcium levels should be supplemented with oral calcium (400–500 mg 2 to 3 times a day), and those who have significant hypocalcemia should receive vitamin D therapy (0.25–0.5 µg once or twice a day) in addition. The effect of vitamin D on serum calcium level should be anticipated after 2 to 3 days and appropriate adjustments in the dose of enteral calcium may become necessary. Patients can be discharged home if normal calcium levels are achieved or if they are asymptomatic and have a rising trend of calcium levels.

Symptomatic patients and those who have severe hypocalcemia require serum calcium estimation every 3 to 6 hours and intravenous infusion of calcium (10–20 mL of 10% calcium gluconate diluted in 200 mL of saline over 20 minutes). Intravenous calcium infusion may be continued until patient symptoms resolve. If serum calcium levels fail to normalize, serum magnesium levels should be evaluated and corrected. In cases of hypocalcemia refractory to treatment or serum calcium below 7 mg/mL, an endocrinologist should be consulted.

The serum calcium level should be monitored at the first postoperative visit 7 to 10 days after discharge and supplementation should be modified accordingly. Gradual tapering of enteral calcium and calcitriol can begin if serum calcium is above 8.5 mg/mL. Supplementation should continue with appropriate adjustment of the dose for patients who maintain their serum calcium level between 7 and 8 mg/mL. Patients who are severely hypocalcemic, with serum calcium below 7 mg/mL, should also have an evaluation of serum parathormone.

Other sequelae of thyroid surgery

Wound infections after thyroid surgery are rare and more common in immunocompromised patients and in patients who have diabetes mellitus. Prophylactic antibiotic therapy does not decrease the rate of infection and should be used only in patients who have diabetes or valvular heart disease or in immunocompromised patients. Minor cellulitis usually is managed with antibiotics directed at *Staphylococcus* and *Streptococcus* species, whereas wound abscess should be treated with drainage and irrigation along with intravenous antibiotics therapy covering aerobic and anaerobic bacteria.

Approximately a third of patients report vocal symptoms during the early period after thyroid surgery, even in the absence of obvious evidence of nerve injury [15]. Half of these patients have persistent symptoms 3 months after the operation. Complaints of a lowered tone, vocal fatigue, and difficulty in high-pitch phonation or projection of voice should alert surgeons to the possibility of SLN injury. Videostroboscopy and laryngeal electromyography may be needed to confirm the diagnosis of SLN palsy [15]. Patients who have significant symptoms should be referred to a speech pathologist in an attempt to improve their speech.

All patients undergoing total thyroidectomy and up to a third of those after thyroid lobectomy require thyroid hormone supplementation [16]. At Memorial Sloan-Kettering Cancer Center, exogenous levothyroxine is administered, based on patient body weight early after surgery, to all patients undergoing total thyroidectomy. In patients who have WDTC requiring RAI scan or treatment, recombinant human thyrotropin administration before scanning prevents the debilitating symptoms of hypothyroidism associated with thyroid hormone withdrawal.

Large goiter and retrosternal extension

If a retrosternal goiter is suspected, radiologic imaging using CT or MRI of the neck and superior mediastinum is required to delineate the inferior extent of the gland and its relation to the great vessels, trachea, and esophagus. Most retrosternal goiters are benign and amenable to surgical resection via the conventional cervical approach. The infrahyoid strap muscles may need to be divided on one or both sides to allow delivery of the gland. After exposure of the superior pole and capsular dissection to preserve the PT glands and RLN (described previously), gentle finger dissection is used to assess intrathoracic extension of the tumor. Retrosternal intrathoracic extension of a benign goiter generally can be mobilized safely by blunt finger dissection and delivered out of the mediastinum into the neck, as the vascular supply to the intrathoracic component almost always originates in the neck. Small vessels along the visceral fascia carefully are divided individually, only after confirming that they are devoid of neural tissue.

With large goiters, the surgeon should be aware of the possibility that the nerve may be displaced several centimeters laterally from the tracheoesophageal groove, making it difficult to identify. In these cases, the RLN may be closely adherent to the posterior capsule of the gland. In some cases, the RLN may be displaced anteriorly, and delivery of the goiter outside of the wound before identifying the RLN places the nerve at significant risk, because it may be located more superficial than its usual location and is encountered early during the dissection (Fig. 14). If the RLN anatomy is unclear, dissection alternatively may be performed in the medial-to-lateral sequence, starting with division of the thyroid isthmus. The superior pole vessels are ligated and the lobe is mobilized laterally. The RLN then can be identified at its entry to the larynx, between the cricoid cartilage and the inferior cornu of the thyroid cartilage. This is a relatively constant anatomic landmark and the course of the RLN is not subject to distortion by the goiter at this location. The RLN then is traced caudally and laterally throughout its course. If appropriate, a benign cyst may be aspirated and it may become necessary to divide a huge benign lobe to prevent stretching and injury to the RLN during delivery of the goiter.

Although the vast majority of retrosternal goiters can be excised adequately and safely via a cervical approach, thoracic exposure is required for these indications: (1) recurrent intrathoracic goiter, (2) previous mediastinal or cardiothoracic surgery, (3) previous radiation to the neck or mediastinum, (4) malignant tumor abutting the great vessels, (5) isolated intrathoracic goiter, and (6) retrotracheal goiter extending below the level of the carina [1]. Median sternotomy allows careful identification of the lower extent of the goiter and its relationship to the great vessels. Readers are referred elsewhere for a detailed description of this approach [17].

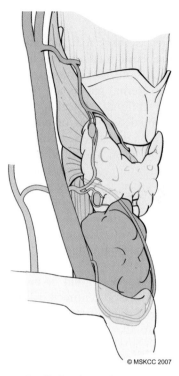

© MSKCC 2007

Fig. 14. The RLN rarely may be displaced anteriorly if a nodule arises from a posterior location on the lower pole. If such a nodule extends retrosternally, attempts at delivery of the goiter outside of the wound before identifying the RLN places the nerve at significant risk, as it may be located more superficial than its usual location and is encountered early during the dissection. (*Courtesy of* the Memorial Sloan-Kettering Cancer Center, New York, NY; with permission.)

Nonrecurrent laryngeal nerve

A non-RLN should be anticipated if the nerve cannot be found inferiorly using the technique described previously. Intraoperatively, a non-RLN can be identified at its entrance to the larynx, lateral to the junction of the cricoid and lower cornu of the thyroid cartilage. This anatomic variant occurs in less than 0.5% of patients, as the RLN may bifurcate directly from the vagus above the level of the ITA [18]. This anatomic variant of the right RLN occurs in patients who have a retroesophageal right subclavian artery. These individuals lack the brachiocephalic artery; their right common carotid artery emerges directly from the aortic arch and the subclavian artery lies posterior to the esophagus (Fig. 15). Suspicion of this vascular anomaly should be investigated before surgery in patients who have a long history of dysphagia that cannot be explained by a large thyroid gland or other causes. The vascular anomaly associated with a nonrecurrent laryngeal nerve can be identified preoperatively using CT, MRI, or modified

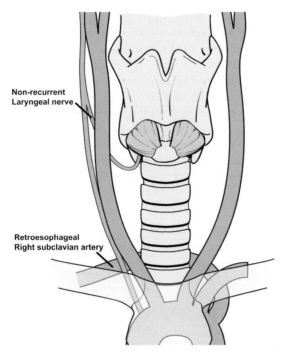

Fig. 15. A nonrecurrent right laryngeal nerve occurs in patients who have a retroesophageal right subclavian artery.

barium swallow test. A left-sided non-RLN is found only in association with situs inversus viscerum (ie, Kartagener's syndrome) [18] and is easier to anticipate preoperatively.

Locally invasive well-differentiated thyroid cancer

Thyroid carcinoma suspected of being locally invasive warrants preoperative evaluation with CT or MRI. These imaging modalities are helpful for evaluating the anatomic relationship of the tumor to adjacent structures to determine the involvement of the thyroid cartilage, trachea, and esophagus before surgery. Although the use of iodinated contrast generally should be avoided in imaging patients who have WDTC, locally aggressive variants tend to be less RAI avid. Contrast-enhanced CT scan, therefore, is acceptable in selected patients, because it provides important anatomic information that may be crucial to the surgeon. In cases of suspected intraluminal extension of the tumor to the trachea or esophagus, imaging should be followed by bronchoscopy and esophagoscopy, respectively. Unilateral vocal cord paralysis is an ominous sign indicative of aggressive biologic behavior of the tumor [19].

If a tumor is adherent to the perichondrium or infiltrates the laryngeal cartilage partly, the perichondrium or cartilage can be resected with the tumor. Minimal invasion of the superficial esophageal musculature may be managed adequately with submucosal resection of gross tumor while maintaining the mucosal conduit of the esophagus. This is done best after inserting a nasogastric tube at the start of the operation, facilitating surgical resection and allowing postoperative tube feeding. Minimal adherence to the tracheal cartilage can be managed with "shaving" the tumor with the tracheal cartilage to ensure total tumor resection. More aggressive surgical resection, including "sleeve resection" of the upper cervical trachea, is required if there is gross invasion of the tracheal wall with or without intraluminal extension. Similarly, total laryngectomy with or without pharyngectomy rarely becomes necessary for more locally advanced tumors. The

Table 1
Summary of surgical technique for thyroidectomy

Positioning and draping	• Reverse Trendelenburg with neck extended
	• Transparent plastic drape helps monitor endotracheal tube and anesthesia circuit
Surgical incision	• Vary location and length depending on body habitus and exposure required
Cutaneous flaps	• Elevate in the subplatysmal plane
Management of strap muscles	• Retraction without division for accessible superior pole
	• Division at superior attachment for inaccessible superior pole
	• Segmental muscle resection if suspected or gross invasion by tumor
	• Division of both strap muscles for huge retrosternal goiter
Superior pole dissection and preservation of ESLN	• Ligate individual branches of the superior thyroid artery anterior to the pole to avoid injury to parathyroid and ESLN
	• Avoid mass ligature of superior pedicle and excise all thyroid tissue
Capsular dissection and preservation of PT glands	• Use fine-tipped clamps for dissection
	• Ligate branches of ITA on the thyroid capsule distal to the PT gland to ensure preservation of the blood supply to the PT glands
Identification of RLN	• Avoid lateral dissection for identification of RLN in paratracheal groove as the initial step
	• Recognize variations in normal anatomy relative to tracheoesophageal groove, branches of the ITA, tuberculum Zuckerkandl, and Berry's ligament
	• Anticipate distortions in normal relationship of RLN to adjoining structures due to tumor
Hemostasis, drains, and wound closure	• Avoid suction drain
	• Layered wound closure
Postoperative care	• Monitor airway
	• Monitor neck wound for hematoma
	• Monitor blood work for hypocalcemia

indications and technical details of these operations are beyond the scope of this article and readers are referred to specialized surgical texts for more information [17,20].

Reoperative thyroid surgery

Reoperation for recurrent cancer in the surgical bed of previously excised thyroid carcinomas is a challenging surgical procedure that carries with it various technical problems. As might be expected, dissection of the RLN in these situations can be difficult and the risk for injury and postoperative dysfunction proportionately higher.

Contrary to the usual approach for identification of the RLN close to the thyroid capsule during subcapsular dissection and preservation of the inferior PT gland, the surgical approach may need to be modified so that the RLN is identified inferiorly and laterally in the paratracheal groove. The RLN then can be traced cephalad but preservation of viable PT tissue becomes virtually impossible in this situation with increased risk for postoperative hypocalcemia. Paradoxically, dissection and preservation of the RLN may be easier if some amount of residual normal thyroid tissue is present, because this often indicates a previously unviolated surgical plane. Intraoperative RLN monitoring may be a useful adjunct [21–23], but it is important to recognize that preservation of anatomic integrity of the nerve does not always result in preservation of vocal cord function. Patients requiring reoperative thyroid bed surgery for recurrent tumor rather than residual normal tissue that is RAI avid should be counseled, therefore, regarding the considerably elevated risk for postoperative RLN and PT gland dysfunction.

Summary

The authors have reviewed their surgical technique for treatment of thyroid cancer and large goiters. The key features of the technique are summarized in Table 1. This technique provides a simple and versatile means of complete extracapsular thyroidectomy for lesions of the thyroid gland and minimizes postoperative complications.

References

[1] Newman E, Shaha AR. Substernal goiter. J Surg Oncol 1995;60(3):207–12.
[2] Johnson JT, Wagner RL. Infection following uncontaminated head and neck surgery. Arch Otolaryngol Head Neck Surg 1987;113(4):368–9.
[3] Friedman M, LoSavio P, Ibrahim H. Superior laryngeal nerve identification and preservation in thyroidectomy. Arch Otolaryngol Head Neck Surg 2002;128(3):296–303.
[4] Skandalakis JE, Droulias C, Harlaftis N, et al. The recurrent laryngeal nerve. Am Surg 1976; 42(9):629–34.

[5] Blumberg NA. Observations on the pyramidal lobe of the thyroid gland. S Afr Med J 1981; 59(26):949–50.

[6] Braun EM, Windisch G, Wolf G, et al. The pyramidal lobe: clinical anatomy and its importance in thyroid surgery. Surg Radiol Anat 2007;29(1):21–7.

[7] Khanna J, Mohil RS, Chintamani, et al. Is the routine drainage after surgery for thyroid necessary? A prospective randomized clinical study [ISRCTN63623153]. BMC Surg 2005; 5:11.

[8] Lee SW, Choi EC, Lee YM, et al. Is lack of placement of drains after thyroidectomy with central neck dissection safe? A prospective, randomized study. Laryngoscope 2006;116(9): 1632–5.

[9] Shaha AR, Jaffe BM. Practical management of post-thyroidectomy hematoma. J Surg Oncol 1994;57(4):235–8.

[10] Lacoste L, Gineste D, Karayan J, et al. Airway complications in thyroid surgery. Ann Otol Rhinol Laryngol 1993;102(6):441–6.

[11] Muller PE, Jakoby R, Heinert G, et al. Surgery for recurrent goitre: its complications and their risk factors. Eur J Surg 2001;167(11):816–21.

[12] Fewins J, Simpson CB, Miller FR. Complications of thyroid and parathyroid surgery. Otolaryngol Clin North Am 2003;36(1):189–206.

[13] Shemen LJ, Strong EW. Complications after total thyroidectomy. Otolaryngol Head Neck Surg 1989;101(4):472–5.

[14] Lin DT, Patel SG, Shaha AR, et al. Incidence of inadvertent parathyroid removal during thyroidectomy. Laryngoscope 2002;112(4):608–11.

[15] Stojadinovic A, Shaha AR, Orlikoff RF, et al. Prospective functional voice assessment in patients undergoing thyroid surgery. Ann Surg 2002;236(6):823–32.

[16] McHenry CR, Slusarczyk SJ. Hypothyroidisim following hemithyroidectomy: incidence, risk factors, and management. Surgery 2000;128(6):994–8.

[17] Shah JP, Patel SG. Head and neck surgery and oncology. 3rd edition. St. Louis (MO): Mosby; 2003.

[18] Henry JF, Audiffret J, Denizot A, et al. The nonrecurrent inferior laryngeal nerve: review of 33 cases, including two on the left side. Surgery 1988;104(6):977–84.

[19] Randolph GW, Kamani D. The importance of preoperative laryngoscopy in patients undergoing thyroidectomy: voice, vocal cord function, and the preoperative detection of invasive thyroid malignancy. Surgery 2006;139(3):357–62.

[20] Grillo HC, Zannini P. Resectional management of airway invasion by thyroid carcinoma. Ann Thorac Surg 1986;42(3):287–98.

[21] Farrag TY, Agrawal N, Sheth S, et al. Algorithm for safe and effective reoperative thyroid bed surgery for recurrent/persistent papillary thyroid carcinoma. Head Neck 2007;29: 1069–74.

[22] Chan WF, Lang BH, Lo CY. The role of intraoperative neuromonitoring of recurrent laryngeal nerve during thyroidectomy: a comparative study on 1000 nerves at risk. Surgery 2006;140(6):866–72.

[23] Yarbrough DE, Thompson GB, Kasperbauer JL, et al. Intraoperative electromyographic monitoring of the recurrent laryngeal nerve in reoperative thyroid and parathyroid surgery. Surgery 2004;136(6):1107–15.

ELSEVIER
SAUNDERS

Surg Oncol Clin N Am
17 (2008) 121–144

SURGICAL
ONCOLOGY CLINICS
OF NORTH AMERICA

Identification and Monitoring of the Recurrent Laryngeal Nerve During Thyroidectomy

Matthew C. Miller, MD, Joseph R. Spiegel, MD*

*Department of Otolaryngology–Head and Neck Surgery, Thomas Jefferson University,
925 Chestnut Street—6th floor, Philadelphia, PA 19107, USA*

Thyroidectomy is a procedure with a rich history that by some accounts spans nearly three millennia. Throughout its evolution, surgery of the thyroid gland has attracted the attention of some of each generation's most revered physicians and surgeons. Moreover, the approach to and technique of thyroidectomy preferred by these individuals often have spurred tremendous disagreement and debate. Spirited discourse regarding the conduct of thyroidectomy continues in the 21st century, and among the most contested discussed topics is that of recurrent laryngeal nerve (RLN) monitoring. But before discussing monitoring in detail, it behooves the reader to understand some of the history and earlier controversies that have led to the topic at hand.

Early concerns regarding surgery of the thyroid gland stem from the fact that operative management of goiter carried not only a high degree of morbidity, but also mortality. Indeed before the 1860s, hemorrhage and infection were commonplace, and the mortality rate for thyroidectomy exceeded 40% [1,2]. By the mid-1800s, the procedure was so feared and marginalized that it was actually banned by the French Academy of Medicine [3]. The modern era of thyroid surgery, however, soon was ushered in by the near-simultaneous development of aseptic technique, general anesthesia, and meticulous hemostasis. Application of these advances to the field of thyroid surgery by pioneers such as Kocher and Billroth brought about a dramatic reduction in the mortality rates associated with thyroidectomy. By the dawn of the 20th century, these numbers had fallen to less than 1% [1].

* Corresponding author.
 E-mail address: joseph.spiegel@jefferson.edu (J.R. Spiegel).

1055-3207/08/$ - see front matter © 2008 Elsevier Inc. All rights reserved.
doi:10.1016/j.soc.2007.10.008
surgonc.theclinics.com

By the 1920s, there was little debate as to whether thyroidectomy could be performed without significant risk to the life of the patient. This allowed for subsequent technical advances to focus on limiting iatrogenic morbidity. Perhaps most notable among these is the potential for injury to the RLN. As early as the 6th century A.D., voice changes after manipulation of the thyroid gland were recognized [2]. As the sciences of anatomy and surgery grew more sophisticated, the role of RLN injury in these changes became better understood. Kocher and his pupils, regarded by many as the fathers of modern-day thyroidectomy, believed that the best way to avoid injury was to avoid the nerve entirely. Thus it became dogmatic among thyroid surgeons that any RLN seen during thyroidectomy was very likely to have been injured. Lahey officially called this practice into question in the 1920s and 1930s [4,5]. Lahey reported his experience with deliberate exposure and identification of the RLN during over 10,000 thyroidectomies. The less than 1% RLN injury rate was significantly lower than any previously published series and led him to advocate the routine identification and dissection of the nerve during thyroid surgery. In essence, it can be said that Lahey was the first surgeon to actively monitor the RLN during thyroidectomy with routine visualization of the structure.

Although Lahey's assertions and practices are accepted widely as a means of reducing the risk of injury to the RLN, the degree to which one uses ancillary tools and techniques for this purpose continues to spark debate. This article was undertaken to better familiarize endocrine surgeons with the development and potential applications of RLN monitoring for thyroid surgery—ultimately helping them to better establish the role that it may or may not play in their own practices. It is not intended to be an endorsement or a criticism of monitoring in this context. In the interest of full disclosure, however, it should be noted that the authors do use intraoperative monitoring for all thyroid and parathyroid surgeries performed at their home institution.

Anatomy of the recurrent laryngeal nerve

In advocating the routine identification of the RLN during thyroidectomy, Lahey essentially devised the earliest system for neuro-monitoring. It is understood that the most basic concept in monitoring is active localization and dissection of the nerve to protect and preserve its function. It follows that a thorough understanding of the anatomy of the recurrent laryngeal nerve is vital to its detection during surgery of the thyroid gland. It is foolhardy to assume that any monitoring technology—regardless of its sensitivity or presumed benefit—can replace the surgeon's fundamental anatomical knowledge and careful technique. This is particularly true when one considers the fact that RLN anatomy renders it particularly vulnerable to iatrogenic injury. Among both novice and expert thyroid surgeons, careful attention to these features and their variations ultimately will assist in the protection of the nerve. This holds equally true for individuals choosing to use monitoring technology and those who do not.

RLNs arise from the vagus nerve at the level of the aortic arch on the left and at the level of the subclavian artery on the right. From this point, they ascend into the tracheoesophageal grooves as the paired inferior laryngeal nerves until terminating within the substance of the larynx. The asymmetry of the RLNs may be accounted for by their differing embryogenesis and relationship to the developing cardiovascular system. The fetal cardiovascular system initially contains six pairs of aortic arches, beneath which the vagus nerves give off branches to the primordial larynx. Development is marked by gradual alterations in these vessels that eventuate in the appearance of mature aortic and pulmonic vessels.

Around week 7 of gestation, the right sixth arch partially involutes. This structure remains intact on the left and becomes the putative proximal aorta. Simultaneously, the fifth arch arteries regress bilaterally. As the fetus continues to grow, the larynx moves cranially, carrying with it what are now the recurrent laryngeal nerves. Proximally, these will become trapped beneath the lowest remaining arches: arch six on the left (the aortic arch) and arch four on the right (the subclavian artery) (Fig. 1) [6]. The result is a more vertical orientation of the RLN on the left and a more oblique orientation of the right RLN in the adult (Fig. 2).

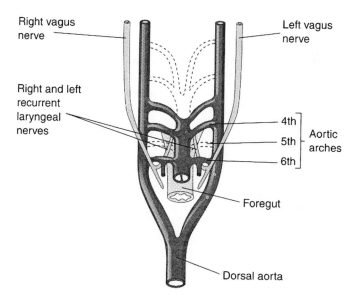

Fig. 1. Embryology of the recurrent laryngeal nerve. The fifth and sixth aortic arches regress on the right. The recurrent laryngeal nerve thereby passes beneath the subclavian artery on the right and the aortic arch on the left. (*From* Moore KL, Persaud TVL. The developing human: clinically oriented embryology. Philadelphia: W.B. Saunders; 1998. p. 387; with permission.)

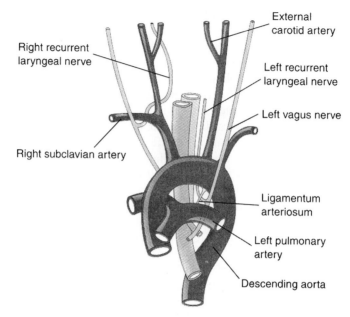

Fig. 2. The position of the recurrent laryngeal nerves relative to the great vessels differs from right to left. This results in a more vertically oriented nerve on the left and a more oblique course of the right recurrent laryngeal nerve. (*From* Moore KL, Persaud TVL. The developing human: clinically oriented embryology. 1998. Philadelphia: W.B. Saunders; 1998. p. 387; with permission.)

This embryology may be used to provide a general framework for localization of the RLN as it courses into the tracheoesophageal groove. It, however, is imprecise and not entirely reliable. Consequently, several authors have attempted to further characterize the relationship of the RLN to the trachea and the esophagus. Although it appears that most inferior laryngeal nerves ascend within the groove, variability is the rule (Table 1) [7–9]. Hence it may not be a safe assumption that the RLN will be found simply by exploring this region.

Additional landmarks have been proposed, but none has proven universally successful. The most widely examined of these is the inferior thyroid artery. Similar to its position relative to the tracheoesophageal groove, the RLN maintains an inconstant relationship to the inferior thyroid artery. It may be found anterior to, posterior to, or even between branches of the artery without a clear predilection (Table 2) [8–14]. In one series examining the recurrent laryngeal nerves of 50 cadaveric specimens (100 nerves), more than 20 different patterns are described [14].

Likewise, attempts have been made at defining relationships between the RLN and other structures along its path toward the larynx. The posterior suspensory (Berry's) ligament, the tubercle of Zuckerkandl, and the

Table 1
Anatomic relationship between recurrent laryngeal nerve, the trachea, and the esophagus

		Tracheoesophageal groove	Paratracheal	Other
Hunt (1968) [7]	Left	77%	22%	1%
	Right	65%	33%	2%
Skandalakis et al (1976) [8]	Left	56%	35%	9%
	Right	41%	49%	10%
Ardito et al (2004) [9]	Left	67%	31%	2%
	Right	61%	38%	1%

cartilaginous framework of the larynx itself have been examined as markers of the position of the RLN.

Not surprisingly, there is disagreement as to the exact relationship between the RLN and Berry's ligament. At least one series [15] found that the RLN passed dorsolateral to this ligament in 100% of cases (over 700 nerves were evaluated). The authors concluded that careful dissection along the capsule of the thyroid gland with separation of the adjacent tissues would assure preservation of the RLN. This should be interpreted with caution, as the RLN also has been found to traverse the ligament in up to 40% of patients and pass through the substance of the gland in up to 10% [8,16].

The tubercle of Zuckerkandl is an embryological remnant of the primordial thyroid that is present in 60% to 90% of adult glands [17]. The tubercle is actually a thickening of the gland located at its most posterolateral extent. These are found most commonly on the right-hand side and are thought to be constant landmarks for the identification of the RLN. The nerve is said to be in a position deep and medial to an enlarged tubercle approximately 95% of the time [17,18]. It has been argued that maintaining a dissection path superficial and lateral to the tubercle of Zuckerkandl will assure preservation of the nerve. Although this assertion may be valid, it should be remembered that a tubercle of Zuckerkandl may be absent or unrecognized in a significant number of patients. As such, it cannot be thought of as a reliable marker for the RLN.

Cartilaginous reference points tend to be more readily identifiable and have been promoted as dependable RLN localizers. Specifically, the RLN has been found to be in close apposition to the cricothyroid joint, in most cases ascending at a 15° to 45° angle [19]. Other geometric relationships between the distal RLN and the surrounding cartilaginous framework of the larynx have been established in cadaveric specimens and are said to be highly predictive of the nerve's position [20]. Detection of the RLN in this fashion, however, requires that a series of measurements be made intraoperatively. This may prove to be cumbersome and less accurate when applied to living patients. Although these approaches may facilitate nerve identification in a rapid and reliable manner, they necessitate that dissection be performed in a retrograde direction. Exposure of the RLN from distal to proximal ultimately may place it at an increased risk of injury. This is

Table 2
Position of the recurrent laryngeal nerve relative to the inferior thyroid artery

	Right recurrent laryngeal nerve (RLN)				Left RLN			
	Nerve anterior to ITA	Nerve posterior to ITA	Nerve between branches	Other	Nerve anterior to ITA	Nerve posterior to ITA	Nerve between branches	Other
Skandalakis, et al (1976) [8]	31%	20%	48%	1%	10%	64%	26%	—
Sturniolo, et al (1999) [11]	22%	31%	29%	18%	19%	37%	22%	22%
Page, et al (2002) [12]	67%	33%	—	—	11%	89%	—	—
Monafred, et al (2002) [13]	21%	28%	50%	1%	21%	50%	28%	1%
Ardito, et al (2004) [9]	12%	61%	27%	—	2%	77%	21%	—
Yalcxin, et al (2006) [14]	40%	34%	26%	—	23%	58%	19%	—

Abbreviation: ITA, inferior thyroid artery.

because extralaryngeal branching is a common occurrence [9,11,12,20,21]. Proximal arborization of the RLN has a reported incidence of 20% to 95%, and the branching patterns are predictably unpredictable. One or more of these branches may be sacrificed inadvertently in the event that the nerve being dissected is not the primary trunk.

Although imperfect, these anatomical relationships serve as valuable tools in the performance of a safe thyroidectomy. Even if a particular landmark was highly predictive of the RLN's position, its utility would be significantly limited in particular cases. Tissue planes may be obscured during revision surgery or following radiation therapy. Anatomy may be distorted as in the case of large goiters or inflammatory processes and carcinomas. Excessive bleeding may limit the surgeon's ability to recognize or use familiar landmarks. Inexperienced surgeons may not have adequate familiarity with the landmarks. These and a host of other reasons explain why even in the hands of a skillful and knowledgeable surgeon, iatrogenic RLN injury does indeed occur.

The recurrent laryngeal nerves at risk

As one discusses monitoring of the RLN, it is important to consider the true risk of iatrogenic injury. This is a difficult question to answer for two primary reasons. First: one must assume that the reporting of RLN injury rates is honest and accurate. There is an inherent risk of bias in any circumstance where complications are being reported, and thyroidectomy is no exception. Second: the definition of RLN injury is applied inconsistently throughout the literature. Much of the data pertaining to RLN injury is a reflection of subjective or observed changes in voice rather than objective assessment of vocal fold motion. Subjective voice complaints and observed hoarseness may not be predictive of a patient's findings on laryngoscopy. As postoperative laryngoscopic examination is not the rule for a great number of thyroid surgeons, the true incidence of RLN injury may be underestimated.

Based upon the existing body of literature, the rate of RLN injury is relatively low. Among patients undergoing thyroidectomy for any reason, the rate of temporary paresis ranges from less than 1% to approximately 6%, while the rates of permanent paralysis are anywhere from 0.05% to about 2.5% [9,11,22–29]. For those patients with thyroid carcinoma, temporary RLN injury occurs in approximately 0.7% to 4% of cases, while paralysis rates range from 1.6% to 10.6% [22–24,27,30]. Likewise, reoperative thyroid surgery carries an increased risk. RLN paresis is seen in up to 10.1% of cases, while permanent injury has been reported up to 8.1% of thyroidectomy patients [24,31–34].

The evolution of recurrent laryngeal nerve monitoring

Although his postoperative voice assessments were subjective rather than laryngoscopic, Lahey presented the first large series of patients with a rate of

RLN injury similar to what is seen today [4,5]. This is in stark contrast to predecessors such as Billroth, who reported a RLN injury rate of around 30% [2]. Much of Lahey's success in reducing the incidence was attributed to the active identification and preservation of the RLN during surgery. Numerous subsequent studies support this practice [24,35–37]. As a consequence, the following becomes the essential question regarding the use of a monitor during thyroidectomy: Can intraoperative monitoring improve a procedure with an already low rate of reported iatrogenic injury? Although the answer to this question continues to be debated (a subject to be discussed in the following sections), its pursuit most certainly has led to significant innovations and technological advances in the field of thyroid and parathyroid surgery.

Early technologies

The first use of technology in an attempt to reduce the risk to the RLN was published by Shedd and Durham [38] in 1965. They argued that despite having "knowledge of anatomy and careful surgical technique," the RLN still might be vulnerable to injury. They cited among the reasons for this vulnerability the presence of anomalous anatomy (ie, nonrecurrent nerves), extralaryngeal branching, displacement or involvement by pathologic processes, and a similar appearance of the nerve to other filamentous structures in the region. Recalling prior experience with intraoperative stimulation of the facial nerve during parotidectomy, an attempt was made at stimulating the RLN and recording a physiologic response. Although facial nerve function could be monitored by observing muscular twitches in response to electrical stimulation, the RLN required an indirect means of monitoring be used. As a result, the authors devised a balloon pressure transducer that was fitted to an endotracheal tube and subsequently placed at the level of the glottis. Initially used in a canine model, this method allowed for the successful identification and confirmation of the RLN. In a follow-up study [39] the technique was employed in people. Again the authors could record vocal cord motion reliably in response to electrical stimulation by pneumatic spirography. They concluded that the use of electrical identification of the RLN increases safety and feasibility of thyroidectomy, particularly in the presence of the aforementioned anatomic distortions. Subsequent authors [40,41] attempted to improve on Shedd's original model, but their success was limited by numerous design flaws. As a consequence, pneumatic monitoring of the vocal folds never gained widespread appeal.

Noting the difficulties experienced with the pneumatic balloon designs, Hvidegaard and colleagues [42] developed a device based upon the acoustic properties of an air column (ie, the trachea) with variable impedance. This instrument consisted of a sound oscillator that was placed into the trachea. The oscillator transmitted a pure tone frequency to a microphone positioned just above the vocal folds. This signal then was amplified and recorded by an external device. During RLN stimulation, the vocal folds close, thereby altering the impedance within the air column and hence, the output signal. Any change in the output signal during stimulation therefore could be interpreted as evidence of functionality of the RLN. Although the initial results were promising, the acoustic impedance monitor did not develop beyond the prototype stages.

These early devices paved the way for many of the electrophysiologic monitoring systems employed today, but the evolution was gradual. In the interim, much attention was given to vocal fold observation as a means of establishing the identity and integrity of the RLN.

Vocal fold visualization

Through his experience with [35] over 1700 thyroidectomies, Riddell noted a reduced risk of postoperative RLN paresis in those patients whose nerves had been identified and dissected deliberately. The author went on to describe a subpopulation of patients (132 patients with 200 nerves at risk) in whom the RLN not only was identified, but also electrically stimulated. Feeling that the glottic pressure transducer was unreliable, Riddell relied upon intraoperative direct laryngoscopy for confirmation of RLN integrity. There was no difference in the rates of RLN paresis between the cases in which it had been stimulated and those in which it simply had been identified. Despite this, the author called intraoperative RLN stimulation "an additional safety measure" that might assist with differentiating ectopic nerve from nearby non-nervous tissue. More importantly, he noted that stimulation, or the absence thereof, was helpful in preventing and identifying a possible bilateral paresis, something he called "an iatrogenic horror, a surgical tragedy, and a disaster likely to be followed by the misery of litigation."

Kratz [43] similarly advocated for vocal fold visualization (using a self-retaining rigid laryngoscope) during surgery as a means of monitoring the RLN. There are inherent limitations to this method, however, including draping, positioning, and a less than ideal view of the larynx and its motion secondary to the presence of an endotracheal tube. Technology has allowed some of these difficulties to be overcome. Premachandra and colleagues [44] described a technique in which intraoperative flexible laryngoscopy was used for this purpose. The flexible laryngoscope is a less cumbersome alternative to rigid laryngoscopy. Positioned beside the endotracheal tube in the hypopharynx, the fiberoptic scope can transmit an image to a video monitor, allowing the surgeon to continuously observe vocal fold motion while dissecting or stimulating the RLN. Again, the limitation in this technique is that an endotracheal tube passed through the glottis reduces the observer's ability to detect vocal fold motion.

The development of the laryngeal mask airway (LMA) in the early 1980's [45] presented an interesting solution to this problem. The LMA is positioned above the vocal folds and allows for positive pressure ventilation in the absence of endotracheal intubation. Tanigawa and colleagues [46] were the first to explore this device for thyroidectomy. Numerous other authors since have described their experience with the method [47–51]. The principal benefit of the LMA in this context is that there is not an endotracheal tube passing through the glottis. A bronchoscope delivered through the lumen of the LMA therefore offers a continuous and unobstructed view of vocal fold motion. Additional benefits of using the LMA for this purpose include relative simplicity of the setup, low capital cost of the monitoring system as compared with other devices, decreased postoperative throat pain, and the lack of instrumentation of the vocal cords, which may in and of itself lead to temporary dysphonia in the postoperative period.

Disadvantages to using the LMA are not necessarily unique to thyroid surgery. The principle concern is that of potential loss of control of the airway. Extrinsic compression, malpositioning of the LMA cuff, or laryngospasm may compromise the security of the airway [51–53]. Indeed up to 10% of patients undergoing thyroidectomy using this form of anesthesia ultimately required endotracheal intubation [47–49]. An additional concern is that of potential aspiration of gastric contents. Certain patients may be more prone to aspiration risk during LMA anesthesia, including those with gastroesophageal reflux disease (GERD), hiatal hernias, and those taking gastroparetic drugs [52–54]. The surgeon choosing to employ an LMA for monitoring purposes must be acutely aware of the potential risks and proceed to endotracheal intubation before issues arise. One creative means at circumventing the difficulties associated with the LMA method of RLN monitoring was presented by Hillerman and colleagues [55]. They proposed a double-intubation technique in which a small (5-0 microlaryngeal) endotracheal tube is passed as a means of securing the airway with simultaneous use of an LMA as a conduit for a flexible laryngoscope. The small-sized tube did not limit the motion of the vocal folds during stimulation. At the same time, it provided a more secure airway than the LMA alone. This and other methods employing laryngeal mask anesthesia have been successful in confirming the identity of the RLN and in predicting postoperative paresis. Many surgeons continue to use them today.

The desire to avoid additional instrumentation and equipment in the operating room has led to the consideration of less cumbersome and expensive approaches to observing vocal fold motion. Spahn and colleagues [56] used a 2 in needle (27 g) placed into the vocal folds through the cricothyroid membrane as a means to observe their movement during electrical stimulation of the RLN. This avoided the inherent difficulty in performing intraoperative laryngoscopy, the poor reliability of the pneumatic balloon, and the extra equipment and cost associated with laryngoscopy or electromyography (EMG).

Simple palpation of the posterior cricoarytenoid (PCA) muscle during stimulation of the RLN also has been promoted as an inexpensive and

accurate means of confirming its identity and integrity [57]. Detection of vocal fold motion by this method has been compared with electromyography
by Randolph and colleagues [58]. In nearly 500 patients studied, it was
found that the stimulus required to elicit a palpable PCA twitch was nearly
identical to that needed to evoke a suprathreshold EMG response. The author concluded that the presence of a palpable twitch at a stimulus of 1 mA
or less was predictive of postoperative vocal fold motion. In the absence of
such a twitch, it is suggested that any efforts at contralateral lobectomy be
deferred pending a formal vocal fold evaluation. Given that palpation is not
a continuous means of monitoring, this technique is advocated as an adjunct
to formal intraoperative EMG.

Electromyographic methods

During the 1950s and 1960s, numerous authors experimented with EMG
of the laryngeal muscles to evaluate their activity during respiration and
phonation. In 1964, Nakamura [59] presented a series of experiments in
dogs, whereby the larynx was dissected, and the laryngeal nerves were cut.
These then were stimulated externally to demonstrate the motor functions
simultaneous with EMG tracing. Flisberg and Lindholm [60] are credited
with bringing this technique into the operating room in 1970.Their initial
work involved placement of EMG recording needles through the cricothyroid membrane and into the vocalis muscle. Muscle action potentials in response to RLN stimulation were recorded successfully in 15 patients. Davis
improved upon this design by taking the recording electrodes out of the operative field and inserting them laryngoscopically [61,62]. The Davis EMG
system was an important advance for two principal reasons. First: it was
an intralaryngeal device. The electrode was not in the operative field and
was less likely to be displaced during dissection. Monitoring thereby could
continue without interruption during the surgery. Second: the recording device was equipped with an audible alert. This helped to eliminate the immediate need for expertise in interpreting EMG, which was required by the
Flisberg/Lindholm model. Successively smaller electrodes were designed
and used for this purpose over the next 10 to 15 years [63–65]. Concurrently,
the NIM-Response system (Medtronic Xomed, Jacksonville, Florida) was
gaining popularity for facial nerve monitoring during parotidectomy. The
availability of commercially prepared electrodes and monitoring equipment
prompted a new interest in electromyographic monitoring during thyroidectomy. As Eisele [66] outlined, however, there were several limitations to be
overcome. Electrode placement was skill- and time-dependent. The electrodes were small and easily displaced, and their replacement often delayed
or prolonged surgery. Likewise, there was a potential risk of foreign body
aspiration.

It was Rea [67] in 1992 who ushered in the modern era of RLN monitoring by adapting an existing postcricoid surface electrode for use during

thyroidectomy. The electrode was designed by Payne and colleagues to evaluate the function of the PCA muscle during phonation and respiration
[68,69]. The original device consisted of two electrodes on the anterior surface that contacted the PCA muscles and a posterior ground electrode that
contacted the posterior hypopharyngeal wall. A long insertion handle was
included in the design for ease of placement during laryngoscopy. Contraction of the PCA muscles in response to electrical stimulation of the RLN resulted in an audible tone on an EMG recording device. Postcricoid surface

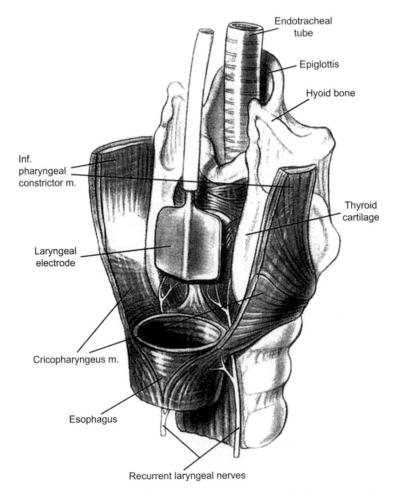

Fig. 3. Postcricoid surface laryngeal electrode. (*From* Rea JL, Khan A. Recurrent laryngeal
nerve location in thyroidectomy and parathyroidectomy: use of an indwelling laryngeal surface
electrode with evoked electromyography. Operative Techn Otolaryngol Head Neck Surg
1994;5:91–6; with permission.)

electrodes are now available commercially (RLN Systems, Incorporated, Jefferson City, Missouri) (Fig. 3).

Recording surface potentials from laryngeal musculature were not an entirely novel idea. In their paper describing laryngoscopically placed needle electrodes, Davis and colleagues [62] remarked that they also had experimented with an endolaryngeal surface electrode consisting of gold foil positioned on the endotracheal tube. EMG potentials were recorded successfully, but the authors found that it was difficult to maintain the position of the electrode during general anesthesia. This concept was revisited in the early 1990s and eventuated in the introduction of fully integrated electrode systems such as the NIM endotracheal tube (Fig. 4) [66,70]. Other endolaryngeal surface electrode types have been designed and validated for use during thyroid and parathyroid surgery [70–76]. Although a discussion of each such device's individual features and merits is beyond the scope of this article, most consist of electrode arrays that are affixed to standard endotracheal tubes, thereby obviating the need for and costs associated with any one particular company's monitor and equipment.

A few series have compared the broader categories of surface electrode monitors (ie, endolaryngeal and postcricoid types) [77,78]. Both types of monitoring system were helpful in identifying and confirming the RLN, and clear superiority of one type was not demonstrated in this regard. Several advantages and disadvantages of each were identified. The postcricoid electrode was found to be less expensive. It may be cut to size so that only one size needs to be stocked by an operating room. A distinct heartbeat artifact could be observed when this array was positioned properly in the postcricoid space, a reassuring finding to the surgeon. This electrode has the disadvantage that it must be placed by an individual familiar with postcricoid anatomy. In addition, it is highly sensitive to downward pressure, and as a result, artifactual EMG activity may be observed during dissection. Furthermore, extralaryngeal tumors potentially can impede proper positioning. The endolaryngeal type electrode was found to be inserted more easily. Proper positioning may be confirmed by either laryngoscopy

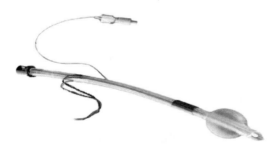

Fig. 4. NIM-II endotracheal tube with integrated electrodes. (*Courtesy of* Medtronic Xomed, Jacksonville, FL; with permission.)

(Fig. 5) or observation of electrode impedances (less than 10Ω is required; less than 1Ω is ideal). Unlike the postcricoid electrode, the endotracheal tube electrode receives input from each vocal fold individually and generates a higher amplitude EMG response for a given stimulus. Disadvantages include the need to stock multiple sizes, the increased cost associated with each disposable tube, and the inability to use the system in circumstances where modified tubes are needed (eg, double lung ventilation, laser surgery) [77].

Sensitivity and specificty of modern monitoring devices

Modern monitoring devices may be used to identify nerve from surrounding tissues, to provide feedback during dissection, to confirm the integrity of a dissected nerve, or any combination thereof. These instruments are designed to record baseline and evoked EMG (eEMG) potentials elicited by dissection or stimulating electrodes for this purpose. But is the absence of an eEMG the sine qua non of vocal fold paresis, and vice versa? To answer this question, one must consider the sensitivity, specificity, and predictive values of monitoring. Sensitivity refers to the ability of monitoring to detect a paralyzed nerve (ie, it is the number of electrically paralyzed nerves as a percentage of the true number [as observed by laryngoscopy] of paralyzed nerves). Tests with high false-negative rates will have a low sensitivity. False negatives suggest neural integrity when in fact it has been compromised. They may result from stimulation distal to an injury or scatter effect to the vocalis muscle from monopolar electrodes [79,80].

Specificity refers to the number of electrically intact nerves as a percentage of those with normal vocal fold motion. Any circumstance in which the false-positive rate is increased (ie, situations in which a functional nerve fails to generate an eEMG when stimulated) can reduce the specificity of the test. Dislodged grounding wires, misplaced electrodes, inadequate

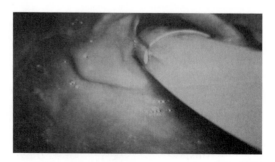

Fig. 5. Proper positioning of the endotracheal electrodes may be confirmed by direct laryngoscopy.

stimulus amplitude, and elevated event threshold voltage settings on the EMG recorder may have this effect. Other potential confounders include temporary neurapraxia, the presence of anesthetic muscle relaxant, or a pseudocholinesterase deficiency [79,80]. Positive predictive value is the probability that in the absence of an eEMG, a patient truly has a vocal fold paresis. Negative predictive value, on the other hand, is the probability that in the presence of an eEMG (or the palpated equivalent), the vocal folds will be mobile.

Several authors have examined evoked stimulation of the RLN as a predictor of postoperative vocal fold motion. Most have found that monitoring possesses a high specificity and negative predictive value [80,81], whereas the sensitivity and positive predictive values are low [81–87]. The message here is that patients who have electromyographically normal nerves are likely to be laryngoscopically normal. Conversely, if a nerve appears to be compromised by eEMG, there is still a greater than 50% probability that the patient will have normal vocal fold motion.

The rationale for and data regarding recurrent laryngeal nerve monitoring

Nerve monitoring

To this point, the anatomy of the recurrent laryngeal nerve has been described; the rates of iatrogenic injury have been presented; the evolution of intraoperative identification and monitoring has been chronicled, and the validity of evoked vocal fold potentials has been characterized. From all of this, it is clear that although complex and potentially capricious in its course toward the larynx, the RLN may be exposed safely and dissected during thyroidectomy with minimal risk of permanent damage. Indeed exposure of the nerve has been shown to reduce this risk [4,5,35,37]. Its identity may be reliably confirmed and its function monitored by numerous methods that involve electrical stimulation and observation of an evoked electromyographic or physical response within the larynx.

This begs the fundamental question regarding RLN monitoring. If identification of the nerve allows for the preservation of its function, does it not follow that any means by which the precise location and identity of the nerve could be confirmed readily might also aid in preserving function?

Several arguments can be made to support a role for monitoring during thyroidectomy. First, identification does not translate necessarily to functional integrity. Eliciting an evoked vocal fold response provides confirmation that the anatomically preserved nerve is also electrophysiologically intact. This in turn may dictate plans for second-side surgery, particularly in the rare circumstance of a patient who presents with a pre-existing vocal fold paresis on the contralateral side. As mentioned previously, there are a host of variables that may lead to unanticipated changes in the expected anatomy of the RLN. The use of continuous, real-time monitoring with audible alerts also provides immediate feedback regarding surgical technique. Gentle and meticulous dissection is in no way assured by an alarming nerve monitor, but it may signal to the surgeon a need to alter his or her current course of action. This may be particularly helpful for resident training purposes [66,88–90].

Potential disadvantages of routine RLN monitoring include the additional costs associated with monitoring equipment, additional setup time at the beginning of surgery, and the potential for false negative EMG [66,88,89,91,92]. In this circumstance, the surgeon mistakenly might sacrifice the RLN based upon its erroneous lack of response to a suprathreshold stimulus. Also worrisome is the theoretical risk of inducing paresis by repeatedly stimulating the RLN [93]. Although not unique to thyroidectomy, one final concern is that surgeons simply will rely upon technology as a means of protecting the RLN rather than using sound anatomical knowledge and careful technique. Indeed the fear that the availability of new technologies and devices will supplant the application of reason and clinical judgment is pervasive throughout medicine today.

Despite the number of arguments in favor of and opposed to RLN monitoring (and the passion with which these positions are held), the collective body of literature has failed to conclusively support or refute its routine use in this regard. Indeed only a handful of reports directly compare the outcomes in between monitored and unmonitored cases. In a 2001 study, Brennan remarked that the rates of RLN paresis observed among 96 monitored nerves at risk compared favorably with historical controls that had undergone appropriate postoperative laryngeal examination [92]. Although this study lacks widespread applicability and is limited by methological flaws, it represents the first attempt at an objective comparison of outcomes between monitored and nonmonitored patients. Subsequent reports were more rigorous in their scientific method and examined increasingly larger patient populations. Robertson and colleagues [94] published a retrospective study that compared RLN injury rates among 116 monitored nerves at risk and an unmatched control group of 120 unmonitored nerves at risk. Although the rates of paralysis and paresis were found to be lower in the monitored group, the differences were not statistically significant. The authors noted that with a larger sample size, more robust differences may very well have been observed.

With this in mind, a multi-institutional prospective trial was undertaken to compare the rates of transient and permanent RLN paralysis among monitored and unmonitored patients with benign goiter [90]. Across 7133 nerves at risk, the rates of transient and permanent RLN palsy were lower for those cases in which monitoring had been employed. These results were highly statistically significant. In a follow-up to this study, Dralle and colleagues [95] analyzed the outcomes of nearly 30,000 nerves at risk. Comparisons were made between cases in which the nerve had not been identified, those in which it had been identified, and those in which it had been identified and monitored. When compared with thyroidectomy without nerve identification, there was a significant difference in paralysis rates favoring visual identification of the RLN, either with or without the addition of a nerve monitor. When comparing neuromonitoring to simple visual identification of the RLN, there was no added benefit. Other significant risk factors for postoperative RLN paralysis included surgical volume (less than 45 nerves at risk per surgeon or less than 275 nerves at risk per hospital annually). Subgroup analysis of patients who had only benign or malignant thyroid disease did not disclose a benefit to monitoring.

Chan similarly found no difference in the incidence of RLN paresis or paralysis when comparing 501 monitored and 499 unmonitored (identified by routine visualization only) nerves [86]. On subgroup analysis, however, monitoring was associated with a reduction in the postoperative paresis/paralysis rate for patients undergoing secondary thyroidectomy. This finding is in contrast to a Mayo Clinic study from 2004 [96]. In it, 52 patients undergoing cervical re-exploration with continuous monitoring for pathology related to a primary thyroid or parathyroid disorder were compared with 59 matched unmonitored controls (151 nerves at risk). The rates of permanent RLN injury were nearly identical (1.4 versus 1.3%, favoring the unmonitored group). The authors felt that monitoring added substantial cost while providing no apparent clinical benefit. Table 3 presents the pertinent findings of the previously mentioned reports.

One of the principal difficulties in substantiating any claim of efficacy rests in the fact that the incidence of thyroidectomy-associated RLN paresis and paralysis is exceedingly low. Given the low prevalence, the amount of statistical power necessary to demonstrate a difference in outcomes attributable to nerve monitoring alone would exceed what is practical for most investigators. This is particularly true, because thyroidectomy is performed for numerous clinically distinct indications, each with differing rates of associated RLN injury. Beldi and colleagues [81] noted that a homogeneous population of over 21,000 nerves at risk would be needed to discern a difference in risk attributable to monitoring alone. Dralle and colleagues [95] further illustrates this point, noting that among patients with thyroid carcinoma, a population of over 39,000 nerves at risk would need to be examined. For benign multinodular goiter, they estimated that this number exceeds nine million. Even more conservative estimates of these numbers exceed the total number of thyroidectomies that many surgeons will perform during their career!

Medicolegal implications

It has been shown that 30% to 50% of endocrine malpractice litigation involves thyroid and parathyroid surgery. Of these, 70% to 90% pertain

Table 3
Rates of temporary and permanent laryngeal nerve paresis in the presence or absence of intraoperative monitoring

Study	Nerve at risk	Temporary paresis			Permanent paresis			Additional risk factors
		Electromyography (EMG)	None	p	EMG	None	p	
Thomusch et al (2001) [90]	7133 (benign goiter)	1.4%	2.1%	< 0.008	0.4%	0.8%	< 0.004	—
Robertson et al (2004) [94]	236	3.45	4.35	NS	0.86	0.62	NS	Advanced T stage
Dralle et al (2004) [95]	29,998	—	—	—	0.21–5.65	0.0–4.74	NS	Absence of nerve identification, low-volume surgeons/hospitals
Yarbrough et al (2004) [96]	151 (reoperative)	12.5%	10.1%	NS	1.4%	1.3%	NS	—
Chan et al (2006) [86]	1000	3.4	4.0	NS	0.8%	1.2	NS	Absence of monitoring in reoperative cases

Additional independent predictors of postoperative paresis are noted for their respective studies.

to RLN injury, with bilateral paresis accounting for nearly 30% of the cases. In the end, only about one in three judgments is in favor of the defendant [97,98]. So despite the lack of clear-cut evidence in support of or against the routine use of RLN monitors for thyroidectomy, there will be ongoing medicolegal questions about the role of this technology in current practice. In an era of evidence-based medicine, do the existing data support RLN monitoring as a standard of care? The answer to this question is not simple and necessitates an understanding of a few basic principles.

The first is the concept of standard of care. This is a legal rather than a medical term. It refers to the level at which the average, prudent provider in a given community would practice. More simply, it is what a similarly qualified physician would have done to manage a given patient under a similar set of circumstances. Moreover, standard of care is an acceptable minimum that may or may not be supported by evidence-based medicine. Malpractice implies that an established standard of care has been breached [99].

One can appreciate therefore the difficulty in defining neuromonitoring of the RLN as a standard of care. Variability in the diseases treated with thyroidectomy, in the experience of the surgeons, and in the patients themselves makes it difficult to apply a standard to thyroidectomy. Additionally, there is variability in the usage patterns of monitoring technology. Although some surgeons only use the monitor as a means to confirm the identity of a visualized nerve, others dissect it completely, stimulating only at the completion of the operation to confirm integrity. Still others may probe the thyroid bed freely in an attempt to electrically uncover the location of the nerve. It is difficult to define a standard of care when there is not a universally accepted method of using the monitor.

It is interesting that in nearly every article written on the subject of nerve monitoring for the thyroid, regardless of the author's conclusions, time is taken to include a sentence or two stating something akin to the following: "Despite any real or perceived benefits of nerve monitoring, it cannot replace experience, sound clinical judgment, and technical skill and should therefore not be considered the standard of care." Each author has crafted these words carefully as to lay the groundwork for his or her own defense or the defense of a physician peer. Going just so far, but not defining it as a gold standard, brings about the concept of best clinical practice.

Contrasted to the standard of care, best clinical practice is a medical term that is qualitative and fluid. It is physician- and circumstance-specific and takes into account one's background and training, knowledge, and experience. Best clinical practice also may be influenced by the severity and complexity of the disease being treated, regulatory bodies, third-party payers, and other outside forces. Implicit in the definition is that a specific physician at a particular time and place is providing the best possible care for a specific patient under a given set of circumstances. Best clinical practice may or may not coincide with what is considered to be the standard of care [99].

A report by Sosa and colleagues [100] sheds some light on this concept. The authors explored the relationship between surgeon experience and outcomes in thyroidectomy in a statewide cross-sectional analysis. They found that the highest volume had the fewest complications (including RLN injury) and the shortest length of stay, even though they were treating the most complicated patients. Similar observations were made by Dralle and colleagues [95].

By the best clinical practice model, one might argue that the expertise of these surgeons might obviate the need to use nerve monitoring. Conversely, less experienced surgeons may be more apt to be assisted by the use of a monitor. Although the issue is certainly more complex than can be described in these few paragraphs, it behooves endocrine surgeons to maintain best clinical practice based on their own experience and results as well as supporting ongoing clinical research in RLN monitoring.

Summary

The recurrent laryngeal nerve is complex and is often in harm's way when performing a thyroidectomy. Visualizing and dissecting the recurrent laryngeal nerve are tantamount to performing a safe thyroid operation. In an attempt to increase the margin of safety, numerous monitoring devices have been developed that are now readily available, of high specificity, and that provide high negative predictive value in confirming the integrity of the RLN. At the same time, data regarding their efficacy in limiting or preventing injury to the nerve are inconclusive. And although it may indeed represent the best clinical practice for a given surgeon to use neuromonitoring for thyroidectomy, it does not necessarily represent the standard of care. In cases where monitors are used, they should be used judiciously and interpreted cautiously. Use of such devices cannot and should not supplant clinical judgment, anatomic knowledge, and meticulous technique.

References

[1] Becker WF. Presidential address: pioneers in thyroid surgery. Ann Surg 1977;185(5): 493–504.

[2] Hegner C. A history of thyroid surgery. Ann Surg 1932;95(4):481–92.

[3] Giddings AEB. The history of thyroidectomy. J R Soc Med 1998;91(Suppl 33):3–6.

[4] Lahey FH. Routine dissection and demonstration of the recurrent laryngeal nerve in subtotal thyroidectomy. Surg Gynecol Obstet 1938;66:775–7.

[5] Lahey FH. Exposure of the recurrent laryngeal nerves in thyroid operations. Further experiences. Surg Gynecol Obstet 1944;194:239–44.

[6] Moore KL, Persaud TVL. The developing human. Clinically oriented embryology. Philadelphia: W.B. Saunders; 1998. p. 349–403.

[7] Hunt PS, Poole M, Reeve TS. A reappraisal of the surgical anatomy of the thyroid and parathyroid glands. Br J Surg 1968;55(1):63–6.

[8] Skandalakis JE, Droulias C, Harlaftis N, et al. The recurrent laryngeal nerve. Am Surg 1976;42(9):629–34.

[9] Ardito G, Revelli L, D'Alatri L, et al. Revisited anatomy of the recurrent laryngeal nerves. Am J Surg 2004;187(2):249–53.

[10] Simon MM. Pitfalls to be avoided in thyroidectomy; a triangle for localization and protection of the recurrent nerve. J Int Coll Surg 1951;15(4):428–42.

[11] Sturniolo G, D'Alia C, Tonante A, et al. The recurrent laryngeal nerve related to thyroid surgery. Am J Surg 1999;177(6):485–8.

[12] Page C, Foulon P, Strunski V. The inferior laryngeal nerve: surgical and anatomic considerations. Report of 251 thyroidectomies. Surg Radiol Anat 2003;25(3–4):188–91.

[13] Monfared A, Gorti G, Kim D. Microsurgical anatomy of the laryngeal nerves as related to thyroid surgery. Laryngoscope 2002;112(2):386–92.

[14] Yalcxin B. Anatomic configurations of the recurrent laryngeal nerve and inferior thyroid artery. Surgery 2006;139(2):181–7.

[15] Sasou S, Nakamura S, Kurihara H. Suspensory ligament of berry: its relationship to recurrent laryngeal nerve and anatomic examination of 24 autopsies. Head Neck 1998;20(8):695–8.

[16] Berlin D. The recurrent laryngeal nerves in total ablation of the normal thyroid gland: an anatomical and surgical study. Surg Gynecol Obstet 1935;60:19–26.

[17] Gauger PG, Delbridge LW, Thompson NW, et al. Incidence and importance of the tubercle of Zuckerkandl in thyroid surgery. Eur J Surg 2001;167(4):249–54.

[18] Costanzo M, Caruso LA, Veroux M, et al. [The lobe of Zuckerkandl: an important sign of recurrent laryngeal nerve]. Ann Ital Chir 2005;76(4):337–40 [in Italian].

[19] Shindo ML, Wu JC, Park EE. Surgical anatomy of the recurrent laryngeal nerve revisited. Otolaryngol Head Neck Surg 2005;133(4):514–9.

[20] Cakir BO, Ercan I, Sam B, et al. Reliable surgical landmarks for the identification of the recurrent laryngeal nerve. Otolaryngol Head Neck Surg 2006;135(2):299–302.

[21] Karlan MS, Catz B, Dunkelman D, et al. A safe technique for thyroidectomy with complete nerve dissection and parathyroid preservation. Head Neck Surg 1984;6(6):1014–9.

[22] Rosato L, Avenia N, Bernante P, et al. Complications of thyroid surgery: analysis of a multicentric study on 14,934 patients operated on in Italy over 5 years. World J Surg 2004;28(3): 271–6.

[23] Lo CY, Kwok KF, Yuen PW. A prospective evaluation of recurrent laryngeal nerve paralysis during thyroidectomy. Arch Surg 2000;135(2):204–7.

[24] Chiang FY, Wang LF, Huang YF, et al. Recurrent laryngeal nerve palsy after thyroidectomy with routine identification of the recurrent laryngeal nerve. Surgery 2005;137(3):342–7.

[25] Kasemsuwan L, Nubthuenetr S. Recurrent laryngeal nerve paralysis: a complication of thyroidectomy. J Otolaryngol 1997;26(6):365–7.

[26] Moulton-Barrett R, Crumley R, Jalilie S, et al. Complications of thyroid surgery. Int Surg 1997;82(1):63–6.

[27] Lacoste L, Gineste D, Karayan J, et al. Airway complications in thyroid surgery. Ann Otol Rhinol Laryngol 1993;102(6):441–6.

[28] Bhattacharyya N, Fried MP. Assessment of the morbidity and complications of total thyroidectomy. Arch Otolaryngol Head Neck Surg 2002;128(4):389–92.

[29] Prim MP, de Diego JI, Hardisson D, et al. Factors related to nerve injury and hypocalcemia in thyroid gland surgery. Otolaryngol Head Neck Surg 2001;124(1):111–4.

[30] Dener C. Complication rates after operations for benign thyroid disease. Acta Otolaryngol 2002;122(6):679–83.

[31] Misiolek M, Waler J, Namyslowski G, et al. Recurrent laryngeal nerve palsy after thyroid cancer surgery: a laryngological and surgical problem. Eur Arch Otorhinolaryngol 2001; 258(9):460–2.

[32] Kupferman ME, Mandel SJ, DiDonato L, et al. Safety of completion thyroidectomy following unilateral lobectomy for well-differentiated thyroid cancer. Laryngoscope 2002; 112(7 Pt 1):1209–12.

[33] Pezzullo L, Delrio P, Losito NS, et al. Postoperative complications after completion thyroidectomy for differentiated thyroid cancer. Eur J Surg Oncol 1997;23(3):215–8.

[34] Chao TC, Jeng LB, Lin JD, et al. Reoperative thyroid surgery. World J Surg 1997;21(6): 644–7.

[35] Riddell V. Thyroidectomy: prevention of bilateral recurrent nerve palsy. Results of identification of the nerve over 23 consecutive years (1946–69) with a description of an additional safety measure. Br J Surg 1970;57(1):1–11.

[36] Hermann M, Alk G, Roka R, et al. Laryngeal recurrent nerve injury in surgery for benign thyroid diseases: effect of nerve dissection and impact of individual surgeon in more than 27,000 nerves at risk. Ann Surg 2002;235(2):261–8.

[37] Jatzko GR, Lisborg PH, Muller MG, et al. Recurrent nerve palsy after thyroid operations—principal nerve identification and a literature review. Surgery 1994;115(2):139–44.

[38] Shedd DP, Durham C. Electrical identification of the recurrent laryngeal nerve. I. Response of the canine larynx to electrical stimulation of the recurrent laryngeal nerve. Ann Surg 1966;163(1):47–50.

[39] Shedd DP, Burget GC. Identification of the recurrent laryngeal nerve. Arch Surg 1966; 92(6):861–4.

[40] Engel PM, Buter HA, Page PS, et al. A device for the location and protection of the recurrent laryngeal nerve during operations upon the neck. Surg Gynecol Obstet 1981;152(6):825–6.

[41] Woltering EA, Dumond D, Ferrara J, et al. A method for intraoperative identification of the recurrent laryngeal nerve. Am J Surg 1984;148(4):438–40.

[42] Hvidegaard T, Vase P, Dalsgaard SC, et al. Endolaryngeal devices for perioperative identification and functional testing of the recurrent nerve. Otolaryngol Head Neck Surg 1984; 92(3):292–4.

[43] Kratz RC. The identification and protection of the laryngeal motor nerves during thyroid and laryngeal surgery: a new microsurgical technique. Laryngoscope 1973;83(1):59–78.

[44] Premachandra DJ, Radcliffe GJ, Stearns MP. Intraoperative identification of the recurrent laryngeal nerve and demonstration of its function. Laryngoscope 1990;100(1):94–6.

[45] Brain AI. The laryngeal mask—a new concept in airway management. Br J Anaesth 1983; 55(8):801–5.

[46] Tanigawa K, Inoue Y, Iwata S. Protection of recurrent laryngeal nerve during neck surgery: a new combination of neutracer, laryngeal mask airway, and fiberoptic bronchoscope. Anesthesiology 1991;74(5):966–7.

[47] Hobbiger HE, Allen JG, Greatorex RG, et al. The laryngeal mask airway for thyroid and parathyroid surgery. Anaesthesia 1996;51(10):972–4.

[48] Shah EF, Allen JG, Greatorex RA. Use of the laryngeal mask airway in thyroid and parathyroid surgery as an aid to the identification and preservation of the recurrent laryngeal nerves. Ann R Coll Surg Engl 2001;83(5):315–8.

[49] Eltzschig HK, Posner M, Moore FD Jr. The use of readily available equipment in a simple method for intraoperative monitoring of recurrent laryngeal nerve function during thyroid surgery: initial experience with more than 300 cases. Arch Surg 2002;137(4):452–6.

[50] Scheuller MC, Ellison D. Laryngeal mask anesthesia with intraoperative laryngoscopy for identification of the recurrent laryngeal nerve during thyroidectomy. Laryngoscope 2002; 112(9):1594–7.

[51] Pott L, Swick JT, Stack BC Jr. Assessment of recurrent laryngeal nerve during thyroid surgery with laryngeal mask airway. Arch Otolaryngol Head Neck Surg 2007;133(3):266–9.

[52] Dolling S, Anders NR, Rolfe SE. Protection of the airway with the LMA during upper airway surgery. Can J Anaesth 2003;50(9):967–8.

[53] Verghese C, Brimacombe JR. Survey of laryngeal mask airway usage in 11,910 patients: safety and efficacy for conventional and nonconventional usage. Anesth Analg 1996; 82(1):129–33.

[54] Keller C, Brimacombe J, Bittersohl J, et al. Aspiration and the laryngeal mask airway: three cases and a review of the literature. Br J Anaesth 2004;93(4):579–82.

[55] Hillermann CL, Tarpey J, Phillips DE. Laryngeal nerve identification during thyroid surgery—feasibility of a novel approach. Can J Anaesth 2003;50(2):189–92.

[56] Spahn JG, Bizal J, Ferguson S, et al. Identification of the motor laryngeal nerves—a new electrical stimulation technique. Laryngoscope 1981;91(11):1865–8.

[57] James AG, Crocker S, Woltering E, et al. A simple method for identifying and testing the recurrent laryngeal nerve. Surg Gynecol Obstet 1985;161(2):185–6.

[58] Randolph GW, Kobler JB, Wilkins J. Recurrent laryngeal nerve identification and assessment during thyroid surgery: laryngeal palpation. World J Surg 2004;28(8):755–60.

[59] Nakamura F. Movement of the larynx induced by electrical stimulation of the laryngeal nerves. In: Brewer DW, editor. Research potentials in voice physiology. Albany (NY): State University of New York Press; 1964. p. 129–40.

[60] Flisberg K, Lindholm T. Electrical stimulation of the human recurrent laryngeal nerve during thyroid operation. Acta Otolaryngol Suppl 1969;263:63–7.

[61] Rea JL, Davis WE, Templer JW. Recurrent nerve locating system. Ann Otol Rhinol Laryngol 1979;88(1 Pt 1):92–4.

[62] Davis WE, Rea JL, Templer J. Recurrent laryngeal nerve localization using a microlaryngeal electrode. Otolaryngol Head Neck Surg 1979;87(3):330–3.

[63] Lipton RJ, McCaffrey TV, Litchy WJ. Intraoperative electrophysiologic monitoring of laryngeal muscle during thyroid surgery. Laryngoscope 1988;98(12):1292–6.

[64] Rice DH, Cone-Wesson B. Intraoperative recurrent laryngeal nerve monitoring. Otolaryngol Head Neck Surg 1991;105(3):372–5.

[65] Maloney RW, Murcek BW, Steehler KW, et al. A new method for intraoperative recurrent laryngeal nerve monitoring. Ear Nose Throat J 1994;73(1):30–3.

[66] Eisele DW. Intraoperative electrophysiologic monitoring of the recurrent laryngeal nerve. Laryngoscope 1996;106(4):443–9.

[67] Rea JL. Postcricoid surface laryngeal electrode. Ear Nose Throat J 1992;71(6):267–9.

[68] Payne J, Higenbottam T, Guindi G. Respiratory activity of the vocal cords in normal subjects and patients with airflow obstruction: an electromyographic study. Clin Sci (Lond) 1981;61(2):163–7.

[69] Guindi GM, Higenbottam TW, Payne JK. A new method for laryngeal electromyography. Clin Otolaryngol Allied Sci 1981;6(4):271–8.

[70] Barwell J, Lytle J, Page R, et al. The NIM-2 nerve integrity monitor in thyroid and parathyroid surgery. Br J Surg 1997;84(6):854.

[71] Mermelstein M, Nonweiler R, Rubinstein EH. Intraoperative identification of laryngeal nerves with laryngeal electromyography. Laryngoscope 1996;106(6):752–6.

[72] Lambert AW, Cosgrove C, Barwell J, et al. Vagus nerve stimulation: quality control in thyroid and parathyroid surgery. J Laryngol Otol 2000;114(2):125–7.

[73] Srinivasan V, Premachandra DJ. Use of a disposable electrode for recurrent laryngeal nerve monitoring. J Laryngol Otol 1998;112(6):561–4.

[74] Djohan RS, Rodriguez HE, Connolly MM, et al. Intraoperative monitoring of recurrent laryngeal nerve function. Am Surg 2000;66(6):595–7.

[75] Horn D, Rotzscher VM. Intraoperative electromyogram monitoring of the recurrent laryngeal nerve: experience with an intralaryngeal surface electrode. A method to reduce the risk of recurrent laryngeal nerve injury during thyroid surgery. Langenbecks Arch Surg 1999;384(4):392–5.

[76] Hemmerling TM, Schmidt J, Bosert C, et al. Intraoperative monitoring of the recurrent laryngeal nerve in 151 consecutive patients undergoing thyroid surgery. Anesth Analg 2001;93(2):396–9.

[77] Khan A, Pearlman RC, Bianchi DA, et al. Experience with two types of electromyography monitoring electrodes during thyroid surgery. Am J Otolaryngol 1997;18(2):99–102.

[78] Rea JL, Khan A. Clinical evoked electromyography for recurrent laryngeal nerve preservation: use of an endotracheal tube electrode and a postcricoid surface electrode. Laryngoscope 1998;108(9):1418–20.

[79] Snyder SK, Hendricks JC. Intraoperative neurophysiology testing of the recurrent laryngeal nerve: plaudits and pitfalls. Surgery 2005;138(6):1183–91.

[80] Otto RA, Cochran CS. Sensitivity and specificity of intraoperative recurrent laryngeal nerve stimulation in predicting postoperative nerve paralysis. Ann Otol Rhinol Laryngol 2002;111(11):1005–7.

[81] Beldi G, Kinsbergen T, Schlumpf R. Evaluation of intraoperative recurrent nerve monitoring in thyroid surgery. World J Surg 2004;28(6):589–91.

[82] Hermann M, Hellebart C, Freissmuth M. Neuromonitoring in thyroid surgery: prospective evaluation of intraoperative electrophysiological responses for the prediction of recurrent laryngeal nerve injury. Ann Surg 2004;240(1):9–17.

[83] Tomoda C, Hirokawa Y, Uruno T, et al. Sensitivity and specificity of intraoperative recurrent laryngeal nerve stimulation test for predicting vocal cord palsy after thyroid surgery. World J Surg 2006;30(7):1230–3.

[84] Thomusch O, Sekulla C, Machens A, et al. Validity of intraoperative neuromonitoring signals in thyroid surgery. Langenbecks Arch Surg 2004;389(6):499–503.

[85] Marcus B, Edwards B, Yoo S, et al. Recurrent laryngeal nerve monitoring in thyroid and parathyroid surgery: the University of Michigan experience. Laryngoscope 2003;113(2):356–61.

[86] Chan WF, Lang BH, Lo CY. The role of intraoperative neuromonitoring of recurrent laryngeal nerve during thyroidectomy: a comparative study on 1000 nerves at risk. Surgery 2006;140(6):866–72.

[87] Chan WF, Lo CY. Pitfalls of intraoperative neuromonitoring for predicting postoperative recurrent laryngeal nerve function during thyroidectomy. World J Surg 2006;30(5):806–12.

[88] Echeverri A, Flexon PB. Electrophysiologic nerve stimulation for identifying the recurrent laryngeal nerve in thyroid surgery: review of 70 consecutive thyroid surgeries. Am Surg 1998;64(4):328–33.

[89] Song P, Shemen L. Electrophysiologic laryngeal nerve monitoring in high-risk thyroid surgery. Ear Nose Throat J 2005;84(6):378–81.

[90] Thomusch O, Sekulla C, Walls G, et al. Intraoperative neuromonitoring of surgery for benign goiter. Am J Surg 2002;183(6):673–8.

[91] Zini C, Gandolfi A. Facial nerve and vocal cord monitoring during otoneurosurgical operations. Arch Otolaryngol Head Neck Surg 1987;113(12):1291–3.

[92] Brennan J, Moore EJ, Shuler KJ. Prospective analysis of the efficacy of continuous intraoperative nerve monitoring during thyroidectomy, parathyroidectomy, and parotidectomy. Otolaryngol Head Neck Surg 2001;124(5):537–43.

[93] Timon CI, Rafferty M. Nerve monitoring in thyroid surgery: is it worthwhile? Clin Otolaryngol Allied Sci 1999;24(6):487–90.

[94] Robertson ML, Steward DL, Gluckman JL, et al. Continuous laryngeal nerve integrity monitoring during thyroidectomy: does it reduce risk of injury? Otolaryngol Head Neck Surg 2004;131(5):596–600.

[95] Dralle H, Sekulla C, Haerting J, et al. Risk factors of paralysis and functional outcome after recurrent laryngeal nerve monitoring in thyroid surgery. Surgery 2004;136(6):1310–22.

[96] Yarbrough DE, Thompson GB, Kasperbauer JL, et al. Intraoperative electromyographic monitoring of the recurrent laryngeal nerve in reoperative thyroid and parathyroid surgery. Surgery 2004;136(6):1107–15.

[97] Lydiatt DD. Medical malpractice and the thyroid gland. Head Neck 2003;25(6):429–31.

[98] Kern KA. Medicolegal analysis of errors in diagnosis and treatment of surgical endocrine disease. Surgery 1993;114(6):1167–73.

[99] Simon RI. Standard-of-care testimony: best practices or reasonable care? J Am Acad Psychiatry Law 2005;33(1):8–11.

[100] Sosa JA, Bowman HM, Tielsch JM, et al. The importance of surgeon experience for clinical and economic outcomes from thyroidectomy. Ann Surg 1998;228(3):320–30.

ELSEVIER
SAUNDERS

Surg Oncol Clin N Am
17 (2008) 145–155

SURGICAL
ONCOLOGY CLINICS
OF NORTH AMERICA

Management of Locally Invasive Well-Differentiated Thyroid Cancer

Nebil Ark, MD, Sessunu Zemo, BA, David Nolen, BA, F. Christopher Holsinger, MD, FACS, Randal S. Weber, MD, FACS*

Department of Head and Neck Surgery, The University of Texas M.D. Anderson Cancer Center, 1515 Holcombe Boulevard, Houston, TX 77030–4009, USA

The proximity of the thyroid gland to the aerodigestive tract (larynx, trachea, pharynx, and esophagus), recurrent laryngeal nerve (RLN), strap muscles, and carotid artery makes them all susceptible to thyroid cancer invasion. Direct invasion of these structures occurs in 7% to 16% of patients who have thyroid cancer [1,2]. Because regional metastasis does not have an impact on overall survival, local invasion is a critical determinant for ultimate disease control and overall morbidity and mortality [3]. Approximately 80% of patients who die of differentiated thyroid cancer have local-regional recurrence. Therefore, every surgeon performing thyroid surgery should be prepared to manage locally invasive disease. A precise understanding of the routes of invasion and surgical management is required to provide the best treatment to those with invasive thyroid cancer.

The surgical management of invasive thyroid carcinoma remains controversial. Some studies support conservative shave procedures, whereas others support total tumor resection with clear margins. Adjuvant treatment modalities, such as radioactive iodine therapy (^{131}I) and external beam radiotherapy, are options to improve local control and reduce the morbidity of these tumors.

The authors review the literature and discuss evaluation and surgical treatment of locally invasive well-differentiated thyroid carcinoma (WDTC) and the role of adjuvant therapy.

---

* Corresponding author.
E-mail address: rsweber@mdanderson.org (R.S. Weber).

1055-3207/08/$ - see front matter © 2008 Elsevier Inc. All rights reserved.
doi:10.1016/j.soc.2007.10.009

Evaluation of disease extent

Signs and symptoms

Any patient who has newly diagnosed or recurrent thyroid cancer should be examined for invasive disease. Invasion of the upper aerodigestive tract and RLN may produce several symptoms. The more common are hoarseness and stridor because of invasion of the RLN and intraluminal invasion of the larynx or trachea, respectively [3]. More threatening symptoms are pain, dysphagia, and hemoptysis, with the latter being associated with intraluminal invasion and ulceration of the laryngeal or tracheal mucosa. Dysphagia is attributable to the tumor compression or invasion of the pharynx and esophagus. On rare occasion, patients may also present asymptomatically.

Physical examination

A thorough physical examination should be performed to confirm clinical suspicion of invasion of the aerodigestive tract. A lump in the base of the neck may indicate tumor recurrence in a patient who has a prior history of thyroid cancer and should be characterized. Extrathyroidal extension can be characterized by firmness, tenderness, and fixation to surrounding structures. Fiberoptic transnasal endoscopy should be performed to visualize the larynx and hypopharynx; this may reveal vocal cord paralysis indicating invasion of the larynx or RLN. Submucosal fullness, ulceration, or mass indicates direct tumor extension into the laryngeal or tracheal lumen. Positive findings on flexible endoscopy should be followed by direct laryngoscopy, bronchoscopy, and rigid esophagoscopy at the time of surgery to provide better visualization and guide surgical management.

Diagnostic imaging

Anatomic diagnostic imaging of the neck should be obtained in all patients who have a history or physical examination suggestive of invasion of the aerodigestive tract. Doppler ultrasonography, although useful in detecting and characterizing a primary thyroid tumor or nodal metastases, is not useful in detecting the subtle signs of invasion. Contrast-enhanced CT and MRI are the tests of choice in evaluating thyroid carcinoma invasion of the aerodigestive tract. Both provide evaluation of the laryngotracheal framework and extension of the tumor beyond the perithyroidal fascia against the trachea, which is pathognomonic for invasive thyroid cancer [4].

In selecting between MRI and CT, one is not proved superior over the other, but some surgeons may prefer the use of MRI for a few reasons. The use of iodine-containing contrast, which is necessary for CT, may interfere with the uptake of radioactive iodine early in the postoperative period and is not required for MRI to visualize vascular structures, thereby not restricting its use in certain patients. MRI can produce large-field images in the coronal plane, thus revealing the neck, cervicothoracic junction, and mediastinum in one or two images. The shoulder artifact is also avoided when using MRI in comparison to CT when imaging the area of the thoracic inlet or thyroid gland [5]. Finally, a barium swallow evaluation may also be used to evaluate intraluminal esophageal invasion.

Histology

Histology is one of the most important factors in invasive thyroid cancer. Ballantyne [6] showed that the histologic type of thyroid cancer is a prime determinant for the duration of survival among patients who underwent surgical resections.

Differentiated thyroid carcinomas, such as papillary and follicular types, account for more than 90% of thyroid carcinomas. When invasion is present in these types of cancer, surgical intervention is amenable for local control even in patients who have known metastatic disease. Most patients die not only because of distant metastasis but because of local disease [1,7]. After resection of local disease, metastatic lesions may respond better to adjuvant treatment.

Poorly differentiated thyroid carcinomas (PDTCs), medullary and anaplastic carcinoma, are rare and aggressive tumors. Although rare in incidence, PDTC has a higher rate of invasion because of its aggressive nature. Surgical resection is recommended for patients who have PDTC only if cervical and mediastinal disease can be resected with limited morbidity [8]. Resections of such organs as the larynx, pharynx, and esophagus should be avoided because of high morbidity. Because of the fact that patients who have anaplastic carcinoma frequently present with advanced disease, they are not candidates for a curative surgical resection, but tracheostomy may be considered to secure the airway. In rare instances in which anaplastic carcinoma is discovered, early surgical resection may be feasible.

Patterns of invasion

Thyroid carcinoma can invade adjacent structures by direct extension from the original tumor or from a paratracheal lymph node containing metastatic tumor.

Primary tumor extension and invasion of anterior or lateral tracheal walls are the initial steps in tracheal invasion (Fig. 1). Peritracheal fascia is continuous with the dense fibrous tissue between the tracheal cartilaginous rings. Between the cartilage plates, there are coursed blood vessels tracking perpendicular to the lumen of the trachea. These penetrating blood vessels allow the tumor to penetrate easily into the airway lumen [9].

Laryngeal invasion may occur through the thyroid cartilage or cricothyroid membrane, both of which are inadequate barriers. Another route of

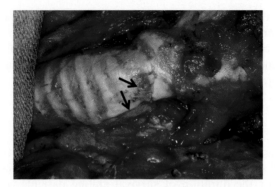

Fig. 1. Airway invasion with thyroid carcinoma (*arrows*) involving the cricotracheal junction.

invasion is direct extension posterior to the thyroid cartilage into the para-glottic space. The latter is also the route for pyriform sinus invasion.

The esophageal mucosa is relatively resistant to thyroid cancer invasion. The tumor is usually confined to the muscular layer of the esophagus, and this facilitates tumor dissection from the mucosa.

The RLN is most susceptible to invasion of thyroid malignancy along the course of the inferior thyroid artery and near its entrance to the larynx at the cricothyroid junction because of its relative fixation at these positions [10].

Surgical management

Total thyroidectomy, regional lymph node dissection, and removal of the disease are the general approaches for invasive thyroid carcinoma. Total thyroidectomy is considered the procedure of choice for most patients who have carcinoma of the thyroid gland. Regional lymph node dissection is also indicated when lymphatic metastases are present or suspected.

Surgical intervention is the preferred method for eradicating invasive thyroid carcinoma, but the extent of resection is still controversial. The main reasons for this debate are two biologic features of differentiated thyroid cancer: slow growth and response of residual microscopic tumor to adjuvant therapy. There are two general approaches. One is resection of the tumor and invaded structures, thus obtaining clear margins, wherein wide margins are not necessary [11–15]. The other approach is shaving or tangential excision of the tumor from the larynx and trachea, followed by adjuvant therapy for the residual disease [6,16,17]. Although the first method seems to be applying sound oncologic principles, function preservation is more successful in the latter.

Management of the aerodigestive tract involvement

Resection of the tumor and invaded parts of the airway with clear margins has many proponents with reasonable supporting data. Park and colleagues [12] found that only 4 of 16 patients remained disease-free among patients in whom cartilage shaving was the primary treatment, followed by adjuvant therapy. Ishihara and colleagues [11] also showed the need for tumor excision without leaving any residual disease in a group of 60 patients, which consisted of complete and incomplete tumor excision groups. In the incomplete group, however, it was not defined whether patients had microscopic or gross residual disease after surgery. Therefore, results of this study cannot be compared with other shave excision/complete resection study results. Bayles and colleagues [18] showed that recurrence occurred in 8 of 8 patients who had WDTC with shave excision, followed by postoperative ^{131}I treatment. The study supports aggressive management at the time of initial surgical resection to be considered, especially when the laryngeal involvement permits partial laryngectomy. Several reports have been published from the series of the Massachusetts General Hospital and Harvard Medical School group [13–15,19]. In their last report, Gaissert and colleagues [15] showed that segmental airway resections for invasive thyroid cancer are safe, preserve speech, and relieve airway obstruction. In the same study, they compared an immediate shave procedure and delayed resection of the airway recurrence group with an early airway resection group and demonstrated better disease-free and overall survival in the latter. Because the comparison was made only with patients who had recurrence in the shave excision group, excluding successfully treated patients of the same group, a fair judgment cannot be made between the two techniques in terms of survival.

Shave or tangential excision seems to be more common and the preferred surgical management for airway invasion without intraluminal extension. Breaux and Guillamondegui [16] define this method as a "reasonable chance of cure." Ballantyne [6] recommends not resecting the trachea or larynx if the tumor is confined to the surface of these structures. Tsang and colleagues [20] reported that microscopic residual disease with adjuvant therapy is not an adverse prognostic factor, whereas macroscopic residual disease is. One of the largest series supporting this technique is from the Mayo Clinic containing 124 patients from 1940 to 2000 with invasive papillary carcinoma with laryngeal or tracheal invasion [17]. These 124 patients were divided into three groups on the basis of the type of surgical resection undertaken: complete tumor excision (frozen section margin control), shave excision (all gross visible disease removed), and incomplete excision (gross residual). Further comparison was made to determine any difference between patients undergoing complete removal versus those undergoing shave excision. No difference was demonstrated; however, when complete and shave groups were compared with the gross residual group, there was a significant decrease of survival in the incomplete resection group ($P < .01$). Based on these results, the McCaffrey [17] recommended conservative procedures designed to preserve function and the sacrifice of airway structures as a means to eradicate all gross tumor. This approach is shown in many other studies to be as effective in locoregional control and survival as complete resection

[21–24]. Although long-term results are good for organ preservation, the proponents of shave procedures refer to a lack of data on quality-of-life issues after adjuvant treatment, such as external beam radiation therapy and radioactive iodine therapy.

Laryngeal and laryngotracheal resections

Extensive invasion of the larynx by differentiated thyroid carcinoma requires operations ranging from partial to total laryngectomy. Conservational laryngeal procedures can be performed in light of the fact that these tumors usually invade one side of the larynx [5,25,26]. Partial vertical hemilaryngectomy and reconstruction with strap muscles or a myocutaneous flap would preserve function in addition to complete excision of the tumor. Reconstruction with a cartilage graft is useful if less than one third of the cricoid circumference is removed [25]. Total laryngectomy is performed in cases of extensive subglottic extension with diffuse cricoid cartilage or cricothyroid membrane destruction.

Tracheal resections

Surgical management differs depending on the extent of tracheal invasion. Shave excision is usually chosen for extraluminal tumor confined to the tracheal cartilage superficially. Cartilage resections are reserved for intraluminal tumors when the tumor is within the lumen of the trachea. When tracheal invasion is identified before surgery, the infiltrated cartilage and paratracheal lymph nodes are resected together with the strap muscles if involved [27]. The extent of the mucosal disease at times exceeds the extent of the extraluminal disease. Therefore, a frozen section is advocated to check for negative airway margins before any reconstruction is performed [28].

If the area of tracheal resection is limited to less than 30% of the circumference of a few tracheal rings, anterior defects can be managed by placing a tracheotomy tube without any reconstruction and later removing the tube in 3 to 5 days. Defects involving more than 30% of the circumference of several tracheal rings may be reconstructed using a rotation flap, such as a sternocleidomastoid myoperiosteal flap [5].

In the case of extensive tracheal cartilage involvement, up to six or seven tracheal cartilage rings can be resected using a primary reanastomosis depending on age and habitus of the patient (Figs. 2 and 3). Circumferential dissection of the trachea is performed only in the area of proposed resection to avoid damage of the blood supply to the remaining trachea. Although additional airway mobilization is rarely required, suprahyoid laryngeal release may be necessary in extensive resections [29].

Esophageal-pharyngeal resections

The outer muscular layer of the esophagus is susceptible to invasion by WDTC. In this case, the tumor may be separated from the submucosa

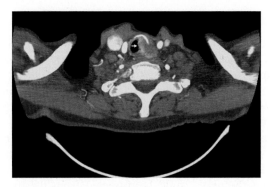

Fig. 2. Axial contrast-enhanced CT shows a large partially exophytic mass (*arrow*) prolapsing into the trachea arising from the paratracheal region.

and mucosal tears are repaired primarily. Resection of this layer is usually sufficient for tumor removal. Even the authors, who advocate more radical resections of the trachea and larynx, prefer this method for extraluminal esophageal invasion [11,15]. Intraluminal involvement requires a full-thickness resection. It is preferable to identify full-thickness invasion of the esophagus before surgery in preparation for an appropriate reconstruction. Small-sized full-thickness defects of the esophagus or pharynx necessitate resection with primary closure. Sometimes, resection of the pyriform sinus by a lateral pharyngotomy that includes a portion of the thyroid lamina can accomplish complete resection without sacrificing voice or swallowing. Extensive tumors of the pharynx with intraluminal invasion might call for total laryngopharyngectomy [25]. Jejunal free flaps may be used for large circumferential defects, whereas myocutaneous or myofascial flaps are appropriate for moderate-sized full-thickness defects. Gastric pull-up reconstruction is also an option for large defects [29].

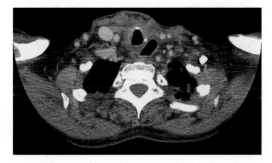

Fig. 3. Axial CT shows status after resection of tumor within the thyroidectomy bed, partial esophagectomy, partial pharyngectomy, tracheal resection, and reconstruction of trachea with primary end-to-end anastomosis.

Management of the recurrent laryngeal nerve involvement

Although vocal cord impairment is an important parameter to predict RLN invasion in locally advanced thyroid cancer, some of the patients with functioning vocal cords may still have RLN invasion. The study by Nishida and colleagues [30] showed 51% RLN involvement among patients who had invasive thyroid carcinoma and had no vocal cord impairment during preoperative evaluations.

The tumor can affect the RLN by direct compression or invasion. In the case of tumor compression without invasion, nerve preservation is recommended regardless of vocal cord function [30,31]. Chiang and colleagues [32] showed that the nerve could be dissected from the thyroid neoplasm in 3 of 16 patients who had paralyzed vocal cords, 2 of whom experienced recovery of nerve function after surgery.

When the RLN is invaded by differentiated thyroid cancer, vocal cord function becomes an important factor in the decision to preserve the nerve. Preservation of RLN invaded with differentiated thyroid cancer does not have an adverse effect on local recurrence and survival rates of patients [30,31]. There is no need for preservation when the vocal cord is paralyzed and the nerve is invaded, however; any return of vocal cord function is unlikely, and the nerve should be resected. With a functioning vocal cord, the involved RLNs should be preserved if not directly invaded or encased. Falk and McCaffrey [31] recommend preserving function of the RLN and removing as much tumor as possible consistent with nerve preservation but not leaving behind gross tumor.

PDTCs are aggressive tumors, and a functioning vocal cord with invasion of the RLN is rarely seen. In general, anaplastic thyroid cancer (ATC) is not a surgically treatable disease; nevertheless, in rare cases, the invaded RLN should be excised without concern for function [31]. In the case of medullary carcinoma, however, RLN preservation with radiation therapy may be an option [31].

Management of the strap muscle involvement

Strap muscles may be invaded by thyroid carcinoma solely or with adjacent structures. Resection of the involved portion of the muscle is sufficient without significant morbidity, although some dysphagia may occur.

Management of the carotid artery involvement

For patients who have carotid artery involvement greater than 270°, surgical resection is not often indicated. Although the common carotid can be ligated and repaired by bypass graft or with a synthetic shunt, patients who have such advanced stage disease are rarely cured. If the laryngopharynx, trachea, or esophagus is also entered during the resection, no concurrent carotid artery resection and vascular reconstructive surgery should be attempted. Thus, an aerodigestive tract repair or anastomosis is a strict contraindication for carotid artery resection.

Adjuvant treatment

Adjuvant therapy for invasive thyroid cancers has an important role in the management of locally invasive WDTC. If there is residual macroscopic disease or a risk for residual microscopic disease after surgery, radioactive iodine with thyroid-stimulating hormone (TSH) suppression is the recommended treatment modality. Mazzaferri [33] reported that postoperative ^{131}I plus thyroid hormone therapy reduces tumor recurrence and mortality adequately to compensate for the increased risks incurred by locally invasive disease. Samaan and colleagues [34] demonstrated that postoperative ^{131}I is the most powerful prognostic indicator for increased disease-free interval and that its use significantly increased survival as well.

In the cases of tumors with limited uptake of ^{131}I or macroscopic residual disease, external beam radiotherapy may be an option. Although Samaan and colleagues [34] could not demonstrate any benefit, Tubiana and colleagues [35] and Brierly and colleagues [36] demonstrated better locoregional control rates with external beam radiotherapy.

Adjuvant chemotherapy is recommended for ATC after surgery by some groups [37,38]. Although the prognosis of most patients who have ATC continues to be poor, case reports of complete resection of ATC combined with postoperative adjuvant chemotherapy and irradiation have resulted in slightly longer survival rates [37].

Summary

Thyroid carcinoma invading the aerodigestive tract accounts for an important portion of the morbidity and mortality associated with differentiated thyroid cancer. Although total excision of the tumor with negative margins is considered to be the best surgical option, leaving residual microscopic tumor followed by adjuvant therapy is an adequate approach for preserving functions with good survival. Because leaving gross residual tumor compromises survival rates, however, radical excision of aerodigestive tract organs may be required to remove disease completely. Radioactive iodine and external beam radiotherapy should be considered to prevent recurrences.

References

[1] McConahey WM, Hay ID, Woolner LB, et al. Papillary thyroid cancer treated at the Mayo Clinic, 1946 through 1970: initial manifestations, pathologic findings, therapy, and outcome. Mayo Clin Proc 1986;61(12):978–96.

[2] Batsakis JG. Laryngeal involvement by thyroid disease. Ann Otol Rhinol Laryngol 1987; 96(6):718–9.

[3] Czaja JM, McCaffrey TV. The surgical management of laryngotracheal invasion by well-differentiated papillary thyroid carcinoma. Arch Otolaryngol Head Neck Surg 1997;123(5): 484–90.

[4] McCaffrey JC. Evaluation and treatment of aerodigestive tract invasion by well-differentiated thyroid carcinoma. Cancer Control 2000;7(3):246–52.

[5] Friedman M. Surgical management of thyroid carcinoma with laryngotracheal invasion. Otolaryngol Clin North Am 1990;23(3):495–507.

[6] Ballantyne AJ. Resections of the upper aerodigestive tract for locally invasive thyroid cancer. Am J Surg 1994;168(6):636–9.

[7] Tollefsen HR, Decosse JJ, Hutter RV. Papillary carcinoma of the thyroid. A clinical and pathological study of 70 fatal cases. Cancer 1964;17:1035–44.

[8] Thyroid Carcinoma Task Force. AACE/AAES medical/surgical guidelines for clinical practice: management of thyroid carcinoma. American Association of Clinical Endocrinologists. American College of Endocrinology. Endocr Pract 2001;7(3):202–20.

[9] Shin DH, Mark EJ, Suen HC, et al. Pathologic staging of papillary carcinoma of the thyroid with airway invasion based on the anatomic manner of extension to the trachea: a clinicopathologic study based on 22 patients who underwent thyroidectomy and airway resection. Hum Pathol 1993;24(8):866–70.

[10] Chan WF, Lo CY, Lam KY, et al. Recurrent laryngeal nerve palsy in well-differentiated thyroid carcinoma: clinicopathologic features and outcome study. World J Surg 2004;28(11):1093–8.

[11] Ishihara T, Kobayashi K, Kikuchi K, et al. Surgical treatment of advanced thyroid carcinoma invading the trachea. J Thorac Cardiovasc Surg 1991;102(5):717–20.

[12] Park CS, Suh KW, Min JS. Cartilage-shaving procedure for the control of tracheal cartilage invasion by thyroid carcinoma. Head Neck 1993;15(4):289–91.

[13] Grillo HC, Zannini P. Resectional management of airway invasion by thyroid carcinoma. Ann Thorac Surg 1986;42(3):287–98.

[14] Hammoud ZT, Mathisen DJ. Surgical management of thyroid carcinoma invading the trachea. Chest Surg Clin N Am 2003;13(2):359–67.

[15] Gaissert HA, Honings J, Grillo HC, et al. Segmental laryngotracheal and tracheal resection for invasive thyroid carcinoma. Ann Thorac Surg 2007;83(6):1952–9.

[16] Breaux GP Jr, Guillamondegui OM. Treatment of locally invasive carcinoma of the thyroid: how radical? Am J Surg 1980;140(4):514–7.

[17] McCaffrey JC. Aerodigestive tract invasion by well-differentiated thyroid carcinoma: diagnosis, management, prognosis, and biology. Laryngoscope 2006;116(1):1–11.

[18] Bayles SW, Kingdom TT, Carlson GW. Management of thyroid carcinoma invading the aerodigestive tract. Laryngoscope 1998;108(9):1402–7.

[19] Grillo HC, Suen HC, Mathisen DJ, et al. Resectional management of thyroid carcinoma invading the airway. Ann Thorac Surg 1992;54(1):3–9 [discussion: 9–10].

[20] Tsang RW, Brierley JD, Simpson WJ, et al. The effects of surgery, radioiodine, and external radiation therapy on the clinical outcome of patients with differentiated thyroid carcinoma. Cancer 1998;82(2):375–88.

[21] Tovi F, Goldstein J. Locally aggressive differentiated thyroid carcinoma. J Surg Oncol 1985; 29(2):99–104.

[22] Segal K, Abraham A, Levy R, et al. Carcinomas of the thyroid gland invading larynx and trachea. Clin Otolaryngol Allied Sci 1984;9(1):21–5.

[23] Melliere DJ, Ben Yahia NE, Becquemin JP, et al. Thyroid carcinoma with tracheal or esophageal involvement: limited or maximal surgery? Surgery 1993;113(2):166–72.

[24] Kowalski LP, Filho JG. Results of the treatment of locally invasive thyroid carcinoma. Head Neck 2002;24(4):340–4.

[25] McCaffrey TV, Lipton RJ. Thyroid carcinoma invading the upper aerodigestive system. Laryngoscope 1990;100(8):824–30.

[26] McCaffrey TV, Bergstralh EJ, Hay ID. Locally invasive papillary thyroid carcinoma: 1940–1990. Head Neck 1994;16(2):165–72.

[27] Zannini P, Melloni G. Surgical management of thyroid cancer invading the trachea. Chest Surg Clin N Am 1996;6(4):777–90.

[28] Ozaki O, Sugino K, Mimura T, et al. Surgery for patients with thyroid carcinoma invading the trachea: circumferential sleeve resection followed by end-to-end anastomosis. Surgery 1995;117(3):268–71.

[29] Gillenwater AM, Goepfert H. Surgical management of laryngotracheal and esophageal involvement by locally advanced thyroid cancer. Semin Surg Oncol 1999;16(1):19–29.

[30] Nishida T, Nakao K, Hamaji M, et al. Preservation of recurrent laryngeal nerve invaded by differentiated thyroid cancer. Ann Surg 1997;226(1):85–91.

[31] Falk SA, McCaffrey TV. Management of the recurrent laryngeal nerve in suspected and proven thyroid cancer. Otolaryngol Head Neck Surg 1995;113(1):42–8.

[32] Chiang FY, Lin JC, Lee KW, et al. Thyroid tumors with preoperative recurrent laryngeal nerve palsy: clinicopathologic features and treatment outcome. Surgery 2006;140(3):413–7.

[33] Mazzaferri EL. Treating high thyroglobulin with radioiodine: a magic bullet or a shot in the dark? J Clin Endocrinol Metab 1995;80(5):1485–7.

[34] Samaan NA, Schultz PN, Hickey RC, et al. The results of various modalities of treatment of well differentiated thyroid carcinomas: a retrospective review of 1599 patients. J Clin Endocrinol Metab 1992;75(3):714–20.

[35] Tubiana M, Schlumberger M, Rougier P, et al. Long-term results and prognostic factors in patients with differentiated thyroid carcinoma. Cancer 1985;55(4):794–804.

[36] Brierley J, Tsang R, Panzarella T, et al. Prognostic factors and the effect of treatment with radioactive iodine and external beam radiation on patients with differentiated thyroid cancer seen at a single institution over 40 years. Clin Endocrinol (Oxf) 2005;63(4):418–27.

[37] Haigh PI, Ituarte PH, Wu HS, et al. Completely resected anaplastic thyroid carcinoma combined with adjuvant chemotherapy and irradiation is associated with prolonged survival. Cancer 2001;91(12):2335–42.

[38] Brignardello E, Gallo M, Baldi I, et al. Anaplastic thyroid carcinoma: clinical outcome of 30 consecutive patients referred to a single institution in the past 5 years. Eur J Endocrinol 2007; 156(4):425–30.

ELSEVIER
SAUNDERS

Surg Oncol Clin N Am
17 (2008) 157–173

SURGICAL
ONCOLOGY CLINICS
OF NORTH AMERICA

Management of the Neck in Differentiated Thyroid Cancer

David M. Cognetti, MD[a,b,*],
Edmund A. Pribitkin, MD[b],
William M. Keane, MD[b]

[a]Department of Otolaryngology–Head and Neck Surgery, University of Pittsburgh Medical Center, Suite 500, Eye and Ear Building, 203 Lothrop Street, Pittsburgh, PA 15213, USA
[b]Department of Otolaryngology-Head and Neck Surgery, Thomas Jefferson University, 925 Chestnut Street, 6th Floor, Philadelphia, PA 19107, USA

The American Cancer Society estimates that there will be 33,550 new cases of thyroid cancer for 2007, representing approximately 2% of all cancers in the United States [1]. Differentiated thyroid carcinoma (DTC) includes papillary thyroid carcinoma (PTC) and follicular thyroid carcinoma (FTC), which are derived from thyroid follicular cells. DTC comprises approximately 90% of all thyroid cancers, and carries an excellent long-term prognosis [2]. In fact, two large database studies involving 15,698 and 53,856 cases of thyroid carcinoma treated in the United States demonstrated a 10-year survival rate for PTC of 98% and 93%, respectively, and a 10-year survival rate for FTC of 92% and 85%, respectively [3,4]. Unlike squamous cell carcinoma of the head and neck, where regional metastases have a definite negative prognostic impact, the effect of cervical nodal involvement on survival in DTC has not been demonstrated clearly. The high survival rate combined with the unclear impact of regional metastases has resulted in inconsistent approaches to the management of the neck in thyroid cancer over the years. Indeed, the relative rarity of the disease, combined with its favorable prognosis, limits the ability to compare different treatment protocols by prospective randomized clinical trials [3]. If long-term survival is the standard metric of all treatment options, then the goal of limiting morbidity and recurrence becomes even more important. Therefore, the management of the neck in DTC must take these factors into account.

* Corresponding author. Department of Otolaryngology–Head and Neck Surgery, Thomas Jefferson University, 925 Chestnut Street, 6th Floor, Philadelphia, PA 19107.
E-mail address: david.cognetti@gmail.com (D.M. Cognetti).

1055-3207/08/$ - see front matter © 2008 Elsevier Inc. All rights reserved.
doi:10.1016/j.soc.2007.10.002   *surgonc.theclinics.com*

In 2006, the American Thyroid Association (ATA) Guidelines Taskforce released updated recommendations for managing DTC, including guidelines for managing neck [5]. This article expands upon those guidelines while discussing the evidence leading to those recommendations and highlighting special considerations and newer techniques proposed for managing the neck in thyroid carcinoma. This review focuses on DTC, which comprises most thyroid cancers.

Pattern of nodal metastasis

Lymph node metastases occur frequently in PTC. A review of 1038 previously untreated patients with DTC who presented to Memorial Sloan-Kettering (New York, New York) over a 55-year period showed the incidence of nodal metastasis in PTC to be 56% [6]. Several more recent studies have confirmed the incidence of nodal metastasis in PTC to be in the range of 60% to 65% [7–10]. Ito and colleagues [11] investigated the rate of nodal metastasis from papillary thyroid microcarcinoma (PTMC), defined as tumor size no more than 10 mm, and still found an incidence close to 50%. Qubain and colleagues [12] investigated the lymph nodes of 80 patients who had DTC that was deemed pathologically N0 by standard hematoxylin and eosin staining. Of the 71 patients who had PTC, 54% had lymph node micrometastases when examined immunohistochemically with cytokeratins (AE1/AE3). Lymph node metastases in FTC occur less frequently. In their 55-year review, Shaha and colleagues [6] reported 21% with cervical metastases at presentation.

Several studies have attempted to define the pattern of lymph node metastases for PTC, as has been demonstrated for squamous cell carcinoma of the head and neck [10,13–16]. Goropoulos and colleagues [10] studied 39 patients in whom a central neck dissection (CND) was performed. Some of these patients also had a lateral neck dissection (LND), and all patients had postoperative I-131 scans. They discovered that metastasis to the central compartment was common (64%), as was metastasis to the ipsilateral cervicolateral compartment (51.2%.) Contralateral cervicolateral metastasis occurred in 33.3% of the patients and never occurred without associated metastases to the central compartment and the ipsilateral side. None of the patients studied had disease in the lateral compartments while lacking metastasis to the central compartment, leading the authors to suggest that the nodal status of the central compartment is a valuable indicator of lymphatic involvement of the lateral compartments.

Gimm and colleagues [13] also demonstrated that the cervicocentral compartment was the most frequent site of metastasis, but differentiated between ipsilateral and contralateral central compartments. Of the 35 patients studied, 24 had metastasis to the ipsilateral cervicocentral compartment, while only five had metastases to the contralateral cervicocentral compartment. All five of these patients had T3 or T4 tumors. Nineteen patients had metastases

to the ipsilateral cervicolateral compartment, while no patients had metastases to the contralateral cervicolateral compartment, and only one patient had
a mediastinal metastasis. Contrary to the suggestion of Goropoulos and
colleagues [10], advocating the central compartment as an indicator of lateral
involvement, Gimm and colleagues [13] discovered ipsilateral cervicolateral
metastases in the absence of central metastases in five patients.

At a Japanese institution where neck dissections are performed routinely
for all sized PTC, a review of 259 cases of PTMC confirmed the preference
of metastases to spread to the central (64%) and ipsilateral nodes (44.5%)
[8]. They did not clarify whether the status of the central compartment
was predictive of the lateral compartment, but they further divided the central compartment to report the incidence of pretracheal (43.2%), ipsilateral
(36.3%), and contralateral (18.9%) positive nodes. Other groups have characterized the pattern of lymph node metastases from PTC to the lateral
nodes further. Kupferman and colleagues [14] reported the distribution of
positive nodes from 44 therapeutic neck dissections, and found levels
2 (52%), 3 (57%), and 4 (41%) to be involved most frequently. The incidence of level 5 nodes (21%) was high enough for the authors to advocate
a comprehensive (levels 2 through 5) neck dissection when lateral metastases
are present. Sivanandan and Soo [16] analyzed specimens from 80 therapeutic neck dissections and had similar results and conclusions.

The rate and number of nodal metastases in PTC have been shown to be
associated with the size of the thyroid tumor [9,15,17]. Ito and colleagues [9]
studied 759 cases of PTC and showed that the frequency of metastasis to the
central compartment was 38.3% for tumors measuring 1 cm or smaller, and
rose significantly to 79.0% for tumors larger than 4 cm. Like Gimm and colleagues [13], they found some patients (11.2%) to be positive for lateral but
negative for central node metastasis, questioning the reliability of the central
compartment as an indicator for lateral involvement.

Effect of nodal metastases on survival

As demonstrated, lymph node metastases in PTC are frequent and have
a predictable pattern. It remains controversial, however, whether the presence of lymph node metastases, either overt or occult, has an impact on
prognosis. It is this fact that has prevented adoption of a universal approach
to management of the neck in thyroid cancer.

Traditionally, it has been suggested that the presence of regional metastases has no effect on survival [18–24]. Hughes and colleagues [19] performed a matched-pair analysis of patients who had differentiated thyroid
cancer and N0 versus N1 neck involvement. There were 100 patients in
each group, and they were matched according to age, tumor size, histology,
and intrathyroidal extent. All lacked distant metastases. There was no significant difference in survival. Shaha and colleagues [18] and McConahey
and colleagues [20] each presented retrospective series of over 800 patients

and also found that the presence of lymph node metastases had no effect on survival. Scheumann and colleagues [17] found that N1 status in PTC did influence survival for patients with T1-T3 status, but not for those with T4 status. A more recent nested case–control study suggests that lymph node metastasis does have an adverse effect on prognosis [25]. Mazzaferri and Jhiang [21] found that cervical metastases carried a higher cancer mortality rate in patients who had FTC, but not in patients who had PTC.

Increasing age, male gender, distant metastases, extrathyroidal spread, and large tumor size all have been shown to be linked more consistently to a worse prognosis [3,4,18,20,21] In fact, when univariate analysis is applied to the presence of regional lymph nodes, some have found it to be a favorable prognostic indicator [19]. Although this appears to be counterintuitive, the finding can be explained by the positive influence of younger age. PTC in younger patients often is associated with nodal metastases. In this instance, age appears to influence survival more than metastatic disease, and therefore biases the results. A study comparing patients of the same age with and without metastatic disease would address this question more properly. Such a study in older patients has demonstrated an adverse impact of nodal disease on survival [26].

Effect of nodal metastases on recurrence

Up to 30% of patients who have DTC develop recurrent metastatic cervical disease with minimal adverse impact on survival [21,23,27]. Patients who have nodal disease at presentation have a higher incidence of recurrent disease in the cervical region. Ito and colleagues [9] evaluated 626 patients with papillary carcinoma whose primary tumor was larger than 1 cm using multivariate analysis. They found that patients who had central node metastasis had an independently significant decreased disease-free survival when compared with those without metastasis. The size and number of the metastatic nodes also were demonstrated to impact recurrence. In McConahey and colleagues' [20] study of 859 patients over a 24-year treatment period, the presence of metastatic nodes at the time of initial examination was associated with a 10-fold increase in the risk of developing a nodal recurrence. Scheumann and colleagues [17] demonstrated that N1 patients had a significant increase in recurrence when compared with N0 patients who had T1-T3 tumors. In Hughes and colleagues' [19] matched-pair analysis, the recurrence rate was higher in N1 patients (17%) than in N0 patients (11%), but did not reach significance. When their analysis was limited to patients over the age of 45, however, the recurrence in N1 patients was 31% and was significantly greater than in the N0 patients (8%).

The effect of metastases, whether occult or overt, on prognosis and recurrence has important implications for the management of the neck. This is discussed further in the context of indications for neck dissection.

Preoperative

Fine needle aspiration

Fine needle aspiration (FNA) is considered the procedure of choice for evaluating thyroid nodules according to the ATA Guidelines Taskforce [5]. The procedure is minimally invasive, accurate, and cost-effective. FNA also plays an important role in the workup of a neck mass. Cervical adenopathy can be the presenting finding in patients who have DTC, especially young people who have PTC [28]. FNA is advocated in the preoperative workup of a neck mass to aid in appropriate diagnosis and preoperative planning. It potentially differentiates metastatic PTC from metastatic squamous cell carcinoma, thus allowing an appropriately directed search and treatment of the respective primary tumor and neck disease. In younger patients, lymphoma often is suspected, and an excisional biopsy of the cervical node may be performed. Cervical metastases are common in younger patients who have PTC, however, and FNA could allow for differentiation from lymphoma before excisional biopsy, thus preventing a potentially inappropriate procedure. Finally, measurement of thyroglobulin in a 1 mL saline wash-out of the needle used for the biopsy has been shown to be an easy, inexpensive, and reliable method of increasing the diagnostic yield of FNA [29,30]. This is especially true of cystic lymph nodes, which frequently result in nondiagnostic cytology [31].

Ultrasound, MRI, CT

Preoperative staging of the neck aids in surgical decision-making for DTC. Physical examination alone can underestimate the involvement of regional lymph nodes, which is quite frequent in PTC. Ultrasonography is noninvasive, well-tolerated, and improves the identification of cervical adenopathy. Kouvaraki and colleagues [27], at the University of Texas MD Anderson Cancer Center, retrospectively reviewed 212 patients with thyroid carcinoma who underwent preoperative ultrasonography. They reported that ultrasonography detected lymph node or soft tissue metastases in neck compartments believed to be uninvolved by physical examination in 39% of the patients. Thus, ultrasonography altered the surgical procedure in these patients, potentially minimizing recurrence in the neck.

Although the specificity of ultrasonography for cervical lymph node metastases is very high, its sensitivity has been shown to be as low as 36.7% for lateral compartments and as low as 10.9% for the central compartments [32–34]. Interestingly, Ito and colleagues [32] examined the usefulness of preoperative ultrasonographic examination of the neck in patients with PTMC and determined that only the lateral compartment nodes that were identified on ultrasound preoperatively had clinical relevance, mitigating the concern for low sensitivity of the technique. They reviewed 590 patients, 67 of whom had evidence of metastases on preoperative ultrasound. These 67 underwent a modified radical neck dissection (MRND) as part of their management. Of the 523 patients without preoperatively detectable metastasis, 249 underwent MRND, and 274 did not. Despite the fact that more than 40% of the patients who underwent MRND had pathologic evidence of metastasis, the MRND and observations groups did not statistically differ in lymph node recurrence rates (less than 1.5% for both) when followed for a mean of over 4 years.

It should be noted that the sonographic criteria for identifying lymph nodes suspicious for metastases is not limited to lymph node size. Architectural features of the lymph node itself that indicate malignancy have been described [27,35]. Benign lymph nodes are typically oval and flattened with a smooth cortex and a central fatty hilum. Features that can indicate malignancy include a rounded bulging shape, replaced fatty hilum, eccentric cortical widening, irregular margins, decreased or heterogeneous echogenicity, alteration in intranodal vascularity, cystic areas, and calcifications. These findings can be present even in small nodes and are not appreciated on simple palpation.

One limitation of ultrasonography is that it is operator-dependant. It is less expensive than CT and MRI, however. Additionally, the 2006 ATA guidelines recommend ultrasound of the thyroid for the workup of all patients who have one or more suspicious thyroid nodules [5]. Preoperative neck ultrasound to evaluate the contralateral thyroid lobe and cervical lymph nodes also is recommended for all patients undergoing thyroidectomy for malignant cytologic findings on biopsy. An experienced sonographer, with appropriate communication from the referring specialist, potentially can extend a diagnostic thyroid ultrasound to include surveillance of the lateral compartments when suspicion for malignancy is heightened by patient history, sonographic features of the thyroid nodule, or preliminary cytologic findings of the thyroid nodule if ultrasound guided FNA is being performed. This would minimize the time required and number of interventions needed during the preoperative workup. Although the ATA guidelines suggest that CT and MRI may be useful in some clinical settings (large, rapidly growing, and invasive tumors), they do not recommend the routine preoperative use of these studies (Box 1) [5]. If CT is used, it is important to remember that iodinated contrast dye can interfere with radioactive iodine uptake; thus it should be avoided when performing a neck CT with suspicion of thyroid cancer.

^{18}F-Fluorodeoxyglucose-positron emission tomography

Positron emission tomography (PET) has gained popularity in the diagnostic workup and post-treatment surveillance of squamous cell carcinoma of the head and neck. Its role in thyroid carcinoma has not been delineated, and the ATA guidelines do not recommend its use preoperatively. Early studies suggest, however, that PET or PET/CT scanning may be useful in patients

---

Box 1. 2006 American Thyroid Association guidelines

Preoperative neck ultrasound for the contralateral lobe and cervical (central and bilateral) lymph nodes is recommended for all patients undergoing thyroidectomy for malignant cytologic findings on biopsy. Routine preoperative use of other imaging studies (CT, MRI, PET) is not recommended.

From Cooper DS, Doherty GM, Haugen BR, et al. Management guidelines for patients with thyroid nodules and differentiated thyroid cancer. Thyroid 2006;16:109–41; with permission from Mary Ann Liebert, Inc.

---

who have an indeterminate FNA of thyroid nodules [36,37]. In this setting, the test has a high negative predictive value, and has been proposed to be a way to reduce the number of hemithyroidectomies for what ultimately is proven to be a benign nodule. Another potential role for PET/CT in thyroid carcinoma is when recurrence is suspected (either clinically or because of elevated thyroglobulin), and radioiodine whole-body scintigraphy (WBS) is negative [38–40]. This situation is difficult from both a diagnostic and therapeutic standpoint. Because the tumor is not radioiodine-avid, it cannot be treated by radioiodine ablation. It also cannot be localized accurately by whole body scintigraphy to allow for surgical excision. In this scenario, the use of PET/CT has been shown to have a high positive predictive value, leading to a change in management in greater than 40% of patients in three different studies [38–40].

As PET imaging gains greater use in other diseases, the prevalence of PET incidentalomas of the thyroid will increase. In a review of 4136 patients who underwent PET imaging for known nonthyroid malignancies, 45 demonstrated focal uptake within the thyroid gland [41]. In 50% of the 32 patients for whom a cytologic diagnosis was available, the tumor was malignant. Given this high prevalence of malignancy, all PET incidentalomas of the thyroid must be evaluated for thyroid carcinoma.

Operative

Central compartment

Metastases from PTC occur frequently in the central compartment. The central compartment generally is defined as the space bounded by the common carotid arteries laterally, the hyoid bone superiorly, and the innominate vessels inferiorly. The recommendation for or against the routine dissection of the central compartment is based upon the risk of lymph node recurrence versus the morbidity of the procedure.

Some authors have suggested that because of the high frequency of central compartment metastases, that elective dissection of the central compartment should be performed in all patients who have PTC [12,13,42]. Others have attempted to actually prove that careful dissection of the central compartment at the time of thyroidectomy can influence patient survival positively [43]. Ito and colleagues [9] reviewed 759 patients and demonstrated that the frequency of central node metastasis increased in relation to tumor size. They also showed that central node metastasis was an independent prognostic factor of disease-free survival in patients who had PTC larger than 1 cm. An argument against the routine performance of a CND in papillary thyroid carcinoma is that it has been shown to be associated with increased morbidity. Both Henry and colleagues [44] and Cheah and colleagues [45] showed that CND was associated with a statistically significant increased risk of both transient and permanent hypocalcemia. Roh and colleagues [7] were able to demonstrate that serum parathyroid hormone levels significantly decreased immediately after neck dissection in patients who had PTC and remained low for several weeks when transient. In this study, the risk of hypocalcemia was increased further when LND was performed in addition to CND. None of these studies showed a statistically increased rate of recurrent laryngeal nerve injury with CND. Another argument for routine CND is that reoperation for recurrence is associated with significantly higher morbidity than an initial operation, and anything that can be done to minimize the risk of recurrence and reoperation should be employed [42].

A 2007 evidence-based review of the literature performed by White and colleagues [46] at the University of Michigan attempted to settle the debate on routine central compartment lymph node dissection. Their goal was to answer these three important questions:

- Does central node dissection decrease recurrence or disease-specific mortality in PTC?
- Does central node dissection increase the risk of hypothyroidism and recurrent laryngeal nerve injury?
- Does reoperation in the central neck compartment for recurrent PTC increase the risk of hypoparathyroidism and recurrent laryngeal nerve injury?

No prospective randomized data exist to answers these questions. After review of 13 studies, which include one prospective study and multiple retrospective cohort studies and case series, White and colleagues [46] concluded that based on the currently available evidence that CND may decrease recurrence and likely improves disease-specific survival. They also found that although CND may be associated with an increased risk of hypoparathyroidism and unintentional nerve injury at initial operation, the increased risk of these complications associated with reoperation for recurrence in the central neck compartment supports the more aggressive initial operation. They concluded that evidence-based recommendations support CND for PTC in the hands of experienced surgeons.

The 2006 ATA guidelines [5] are in accordance with the University of Michigan literature review. They recommend that routine central compartment neck dissection should be considered for patients who have PTC and suspected Hurthle cell carcinoma (Box 2). Because of the low rate of metastases in FTC, they suggest that near-total or total thyroidectomy without CND may be appropriate for that diagnosis. Finally, they offer thyroidectomy without CND and followed by radioactive iodine (RAI) therapy as alternative approach for papillary and Hurthle cell cancers.

Lateral compartments

In PTC, lymph node metastases are also common in the lateral neck, specifically the ipsilateral side. Because these metastases are frequently occult, discussion of the management of the lateral neck must be framed in the context of clinically negative and clinically positive.

The approach to the clinically negative neck traditionally has differed in Japan as compared with the United States. Studies from Japan indicate that patients were more likely to undergo a lateral neck dissection as part of the elective management for DTC [8,22,32,47]. A contributing factor to this is that postoperative RAI therapy rarely is employed in Japan. Because of this, Japanese centers have provided insight into the effect of an elective neck dissection for DTC in the absence of RAI, specifically for PTMC (tumor size less than 1 cm). Wada and colleagues [8] compared 235 patients who underwent prophylactic neck dissection for PTMC with 155 patients who underwent thyroidectomy for presumably benign disease and were discovered to have PTMC postoperatively. These 155 patients, therefore, did not undergo a neck dissection as part of their management and served as controls. Both groups were similar in regards to age, gender, and length of follow-up (greater than 53 months mean for both). They discovered that the recurrence rate did not differ between the prophylactic group and

---

Box 2. 2006 American Thyroid Association guidelines

Routine central compartment (level 6) neck dissection should be considered for patients who have papillary thyroid carcinoma and suspected Hurthle carcinoma. Near-total or total thyroidectomy without central node dissection may be appropriate for follicular cancer, and when followed by radioactive iodine therapy, may provide an alternative approach for papillary and Hurthle cell cancers.

From Cooper DS, Doherty GM, Haugen BR, et al. Management guidelines for patients with thyroid nodules and differentiated thyroid cancer. Thyroid 2006;16:109–41; with permission from Mary Ann Liebert, Inc.

the observation group (0.43% versus 0.65%) and that it was low for both groups. They concluded that prophylactic neck dissection is not beneficial in patients who have PTMC. Ito and colleagues [32] investigated 523 patients with PTMC who did not have detectable lateral node metastasis on ultrasonography. Of these patients, 249 underwent prophylactic LND, and 274 did not. After a mean follow-up of over 4 years, there was no statistical difference in regards to lymph node recurrence-free survival. They also concluded that LND is not necessary in patients who have PTMC without lymph node metastases detected on ultrasonography preoperatively.

Indeed, PTMC has a benign course. It frequently is found incidentally at autopsy, and its discovery is a situation where completion thyroidectomy may be unnecessary according to the ATA guidelines [5,48]. The prevalence of ultrasound-guided FNA biopsy has led to an increase in its diagnosis, thus forcing further consideration of its clinical significance. In another study, Ito and colleagues [33] offered a trial of observation for patients with PTMC. Of 732 patients, 162 opted for observation. During follow up, more than 70% of the primary tumors either did not change or decreased in size, and lateral compartment metastasis appeared in only 1.2% of patients. This is despite the fact that metastases were confirmed histologically in 50% of the patients in the surgically treated group. This again questions the clinical significance of occult nodal metastasis in PTMC. One limitation of the study is that the mean follow-up time was only approximately 4 years, which perhaps does not allow enough time for subclinical metastasis to become overt.

When PTC is larger than 1 cm, the risk of nodal metastases is higher [9]. Although there is arguably no effect on survival with nodal metastasis, there is the concern of an increased risk of recurrence. Some authors use the presence of the central compartment lymph nodes as an indication of a comprehensive approach to the lateral neck [10,15]. The recommendations are made with the goal of reducing recurrence, but these studies have not yet completed the follow-up to prove that an aggressive approach with ipsilateral modified radical neck dissection (MRND) actually results in lower recurrences. No prospective, randomized trials exist to identify the best management of the lateral neck in thyroid cancer because of the limitations discussed earlier [49]. And, unfortunately, the largest retrospective studies examining prognostic factors in DTC do not provide adequate detail to draw conclusions about the management of the neck [3,4,6,20,24].

The NCDB report of 53,856 cases of thyroid cancer treated in the United States between 1985 and 1995 was able to observe that most patients who had DTC did not undergo lymph node dissection and that lymph node sampling was more popular than formal, comprehensive lymph node dissection [3]. For PTC, for example, 14.6% of all patients underwent a limited lymph node dissection as part of their treatment, whereas 7.2% of patients had a radical or modified radical neck dissection. Another observation was that 38.3% of patients who had PTC within this population received radiotherapy (usually RAI) after surgery. The reported 10-year overall relative survival for PTC in this study was 93%. Without a means of identifying the indications for the previously mentioned treatments and analysis of who received which combinations of surgery and radioactive iodine, however, there is no way to make meaningful conclusions on how the treatments affected outcomes. The Surveillance, Epidemiology and End Results (SEER) program is another large database (15,698 patients) that is similarly limited by lack of treatment-based analysis and controls [4].

When lateral lymph node metastases are clinically apparent, the need for surgical excision is more obvious. In the past, lateral lymph nodes simply have been excised by means of node-picking procedures, but these procedures seldom are advocated today. The current recommendation of the ATA guidelines [5] is for functional compartmental en bloc dissection for clinically positive nodes. Although this approach seems to be more oncologically sound, there are limited data to prove that it truly improves outcomes. In fact, in a group of 859 patients treated for PTC at the Mayo Clinic (Rochester, Minn.) between 1946 and 1970, when node picking was the more popular approach for cervical nodes and postoperative iodine was used only in 3% of patients, the nodal recurrence rate was only 6% [20]. The overall mortality observed at 30 years was only 3% above that expected, with 6.5% of the patients dying from PTC. Unfortunately, this study failed to compare the effect of node picking (245/400) versus MRND (125/400) in regards to recurrence or mortality in their patients with cervical node excisions.

On the other hand, although only 6.5% of patients dying from the disease may look good compared with other types of cancer, a more aggressive approach that does not increase morbidity significantly would be warranted to further minimize mortality in this typically curable disease. In two studies looking at small groups of patients who had DTC, Kupferman and colleagues [14,50] indicated that the pattern of lymph node metastases in patients with clinically positive necks warranted a comprehensive neck dissection with inclusion of levels 2 through 5 and that this procedure can be performed with acceptable morbidity.

In 2004, Wang and colleagues [51] reported a series of patients with DTC who were managed using the previously suggested approach: LND only for clinically palpable nodes, and MRND with preservation of the submandibular triangle when these nodes were excised. Of the 508 patients, 44 required a neck dissection for clinically palpable lateral nodes. Only 3% of the 464 patients who did not undergo initial neck dissection recurred in the lateral cervical nodes. They discovered that recurrence was more likely when the initial tumor is larger than 4 cm. Of the 16 patients who recurred in the lateral neck, five were younger than 45 years and were alive and free of disease. Of the 11 who recurred and were over 45 years, however, five had died of their thyroid cancer. This led the authors to conclude that aggressive attempts to detect and treat occult lateral cervical nodes was for the most part unnecessary, but could be considered in older patients with large primary tumors. Leboulleux and colleagues [23] examined 148 patients with lymph node metastases (140 patients) or extrathyroidal extension (8 patients) who underwent total thyroidectomy with central and ipsilateral en bloc neck dissection of levels 3 and 4 followed by RAI. The neck dissection was extended to include levels 2 and 5 if frozen sections of the levels 3 and 4 showed metastatic involvement. Of these high-risk patients, 22% had persistent disease on the postablation WBS. This allowed the authors to identify significant risk factors for persistent disease, which include greater than 10 lymph node metastases, lymph nodes with extracapsular extension, and tumor size greater than 4 cm. Still, the 10-year disease specific survival was 99%, and the recurrence rate for the patients with a normal postablation WBS was 7% with an 8-year mean follow up.

The ATA guidelines agree with the findings and recommendations of these two studies [5]. They suggest that a compartmental lymph node dissection should be performed for patients who have biopsy-proven metastatic cervical lymphadenopathy, especially when they are likely to fail radioactive iodine (Box 3).

Dissection of the lateral compartment can be accomplished through a single transverse incision by extending the thyroidectomy incision laterally to the anterior border of the trapezius. A second transverse incision (MacFee incision) may be added superiorly, when necessary, to facilitate exposure of the upper neck nodes. Alternatively, a modified apron incision that incorporates the thyroidectomy incision can be used.

Sentinel node biopsy

Sentinel lymph node (SLN) biopsy is a technique that has gained wide acceptance in the management of breast cancer and melanoma. Recently, it has been offered as an option in the management of DTC. Fukui and colleagues [52] performed SLN biopsy in 22 patients by injecting methylene blue around the primary tumor site at the time of surgery. They proceeded

---

Box 3. 2006 American Thyroid Association guidelines

Lateral neck compartmental lymph node dissection should be performed for patients who have biopsy-proven metastatic cervical lymphadenopathy detected clinically or by imaging, especially when they are likely to fail radioactive iodine treatment based on lymph node size, number, or other factors, such as aggressive histology of the primary tumor.

From Cooper DS, Doherty GM, Haugen BR, et al. Management guidelines for patients with thyroid nodules and differentiated thyroid cancer. Thyroid 2006;16:109–41; with permission from Mary Ann Liebert, Inc.

to perform MRND in all of the patients. They reported a 90.5% concordance rate between the SLN findings and the regional lymph node status. Dzodic [53] offered the SLN biopsy as means to determine which patients who had clinically negative necks could benefit from MRND. He performed the procedure in 40 patients with DTC and had a 92.5% SLN identification rate. Although the procedure can be done, it is unclear if it would be beneficial in DTC. Breast cancer and melanoma differ from DTC in that lymph node metastasis has a definite and important impact on prognosis for these tumor types. Additionally, regional lymphadenectomy for these cancers is associated with significant morbidity. Currently, neck dissection is recommended only for clinically or ultrasound apparent nodal metastases in patients who have DTC [5]. Because the impact of occult lymph node metastasis on survival in DTC has been shown to be low and possibly insignificant, it is unclear whether SLN biopsy would alter outcomes. The influence of occult lymph node metastasis on recurrence is likely higher, however, and if occult cervical metastases could account for the small percentage of patients who die of DTC, then their identification would be beneficial. The ATA guidelines [5] suggest that future research must be aimed at developing techniques to identify small cervical metastases in DTC for these reasons. SLN biopsy has potential to fulfill that goal. A large study demonstrating not only its feasibility and accuracy, but more importantly its benefit, must be performed before SLN is adopted in the workup of DTC.

Minimally invasive/endoscopic neck dissection

SLN biopsy was developed as a method to minimize morbidity by preventing unnecessary en bloc lymph node dissections. Minimally invasive and endoscopic techniques are proposed as methods to minimize morbidity when lymph node dissections are necessary. Additionally, a minimally invasive approach to thyroidectomy is gaining in popularity, which likely will lead to increased patient awareness and demand for the technique within this patient population. Terris and colleagues [54] demonstrated the feasibility of an endoscopic selective neck dissection using a porcine model. Lombardi and colleagues [55] recently described a minimally invasive technique using video assistance for performing a lateral neck dissection, which they employed in two patients who had PTC. Additionally, the combination of SLN biopsy with an endoscopic approach has been offered as an initial low-morbidity staging procedure [56]. This would allow for an easy conversion to an endoscopic neck dissection if the sentinel node proves to be positive. As with SLN biopsy, however, the role of this technique in DTC is limited because of the apparent lack of significance of occult lymph node metastasis. Therefore, minimally invasive techniques must be proven to be safe and effective for N+ necks, or prophylactic dissection of the lateral neck in DTC must be proven to be beneficial before endoscopic-assisted neck dissection can be considered useful in the management of DTC.

Indeed, if occult metastases are proven to affect prognosis, then SLN biopsy and minimally invasive techniques could play an important role in the future management of the neck in DTC.

Summary

DTC is a relatively rare malignancy carrying a favorable prognosis. Despite a high long-term survival rate, recurrences are common, and death from DTC does occur, even if in less than 10% of patients. An appropriately aggressive treatment of DTC must limit the risk of recurrence and death while minimizing treatment morbidity and recognizing the indolent course that DTC follows in most patients. This is especially true of the management of the neck, where lymph node metastases occur frequently and are associated with an unclear effect on prognosis. The 2006 updated treatment guidelines by the ATA are based on the currently available data, and make an effort to reach that treatment balance. An aggressive compartment-oriented neck dissection is recommended for patients who have evidence of cervical lymph node metastasis on physical examination or ultrasonography, but elective dissection of the negative lateral neck is not.

The ATA guidelines are based largely on retrospective reviews, because the infrequency of the disease, combined with its high survival rate, limits the practicality of a large randomized prospective trial. Although a randomized prospective trial would provide the best evidence for management protocols, the ATA guidelines are a valuable interpretation of the current evidence, which at times is conflicting. A uniform approach to the management of DTC should limit the chance of undertreatment and should improve the ability to analyze outcomes in the future. Both would aid in further lowering the risk of recurrence and death from thyroid cancer.

References

[1] American Cancer Society. Cancer facts and figures 2007. Atlanta (GA): American Cancer Society; 2007.

[2] Shaha AR. Implications of prognostic factors and risk groups in the management of differentiated thyroid cancer. Laryngoscope 2004;114:393–402.

[3] Hundahl SA, Fleming ID, Fremgen AM, et al. A national cancer data base report on 53,856 cases of thyroid carcinoma treated in the U.S., 1985–1995. Cancer 1998;83:2638–48.

[4] Gilliland FD, Hunt WC, Morris DM, et al. Prognostic factors for thyroid carcinoma: a population-based study of 15,698 cases from the Surveillance, Epidemiology, and End Results (SEER) program 1973–1991. Cancer 1997;79:564–73.

[5] Cooper DS, Doherty GM, Haugen BR, et al. Management guidelines for patients with thyroid nodules and differentiated thyroid cancer. Thyroid 2006;16:109–41.

[6] Shaha AR, Shah JP, Loree TR. Patterns of nodal and distant metastasis based on histologic varieties in differentiated carcinoma of the thyroid. Am J Surg 1996;172:692–4.

[7] Roh JL, Park JY, Park CI. Total thyroidectomy plus neck dissection in differentiated papillary thyroid carcinoma patients: pattern of nodal metastasis, morbidity, recurrence, and postoperative levels of serum parathyroid hormone. Ann Surg 2007;245:604–10.

[8] Wada N, Duh QY, Sugino K, et al. Lymph node metastasis from 259 papillary thyroid microcarcinomas: frequency, pattern of occurrence and recurrence, and optimal strategy for neck dissection. Ann Surg 2003;237:399–407.

[9] Ito Y, Jikuzono T, Higashiyama T, et al. Clinical significance of lymph node metastasis of thyroid papillary carcinoma located in one lobe. World J Surg 2006;30:1821–8.

[10] Goropoulos A, Karamoshos K, Christodoulou A, et al. Value of the cervical compartments in the surgical treatment of papillary thyroid carcinoma. World J Surg 2004;28:1275–81.

[11] Ito Y, Tomoda C, Uruno T, et al. Clinical significance of metastasis to the central compartment from papillary microcarcinoma of the thyroid. World J Surg 2006;30:91–9.

[12] Qubain SW, Nakano S, Baba M, et al. Distribution of lymph node micrometastasis in pN0 well-differentiated thyroid carcinoma. Surgery 2002;131:249–56.

[13] Gimm O, Rath FW, Dralle H. Pattern of lymph node metastases in papillary thyroid carcinoma. Br J Surg 1998;85:252–4.

[14] Kupferman ME, Patterson M, Mandel SJ, et al. Patterns of lateral neck metastasis in papillary thyroid carcinoma. Arch Otolaryngol Head Neck Surg 2004;130:857–60.

[15] Machens A, Hinze R, Thomusch O, et al. Pattern of nodal metastasis for primary and reoperative thyroid cancer. World J Surg 2002;26:22–8.

[16] Sivanandan R, Soo KC. Pattern of cervical lymph node metastases from papillary carcinoma of the thyroid. Br J Surg 2001;88:1241–4.

[17] Scheumann GFW, Gimm O, Wegener G, et al. Prognostic significance and surgical management of locoregional lymph node metastases in papillary thyroid cancer. World J Surg 1994; 18:559–68 [discussion: 567–8].

[18] Shaha AR, Shah JP, Loree TR. Risk group stratification and prognostic factors in papillary carcinoma of thyroid. Ann Surg Oncol 1996;3:534–8.

[19] Hughes CJ, Shaha AR, Shah JP, et al. Impact of lymph node metastasis in differentiated carcinoma of the thyroid: a matched-pair analysis. Head Neck 1996;18:127–32.

[20] McConahey WM, Hay ID, Woolner LB, et al. Papillary thyroid cancer treated at the mayo clinic, 1946 through 1970: initial manifestations, pathologic findings, therapy, and outcome. Mayo Clin Proc 1986;61:978–96.

[21] Mazzaferri EL, Jhiang SM. Long-term impact of initial surgical and medical therapy on papillary and follicular thyroid cancer. Am J Med 1994;97:418–28.

[22] Moley JF, Wells SA. Compartment-mediated dissection for papillary thyroid cancer. Langenbecks Arch Surg 1999;384:9–15.

[23] Leboulleux S, Rubino C, Baudin E, et al. Prognostic factors for persistent or recurrent disease of papillary thyroid carcinoma with neck lymph node metastases and/or tumor extension beyond the thyroid capsule at initial diagnosis. J Clin Endocrinol Metab 2005;90:5723–9.

[24] Shaha AR, Shah JP, Loree TR. Low-risk differentiated thyroid cancer: the need for selective treatment. Ann Surg Oncol 1997;4:328–33.

[25] Lundgren CI, Hall P, Dickman PW, et al. Clinically significant prognostic factors for differentiated thyroid carcinoma: a population-based, nested case–control study. Cancer 2006; 106:524–31.

[26] Sellers M, Beenken S, Blankenship A, et al. Prognostic significance of cervical lymph node metastases in differentiated thyroid cancer. Am J Surg 1992;164:578–81.

[27] Kouvaraki MA, Shapiro SE, Fornage BD, et al. Role of preoperative ultrasonography in the surgical management of patients with thyroid cancer. Surgery 2003;134:946–55.

[28] Sanders LE, Rossi RL. Occult well-differentiated thyroid carcinoma presenting as cervical node disease. World J Surg 1995;19:642–6.

[29] Frasoldati A, Toschi E, Zini M, et al. Role of thyroglobulin measurement in fine-needle aspiration biopsies of cervical lymph nodes in patients with differentiated thyroid cancer. Thyroid 1999;9:105–11.

[30] Cunha N, Rodrigues F, Curado F, et al. Thyroglobulin detection in fine-needle aspirates of cervical lymph nodes: a technique for the diagnosis of metastatic differentiated thyroid cancer. Eur J Endocrinol 2007;157:101–7.

[31] Cignarelli M, Ambrosi A, Marino A, et al. Diagnostic utility of thyroglobulin detection in fine-needle aspiration of cervical cystic metastatic lymph nodes from papillary thyroid cancer with negative cytology. Thyroid 2003;13:1163–7.

[32] Ito Y, Tomoda C, Uruno T, et al. Preoperative ultrasonographic examination for lymph node metastasis: usefulness when designing lymph node dissection for papillary microcarcinoma of the thyroid. World J Surg 2004;28:498–501.

[33] Ito Y, Uruno T, Nakano K, et al. An observation trial without surgical treatment in patients with papillary microcarcinoma of the thyroid. Thyroid 2003;13:381–7.

[34] Shimamoto K, Satake H, Sawaki A, et al. Preoperative staging of thyroid papillary carcinoma with ultrasonography. Eur J Radiol 1998;29:4–10.

[35] Hoang JK, Lee WK, Lee M, et al. US features of thyroid malignancy: pearls and pitfalls. Radiographics 2007;27:847–60.

[36] de Geus-Oei LF, Pieters GFFM, Bonenkamp JJ, et al. 18F-FDG PET reduces unnecessary hemithyroidectomies for thyroid nodules with inconclusive cytologic results. J Nucl Med 2006;47:770–5.

[37] Mitchell JC, Grant F, Evenson AR, et al. Preoperative evaluation of thyroid nodules with 18FDG-PET/CT. Surgery 2005;138:1166–75.

[38] Palmedo H, Bucerius J, Joe A, et al. Integrated PET/CT in differentiated thyroid cancer: diagnostic accuracy and impact on patient management. J Nucl Med 2006;47:616–24.

[39] Nahas Z, Goldenberg D, Fakhry C, et al. The role of positron emission tomography/computed tomography in the management of recurrent papillary thyroid carcinoma. Laryngoscope 2005;115:237–43.

[40] Shammas A, Degirmenci B, Mountz JM, et al. 18F-FDG PET/CT in patients with suspected recurrent or metastatic well-differentiated thyroid cancer. J Nucl Med 2007;48:221–6.

[41] Kim TY, Kim WB, Ryu JS, et al. 18F-fluorodeoxyglucose uptake in thyroid from positron emission tomogram (PET) for evaluation in cancer patients: high prevalence of malignancy in thyroid PET incidentaloma. Laryngoscope 2005;115:1074–8.

[42] Shindo M, Wu JC, Park EE, et al. The importance of central compartment elective lymph node excision in the staging and treatment of papillary thyroid cancer. Arch Otolaryngol Head Neck Surg 2006;132:650–4.

[43] Tisell LE, Nilsson B, Molne J, et al. Improved survival of patients with papillary thyroid cancer after surgical microdissection. World J Surg 1996;20:854–9.

[44] Henry JF, Gramatica L, Denizot A, et al. Morbidity of prophylactic lymph node dissection in the central neck area in patients with papillary thyroid carcinoma. Langenbecks Arch Surg 1998;383:167–9.

[45] Cheah WK, Arici C, Ituarte PHG, et al. Complications of neck dissection for thyroid cancer. World J Surg 2002;26:1013–6.

[46] White ML, Gauger PG, Doherty GM. Central lymph node dissection in differentiated thyroid cancer. World J Surg 2007;31:895–904.

[47] Noguchi M, Kumaki T, Taniya T, et al. Impact of neck dissection on survival in well-differentiated thyroid cancer: a multivariate analysis of 218 cases. Int Surg 1990;75:220–4.

[48] Yamamoto Y, Maeda T, Izumi K, et al. Occult papillary carcinoma of the thyroid. A study of 408 autopsy cases. Cancer 1990;65:1173–9.

[49] Shaha AR. TNM classification of thyroid carcinoma. World J Surg 2007;31:879–87.

[50] Kupferman ME, Patterson DM, Mandel SJ, et al. Safety of modified radical neck dissection for differentiated thyroid carcinoma. Laryngoscope 2004;114:403–6.

[51] Wang TS, Dubner S, Sznyter LA, et al. Incidence of metastatic well-differentiated thyroid cancer in cervical lymph nodes. Arch Otolaryngol Head Neck Surg 2004;130:110–3.

[52] Fukui Y, Yamakawa T, Taniki T, et al. Sentinel lymph node biopsy in patients with papillary thyroid carcinoma. Cancer 2001;92:2868–74.

[53] Dzodic R. Sentinel lymph node biopsy may be used to support the decision to perform modified radical neck dissection in differentiated thyroid carcinoma. World J Surg 2006;30:841–6.

[54] Terris DJ, Monfared A, Thomas A, et al. Endoscopic selective neck dissection in a porcine model. Arch Otolaryngol Head Neck Surg 2003;129:613–7.

[55] Lombardi CP, Raffaelli M, Princi P, et al. Minimally invasive video-assisted functional lateral neck dissection for metastatic papillary thyroid carcinoma. Am J Surg 2007;193:114–8.

[56] Malloy KM, Cognetti DM, Wildemore BM, et al. Feasibility of endoscopic sentinel node biopsy in the porcine neck. Otolaryngol Head Neck Surg 2007;136:806–10.

SURGICAL
ONCOLOGY CLINICS
OF NORTH AMERICA

Surg Oncol Clin N Am
17 (2008) 175–196

Vocal Fold Paresis and Paralysis: What the Thyroid Surgeon Should Know

Adam D. Rubin, MD[a,b,*],
Robert T. Sataloff, MD, DMA[c]

[a]*Lakeshore Professional Voice Center, Lakeshore Ear, Nose, and Throat Center,
21000 East 12 Mile Road, Suite 111, St. Clair Shores, MI 48081, USA*
[b]*Department of Otolaryngology, University of Michigan, University of Michigan Medical
Center, 1904 Taubman Center, 1500 E. Medical Center Drive, Ann Arbor, MI 48109, USA*
[c]*Department of Otolaryngology–Head and Neck Surgery, Drexel University College
of Medicine, 1721 Pine Street, Philadelphia, PA 19103, USA*

Superior laryngeal nerve

The superior laryngeal nerve (SLN) and recurrent laryngeal nerve (RLN) are at risk during thyroid surgery. Injury to one or more of these nerves may disturb voice, airway, and swallowing function. The thyroid surgeon must be familiar with laryngeal neuroanatomy and various manifestations of vocal fold paresis or paralysis. Recognition of preoperative vocal fold dysfunction is important in treatment planning, whereas early recognition of postoperative vocal fold hypomobility may prevent further complications. Patients must be made aware of the risk to these nerves before surgery. The informed consent discussion is extremely important, especially if the patient depends on the voice professionally. If thyroid surgery is to be performed by a general surgeon, collaboration with an otolaryngologist is extremely important for voice assessment and management. This article reviews pertinent anatomy, differential diagnosis, prevention, and treatment of vocal fold paresis and paralysis.

Anatomy

Central innervation of vocal fold motion involves the pyramidal and extrapyramidal systems. Cortical innervation is bilateral, which is why

---

* Corresponding author. Lakeshore Professional Voice Center, Lakeshore Ear, Nose, and Throat Center, 21000 East 12 Mile Road, Suite 111, St. Clair Shores, MI 48081.

E-mail address: rubinad@sbcglobal.net (A.D. Rubin).

a unilateral cortical stroke does not usually result in vocal fold paralysis. Upper motor neurons relay cortical input to the cell bodies of the laryngeal nerves in the brain stem. The cerebellum and basal ganglia are involved in the coordination and fine-tuning of laryngeal function. More primitive visceromotor pathways are also involved. Complex involuntary protective and swallowing reflexes are coordinated within the brain stem [1].

Recurrent laryngeal nerve

The incidence of RLN injury during thyroid surgery has been reported to range from 0.3% to 13.2% [2–5]. Deliberate identification of the RLN minimizes the risk for injury during thyroid surgery. Intraoperative hemostasis and a thorough understanding of the anatomy are essential for nerve identification and preservation.

The nuclei of the RLN axons lie within the nucleus ambiguus in the medulla of the brain stem. The RLN axons travel with the vagus nerve down the neck until they branch off at the level of the aortic arch on the left and the subclavian artery on the right. On the left, the nerve passes inferior and posterior to the aortic arch and reverses its course to continue superiorly into the visceral compartment of the neck. The right RLN loops behind the right subclavian artery and ascends superomedially toward the tracheo-esophageal groove. Both RLNs travel just lateral to or within the tracheo-esophageal groove and enter the larynx posterior to the cricothyroid (CT) joint. The positions of the nerves in the neck make them susceptible to iatrogenic injury during surgery. Low in the neck, the course of the right recurrent nerve is more oblique, lateral, and probably more prone to injury than that of the left RLN [6].

The inferior thyroid artery has been described as an important landmark for identifying the RLN. The nerve is always in close proximity to the artery, but there is much variation in its exact relation. Therefore, the inferior thyroid artery is not a dependable landmark for identifying the nerve. The inferior cornu of the thyroid cartilage has also been described as a reliable landmark for identification of the nerve. The nerve may be identified 0.5 cm below the inferior cornu [7–9].

Perhaps the most efficient way to identify the nerve is to locate it within the carotid triangle. The carotid artery and trachea make up the lateral and medial sides of the triangle, respectively. The tissue within this triangle is spread gently, parallel to the direction of the nerve, and one layer at a time, until the nerve is identified. Care must be taken not to disrupt the surrounding vascular network of the nerve.

The thyroid is attached to the trachea by thick connective tissue called Berry's ligament at the level of the second or third tracheal ring [6]. This is the most common site of injury to the nerve. The nerve may run deep to the ligament, pass through it, or even penetrate the gland a short distance at this level [3]. Great care must be taken in this area during surgery.

Retraction of the thyroid lobe may result in traction injury and make the nerve more susceptible to transection. The path of the nerve must be clearly identified.

Approximately 5 in 1000 people have a non-RLN on the right. A non-RLN occurs only on the right, except in the rare case of situs inversus. It branches from the vagus nerve at the level of the cricoid cartilage and enters the larynx directly, without looping around the subclavian artery. This anomaly occurs in conjunction with a retroesophageal right subclavian artery [6]. The surgeon must be aware of this variant, particularly when he or she is having difficulty in identifying the nerve in its usual location.

The RLN innervates four of the intrinsic muscles of the larynx: the thyroarytenoid (TA), posterior cricoarytenoid (PCA), lateral cricoarytenoid (LCA), and interarytenoid (IA) muscles. Muscle innervation is unilateral, except for the IA muscle, which receives contributions from both RLNs [10]. The TA and LCA muscles are vocal fold adductors. Unilateral denervation of these muscles results in an inability to close the glottis, with resulting breathy voice and possible aspiration.

The PCA is the main vocal fold abductor. Paralysis of this muscle results in an inability to abduct during inspiration. Denervation of the PCA usually causes the arytenoid cartilage to subluxate anteromedially in unilateral vocal fold paralysis. The denervated PCA no longer counters the anterior pull on the arytenoid cartilage by the vocal ligament [10]. If both PCA muscles are denervated, as in the case of bilateral RLN paralysis, airway obstruction may occur.

The IA muscle is actually made up of three muscles, including the transverse arytenoideus muscle and two oblique arytenoideus muscles. The function of the IA muscle is not completely understood; however, it may assist in vocal fold adduction [10] and provide medial compression to close the posterior glottis.

Superior laryngeal nerve

The SLN branches from the vagus nerve just inferior to the nodose ganglion, which contains the sensory cell bodies of the SLN. The nerve travels inferiorly along the side of the pharynx, medial to the carotid artery, and splits into two branches about the level of the hyoid bone. The internal division of the SLN penetrates the thyrohyoid membrane with the superior laryngeal artery and supplies sensory innervation to the larynx. It should not be at risk during most thyroid surgical procedures.

The external division of the SLN provides motor innervation to the CT muscle and is at risk during thyroid surgery. Incidence of injury to this nerve has been reported to range from 0% to 25% [11,12]. The CT muscle changes vocal fold tension by elongating the fold. It is responsible for increasing the fundamental frequency (pitch) of the voice. Clinical presentation of SLN injury is more subtle and likely underreported. Jansson and colleagues

[13] performed pre- and postoperative electromyography (EMG) on 20 patients undergoing thyroid surgery. Nine patients had postoperative SLN paresis as demonstrated by EMG. Additionally, 3 patients who had goiters had preoperative SLN paresis that worsened after surgery. Fifty-eight percent of the SLN pareses were present at 1 year of follow-up, although most cases had had some nerve recovery.

The external division of the SLN lies close to the superior thyroid artery, although its exact relation to the artery is variable. A critical area of 1.5 to 2.0 cm from the thyroid capsule has been described through which the external branch of the SLN is most intimately involved with the branches of the superior thyroid artery [11,12]. It is often difficult to identify the SLN. One can usually avoid injury by ligating the terminal branches of the superior thyroid artery as close to the thyroid capsule as possible. Care also must be taken not to cauterize the CT muscle itself, because this can cause fibrosis and similar manifestations of an SLN injury.

Presentation

A unilateral immobile vocal fold typically presents as a breathy voice. Diplophonia (two pitches during phonation) and aspiration may occur. Bilateral vocal fold immobility typically presents with airway obstruction. Vocal fold immobility after thyroid surgery is usually the result of injury to the RLN, although the possibility of arytenoid cartilage dislocation should be considered [14].

A unilateral vocal fold paralysis may not be immediately apparent after surgery, because vocal fold edema secondary to intubation may actually assist in glottic closure. In addition, hoarseness during the first several days after intubation is not unusual and may not raise suspicion. The degree of voice impairment later on depends on the relative position of the immobile vocal fold and the ability of the contralateral vocal fold to compensate by crossing the midline of the glottis.

Bilateral vocal fold paralysis may present acutely with an airway emergency. This may require urgent reintubation or tracheostomy. Bilateral vocal fold paralysis may also present weeks to months later with exertional dyspnea or airway obstruction during an upper respiratory infection. Voice quality is often fairly good in the setting of bilateral vocal fold paralysis, given the paramedian position of both vocal folds.

The prognosis for regaining nerve function and vocal fold mobility depends on the mechanism and degree of injury. The nerve may be injured by transection, crush, traction, inadvertent ligature placement, and thermal injury. The Sunderland classification system describes different degrees of nerve injury. First-degree injury means neurapraxia. Nerve function should recover completely. Second-degree injury means that Wallerian degeneration has occurred distal to an injured site (axonotmesis). Second-degree injury usually occurs after a crush injury and also results in complete recovery. Because the endoneural sheaths remain intact in a second-degree injury, synkinesis does not occur. Third-degree injury includes endoneural scarring, which can cause misdirected regeneration. Fourth-degree injury involves scarring, which may block regenerating axons. Fifth-degree injury signifies complete transection of the nerve [15,16].

Although vocal fold paralysis implies complete denervation, with lack of muscle fiber recruitment during voluntary attempts at motion, this is not often the case except immediately after nerve transection. In fact, even after nerve transection, reinnervation of the affected laryngeal musculature usually occurs. The source of the reinnervation is not known but may include regenerating fibers from the transected RLN, the SLN, cervical autonomic nerves, and nerve branches innervating pharyngeal constrictors. If reinnervation occurs, it typically is not identifiable for approximately 4 months [17].

Unfortunately, although reinnervation prevents muscle atrophy, it usually does not restore useful movement to the vocal fold because of synkinesis. Synkinesis results from nonselective innervation of adductor and abductor muscles. As a result, muscles that perform opposite functions contract simultaneously, resulting in immobility or hypomobility of the vocal fold. The clinical picture depends on the proportion of adductor and abductor fibers reinnervated [18].

Crumley [19] describes a classification system for laryngeal synkinesis. In type I synkinesis, or favorable synkinesis, there is little or no vocal fold movement. The patient's airway and voice are fairly normal. Types II, III, and IV are considered unfavorable synkinesis. A spastic vocal fold that may twitch without control characterizes type II. Voice quality is poor. In type III synkinesis, there is tonic adduction of the vocal fold. This results in a reasonable voice, but the airway may be compromised. Finally, type IV synkinesis involves tonic abduction of the vocal fold, resulting in a breathy voice and greater risk for aspiration. Type III synkinesis probably results from greater reinnervation of the LCA fibers in comparison to the PCA fibers, whereas in type IV, the opposite likely occurs [19].

Vocal fold paresis (incomplete paralysis) results in a hypomobile vocal fold. This may result from injury to the SLN or a less severe injury to the RLN. Classically, paralysis of the SLN results in loss of a patient's upper pitch register [20,21]. Normally, the CT muscle contracts briskly in falsetto or modal phonation to increase tension in the vocal fold [22]. The inability to increase vocal tension results in poor vocal performance, especially at higher pitches [20,21]. The clinical manifestations specific to SLN paralysis are likely to be more troublesome for singers and professional speakers [23].

More subtle paresis of the SLN or RLN may cause numerous voice complaints, including vocal fatigue, hoarseness, impairment of volume, loss of upper range, loss of projection, and breathiness. Vocal fatigue may be caused by the additional effort required to raise vocal pitch and projection, and by hyperfunctional compensatory gestures. Patients who have RLN or SLN paresis often develop muscle tension dysphonia to generate a "stronger" voice [24].

Such tension may lead to the development of additional vocal pathologic conditions, such as vocal nodules, polyps, cysts, and scar.

Other symptoms may occur with injury to the vagus or the laryngeal nerve branches. Dysphagia often occurs with vocal fold paralysis and paresis. Although isolated RLN injury seldom causes significant aspiration risk, inefficient glottic closure can affect swallowing function. Also, recent evidence suggests that the external division of the SLN may supply innervation to the cricopharyngeus. Denervation may result in cricopharyngeal dysfunction and subsequent dysphagia [25]. Neuralgia or paresthesia of the laryngeal nerves may also manifest as or contribute to chronic cough, globus, or laryngeal pain syndromes [26,27].

Evaluation

The thyroid surgeon should inquire about voice and swallowing difficulties before and after surgery. Any suspicion of vocal fold paresis or paralysis should prompt referral to an otolaryngologist, preferably a voice specialist (laryngologist). Routine preoperative laryngoscopy on any patient contemplating thyroid surgery is prudent. It is essential if the patient has already had thyroid surgery (eg, if a patient is returning for completion thyroidectomy after a hemithyroidectomy). Preoperative recognition of a hypomobile vocal fold may raise suspicion of a malignant thyroid lesion [28] or traction injury from a thyroid goiter or benign lesion [29]. Laryngeal nerve injury in the setting of a goiter should alert the surgeon that the nerve is likely being displaced from its normal path. Moreover, if a total thyroidectomy is required in a patient who has preoperative unilateral vocal fold paralysis, the patient needs to be informed of the increased risk for postoperative bilateral vocal fold paralysis or airway obstruction and the possible need for tracheostomy and further surgery.

Preoperative documentation of hypomobility may also spare the surgeon potential medical-legal issues after surgery. Furthermore, the laryngologist can address other issues that might be affecting voice and swallowing, such as muscle tension dysphonia, reflux, and nodules. Early treatment of such problems can optimize the patient's chance of good vocal and swallowing function after surgery.

Early recognition of postoperative voice changes is critical as well. A common mistake is for a surgeon to ignore such changes because the surgeon knows that he or she did not transect the nerve. Neuropraxia may occur even with excellent surgical technique. Time to recovery of normal vocal fold motion is unpredictable. Patients may develop hyperfunctional compensatory vocal behavior that can be detrimental and difficult to eliminate even after nerve recovery. This problem can be avoided by early treatment. In addition, without treatment, patients may be forced to live and function with a suboptimal voice, which can affect their livelihoods and quality of life.

Inquiries about other potential causes of vocal fold paresis should be made, particularly when the history is not completely suggestive of postoperative vocal fold paralysis. Other potential iatrogenic causes include intubation itself; cervical spine, carotid artery, or thoracic surgery; radiation; and even I-131 therapy [30–32]. Other potential causes to consider include nonthyroid malignancies, such as the classic "Pancoast" lung tumor, idiopathic vocal fold paralysis [33], neurologic disease [34–44], infection [24,45–48], endocrinologic disease [49,50], and collagen-vascular disease [41–54]. Finally, one must consider other possible causes of vocal fold immobility and hypomobility, such as cricoarytenoid joint fixation [55], posterior glottic stenosis [56,57], and arytenoid cartilage dislocation [14].

Physical examination should include a subjective evaluation of the patient's voice (with a note documenting vocal quality), a complete head and neck evaluation, and laryngeal visualization. Endoscopic visualization of the larynx is a critical part of the assessment of any patient who has a voice complaint. A dynamic voice assessment is best performed with a flexible rhinolaryngoscope to allow the patient to be in as physiologic a position as possible. Rigid videostroboscopy is essential as well to look for vibratory abnormalities, to assess vocal fold tone, and to assess discrepancies in vocal process height. Protrusion of the tongue during rigid videostroboscopy creates a nonphysiologic position for vocalization; therefore, transoral evaluation is less useful in detecting subtle movement abnormalities of the larynx [23,58].

The patient should be asked to perform a variety of vocal tasks to observe the gross movement of the vocal folds [23,58–61]. One should inspect for asymmetry in motion, hyperfunction, tremor, spasms, dysdiadokinesia, and other irregular motions. Vocal fold paresis may be subtle. Rapid repetitive phonatory tasks are useful for eliciting subtle vocal fold lag, which can be a sign of vocal fold paresis. Repeated maneuvers alternating a sniff with the sound /i/ are particularly helpful in unmasking mild PCA paresis. Repeated rapid phonation on /i/ with a complete stop between each phonation during the task /i/-/hi/-/i/-/hi/-/i/-/hi/... frequently causes increased vocal fold lag, because the pathologic side fatigues more rapidly than the normal side. Having the patient repeat /pa/-/ta/-/ka/-/pa/-/ta/ka/-pa/ta/ka is analogous to rapid alternating maneuvers performed in a general neurologic examination. It is useful for identifying dysdiadokinesia. Vocal fold lag is sometimes easier to see during whistling. Moreover, whistling may help to distinguish lag resulting from a true paresis from asymmetry created from muscle tension. Laryngeal posture during this maneuver provides particularly good visibility of rapid vocal fold motions [23,58].

A glissando maneuver, asking the patient to slide slowly from his or her lowest to highest note and then to slide back down, is invaluable for assessing SLN function. If an SLN is injured, longitudinal tension does not increase as effectively on the abnormal side, disparities in vocal fold length are apparent at higher pitches, and the vocal folds may actually scissor slightly with the normal fold being higher. This height discrepancy is easier to observe with rigid videostroboscopy. The classic finding of rotation of the posterior larynx to the side of SLN injury is likely to occur only with complete and isolated unilateral SLN paralysis [23,58–61].

The patient should also be asked to use his or her voice as he would in the work environment. Singers should be asked to demonstrate their vocal range, whereas professional speakers or teachers should give a sample of their day-to-day vocal demands. This gives more insight to the patient's capability of performing in the workplace and reveals how much he or she is compensating to meet vocal demands.

Laryngeal electromyography

Laryngeal electromyography (LEMG) evaluates the integrity of the nerves and muscles of the larynx (Fig. 1). Although its usefulness remains unproven by evidence-based data, it remains the most objective means of evaluating neuromuscular function of the larynx and is an accepted component of laryngeal evaluation [62]. Its usefulness in the evaluation of postoperative vocal fold immobility is several fold. In the first place, it can distinguish paralysis from arytenoid fixation. Arytenoid dislocation, although rare, requires early intervention for the best chance to restore mobility [14]. Moreover, LEMG can provide prognostic information as to nerve recovery, which can guide timing of surgical management [63].

LEMG can confirm or refute clinical suspicions on examination. Asymmetric vocal fold motion seen on flexible examination may suggest the presence of a mild vocal fold paresis. Even if a paresis is present, however, the examiner may predict the nerve or side involved incorrectly. A recent study by Rubin and colleagues [59] demonstrated that 25% of the time when a unilateral mild paresis was suspected in patients who had mobile vocal folds on endoscopic examination, laryngeal EMG disagreed with the side of paresis predicted. In addition, in some cases in which the laryngeal examination was thought to be normal, LEMG demonstrated bilateral paresis. The failure to predict paresis on examination in these cases was likely because movement was fairly symmetric, because both sides were affected. Heman-Ackah and Barr [60,61] found that LEMG agreed with the nerve predicted to be involved in only 64% of cases. In both of these studies, however, LEMG confirmed the presence of neuropathy in more than 85% of suspected cases.

LEMG can be helpful for management of patients who have movement abnormalities on examination. Voice therapy routines can be created to focus on strengthening muscles specifically affected by the paresis. For example, for isolated SLN injury, exercises like glissando can be performed to strengthen the CT muscles, taking care to avoid compensatory hyperfunction in other muscles. Moreover, the information obtained can give clinical insight for surgical planning. For example, a patient who seems to have

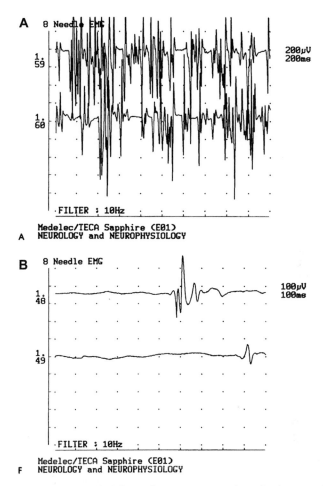

Fig. 1. (*A*) Normal LEMG with full recruitment pattern and maximal contractions. (*From* Sataloff RT, Mandel S, Heman-Ackah YD, et al. Laryngeal electromyography. 2nd edition. San Diego (CA): Plural Publishing; 2006. p. 81; with permission.) (*B*) LEMG with maximal contraction approximately 1 year after RLN injury. There is essentially 100% reduced recruitment, and a single polyphasic motor unit potential can be seen. (*From* Sataloff RT, Mandel S, Heman-Ackah YD, et al. Laryngeal electromyography. 2nd edition. San Diego (CA): Plural Publishing; 2006. p. 84; with permission.)

a unilateral paresis on examination may benefit from bilateral thyroplasty if a bilateral paresis is noted on LEMG.

Some surgeons use electrophysiologic monitoring of the RLN during thyroid surgery [2]. An endotracheal tube has been designed with EMG electrodes that are exposed at the glottis to contact the vocal folds. EMG monitoring may be particularly beneficial during revision thyroid surgery, in previously radiated necks, or in large masses when the nerve is at increased risk. Standard techniques to visualize the nerve combined with expert electrophysiologic monitoring optimize the surgeon's chances of preventing laryngeal nerve injury.

Treatment

Treatment for unilateral vocal fold paralysis is designed to eliminate aspiration, improve voice, and avoid the development of other complications (eg, muscle tension dysphonia). When there is no aspiration, treatment depends on the patient's need and desire for improved voice quality. It is well recognized that recovery of laryngeal nerve function is common if the injury was not caused by transection of the nerve. Consequently, it is best to delay permanent surgical intervention for approximately 1 year, if possible, unless the nerve is known to have been divided or resected. This does not mean that therapy should be delayed, however, only irreversible surgery. The collaboration of an excellent voice pathologist is invaluable.

Voice therapy

Objective voice analysis, assessment, and therapy by speech-language pathologists specializing in voice are helpful in the treatment of postoperative vocal fold paresis and paralysis. Voice therapy often obviates the need for surgical intervention. Heuer and colleagues [64] studied 19 female patients and 22 male patients who had unilateral recurrent nerve paralysis and found that after excellent voice therapy, 68% of the female patients and 64% of the male patients considered their voices satisfactory and elected not to have surgery. Final outcome satisfaction data were similar for surgical and nonsurgical patients. Even when surgery is eventually required, preoperative voice therapy helps the patient while surgical decisions are pending, provides training for optimal postoperative phonation, and prepares the patient psychologically for surgery with the knowledge that everything possible has been done to avoid unnecessary operative intervention. This results in superior patient cooperation, motivation, and understanding through educated participation in the voice restoration process. The importance of this factor should not be overlooked in terms of the art of medicine and medical-legal prudence.

In people with unilateral vocal fold paralysis, initial assessment not only quantitates and documents vocal dysfunction but explores a wide range of potentially useful compensatory strategies. In addition, the speech-language pathologist identifies spontaneous compensatory behaviors that may be counterproductive. For example, although speech pathology textbooks generally classify and treat vocal fold paralysis as a "hypofunctional" disorder [65,66], undesirable compensatory hyperfunctional behavior is common in these patients. This is responsible for most of the voice strain, neck discomfort, and fatigue that may accompany unilateral vocal fold paralysis. Such gestures often can be eliminated even during the first assessment and trial therapy session, increasing vocal ease and endurance. Moreover, if the assessment reveals improved voice with a different pitch, training in safe pitch modification in combination with other techniques may also provide rapid improvement. Indeed, under good guidance, therapy sometimes produces astonishingly rapid improvements in voice quality despite persistence of the neurologic deficit. Therapy is directed toward avoidance of hyperfunctional compensation and progressive development of optimal breathing, abdominal support, and intrinsic laryngeal muscle strength and agility. Training includes head and neck muscle relaxation exercises, aerobic conditioning, abdominal and thoracic muscle strength and control exercises, attention to respiration, and various voice exercises that build limb strength through multiple repetitions with light weights. Forced adduction exercises, often recommended in speech pathology texts, such as pushing or pulling on chairs, must be avoided or monitored closely and used with extreme caution. Although such exercises are still in fairly common use, other techniques may be more effective and have less potential for harm [23].

Like surgery, therapy is least successful in combined paralysis. In most patients who have unilateral vocal fold paralysis, therapy results in improvement. In many cases, the improvement is sufficient for the patient's needs. When the patient has complied with voice therapy, improvements have reached a plateau, and he or she believes that his or her voice quality is not satisfactory, surgery may be indicated.

If preoperative voice therapy has been optimal and if surgery has been successful, the postoperative voice therapy course should be short. Nevertheless, the patient is working with a "new voice." At least a few sessions with a speech-language pathologist generally helps the patient to apply effective principles learned in preoperative therapy. It is particularly important for the voice therapist and speech-language pathologist to monitor the patient, avoiding development of abusive habits and stressing the importance of vocal hygiene measures [23].

Surgical therapy

The two main surgical options for patients who have unilateral vocal fold paralysis are medialization and reinnervation [67–87]. Medialization procedures include injection laryngoplasty (Fig. 2) and laryngeal framework surgery. Several materials have been injected to medialize the vocal fold and improve glottic competence. These include Teflon [68,69], Gelfoam [70,71], fat [72,73], collagen [74,75], hydroxylapatite [76,77], and hyaluronic acid [78,79].

Teflon used to be the most popular choice; however, it has few (if any) indications today. Teflon is permanent and leads to a chronic granulomatous inflammatory response. Teflon can also migrate and may even spread to other

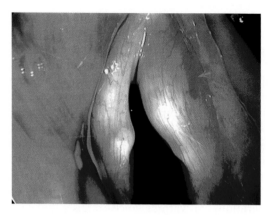

Fig. 2. Intraoperative photograph after right autologous fat injection, illustrating 30% to 40% overcorrection. The white arrow illustrates the injection site. In general, the injection should be performed at this location or more posteriorly. Injection further anteriorly increases the risk for anterior overcorrection and producing a "strained" voice. (*From* Sataloff RT, Hawkshaw MJ, Eller RL. Atlas of laryngoscopy. 2nd edition. San Diego (CA): Plural Publishing; 2006. p. 203; with permission.)

parts of the body. Teflon granulomas are difficult to remove and often result in a poor vocal outcome [80,81]. Other injectables are used as temporary measures, typically when future return of vocal fold function is possible but the patient needs or wants immediate symptomatic improvement.

Laryngeal framework surgery

Type I thyroplasty was popularized by Isshiki and colleagues [82]. Arytenoid adduction surgery was designed by Isshiki and colleagues [83] as well to improve closure of the posterior glottis. During thyroplasty, a window is drilled from the thyroid cartilage lamina. A prosthesis is designed to push the paralyzed vocal fold toward the midline to improve glottic closure (Figs. 3 and 4) [82,84]. Arytenoid adduction surgery and its variations permanently rotate the arytenoid cartilage to improve posterior glottic closure and the height of the vocal process [83,85].

Some laryngologists believe that after a long duration of vocal fold paralysis, the cricoarytenoid joint scars and becomes fixed. In this case, the ankylosis often must be addressed for a medialization procedure to be effective. Several animal and cadaver studies suggest that the cricoarytenoid joint remains normal for as long as 17 years after RLN injury [86,87].

Reinnervation

Several reinnervation procedures for the paralyzed vocal fold have been described using the ansa cervicalis [88], phrenic nerve [89,90], preganglionic

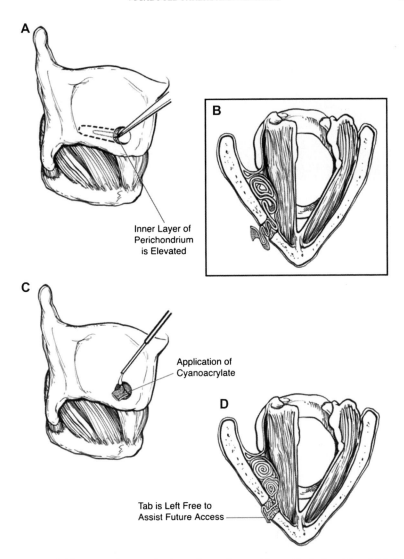

Fig. 3. (*A*) Minithyrotomy is created using a 5-mm diamond burr. Limited perichondrial eleva-tion is performed. (*B*) Gore-Tex (W.L. Gore and Associates Incorporated, Newark, Delaware) is layered into the space between the cartilage and perichondrium. The patient is asked to pho-nate, and Gore-Tex is adjusted until phonatory output is optimal. (*C*) Cyanoacrylate is used to seal the thyrotomy. (*D*) Small amount of Gore-Tex is left externally. (*From* Sataloff RT. Pro-fessional voice: the science and art of clinical care. 3rd edition. San Diego (CA): Plural Publish-ing; 2005. p. 1190; with permission.)

sympathetic neurons [91], hypoglossal nerve [92], and nerve-muscle pedicles [93,94]. The main purpose of reinnervation procedures is to prevent dener-vation atrophy of laryngeal muscles. Crumley [88] reports improved vocal quality and restoration of the mucosal wave after reinnervation using the

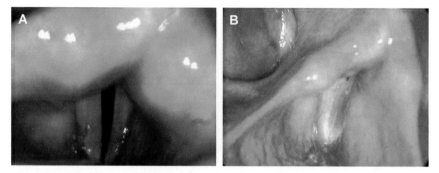

Fig. 4. Vocal fold adduction with left vocal fold paresis. Note the glottic gap. Vocal fold adduction after left Gore-Tex thyroplasty. The patient has excellent glottic closure and voice, although she still has some left false vocal fold hyperfunction.

ansa cervicalis. The ansa cervicalis provides weak tonic innervation to the intrinsic laryngeal muscles. Reinnervation of the TA muscle restores tension, resulting in a more normal mucosal wave. Reinnervation of the PCA and LCA muscles stabilizes the arytenoids and prevents inferior displacement of the vocal process, which may occur in some patients. Crumley [88] reports additionally that the ansa cervicalis–RLN anastomosis is particularly useful in cases of synkinesis after nerve injury resulting in jerky movements of the vocal folds. Although there is still synkinesis after ansa cervicalis–RLN anastomosis, the weak tonic innervation supplied by the ansa produces a vocal fold that is less spastic.

Attempts to design reinnervation techniques that might avoid synkinesis and restore movement to the paralyzed vocal fold have been reported [95–97]. Hogikyan and colleagues [97] examined muscle-nerve-muscle neurotization in the cat. In this technique, the paralyzed TA muscle is reinnervated by means of axons that sprout from the contralateral innervated TA muscle through an interposed nerve graft. These investigators demonstrated histologic and EMG evidence of this specific reinnervation pathway in more than half of the cats used. Actual return of vocal fold adduction was demonstrated in one cat. This technique of motion-specific reinnervation is promising for restoration of physiologic movement after vocal fold paralysis.

Tucker [98] has reported improvement in voice quality and restoration of adduction of the unilateral paralyzed vocal fold after nerve-muscle pedicle transfer. This technique involves implanting a piece of strap muscle innervated by nerve terminals from the ansa cervicalis into one of the denervated laryngeal muscles, usually the LCA or TA. Tucker [98] also reports better vocal quality in patients who have unilateral vocal fold paralysis (UVFP) when they are treated with nerve-muscle pedicle and medialization than when they are treated with medialization alone.

Bilateral vocal fold paralysis

Although voice quality is typically good in the presence of bilateral vocal fold paralysis (BVFP), airway patency is jeopardized commonly by the paramedian position of the vocal folds. Tracheotomy may be required acutely, followed by surgery, to improve the size of the glottic airway. Surgical techniques are designed to lateralize one or both vocal folds to improve airway patency and assist with decannulation. Voice quality is impaired when the paralyzed vocal fold is lateralized.

Cordotomy and partial or total arytenoidectomy are the most commonly performed lateralization procedures to treat BVFP [99–101]. During a cordotomy, the vocal fold is detached from the vocal process (Fig. 5). The goal of procedures to treat bilateral vocal fold paralysis is to widen the posterior airway without compromising airway protection. Patients must be aware that the voice might be weakened.

These procedures are typically performed endoscopically with use of the carbon dioxide (CO_2) laser. The advantages of using the CO_2 laser include arguably increased precision through the narrow endoscope and improved hemostasis requiring less need for tissue manipulation [99]. Potential complications include granuloma formation, scar, perichondritis, and endotracheal tube fire. Patients should be put on antireflux medication after surgery to reduce the risk for scar and granuloma formation [99]. Several reinnervation procedures to the PCA muscle have been described [90,91], although none with clinical success. The phrenic nerve is an obvious candidate for anastomosis, given its inspiratory activity.

The use of botulinum toxin injection in the treatment of BVFP has been explored in animal models [102,103]. Injection of toxin into the CT muscle results in decreased tension in the vocal fold and subsequent lateralization with airway improvement. One of the authors (RTS) has also used botulinum toxin injections in the adductor muscles (TA and LCA) for bilateral

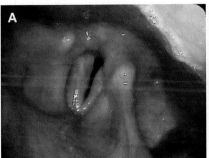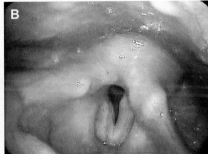

Fig. 5. Bilateral vocal fold paralysis. Bilateral vocal fold paralysis after right cordotomy. Notice the wider posterior airway, which was sufficient for decannulation of the patient's tracheostomy tube.

severe paresis to eliminate synkinesis and permit unopposed action of the PCA to abduct the vocal folds so as to improve breathing.

When both vocal folds are paralyzed in the cadaveric position, as from a high vagal lesion, the airway may be fine, although voice and swallowing may be impaired. In this setting, conservative unilateral or bilateral medialization procedures may be useful.

Laryngeal pacing

Functional electrical stimulation (FES) of the larynx or laryngeal pacing continues to be explored as a potential therapeutic option for unilateral and bilateral paralysis [104–112]. FES systems have been used to restore motor function to patients who have spinal cord injury, to control heart rhythms in cardiac disease, and to restore sensory function (eg, cochlear implant).

Unlike cardiac pacemakers, laryngeal pacers require an efferent and afferent limb. An afferent limb is needed to provide information to enable effective timing of muscle contracture. For example, in the setting of UVFP, if the paralyzed side is stimulated to adduct when the innervated side is abducted, this does not result in improvement of glottic competence or voice. In the setting of BVFP, firing of the phrenic nerve, a change in intrathoracic pressure, or chest wall expansion can provide the afferent input signaling inspiration. This would result in stimulation of the PCA muscles to abduct the vocal folds. In the setting of UVFP, the contralateral TA or LCA muscles would be the best candidates for afferent input.

The efferent limb of the system may be connected to a nerve, the vagus, or RLN if it is still intact, to the nerve of a nerve-muscle pedicle, or to the denervated muscles themselves. After an RLN transection, axons may fail to regrow through a neurorrhaphy or other reinnervation procedure. By placing the electrodes in the denervated muscles themselves, the system would bypass this potential pitfall. In addition, one would not have to wait for axons to regenerate for the system to function.

There have been some implantations of laryngeal pacers done around the world in patients who have bilateral vocal fold paralysis. More than half of the patients have been decannulated. Patients must turn on the device manually and train themselves to breathe synchronously with the device. In the future, pressure-sensing devices may be added to stimulate abduction with inspiration [113].

Gene therapy

Gene therapy may offer future treatment options for RLN injury. Several growth factors have been identified that promote neuronal survival and sprouting. Delivery of genes encoding such growth factors into host tissue may protect against neuronal degeneration and stimulate regeneration after nerve injury. Shiotani and colleagues [114] delivered the gene for insulin-like growth factor-I (IGF-I) in a nonviral vector to the rat TA muscle after RLN transection. Rats that received the gene demonstrated greater reinnervation and less muscle atrophy than rats that did not receive the treatment.

Viral vectors carrying gene products can be delivered to the central nervous system (CNS) by retrograde transport after peripheral injection into nerve or muscle. Rubin and colleagues [115,116] demonstrated that delivery of viral vectors to the CNS is possible through the RLN. This technique could be particularly useful in the treatment of neurodegenerative diseases, such as amyotrophic lateral sclerosis, or for RLN injury with a partially intact nerve.

Summary

The thyroid surgeon must have a thorough understanding of laryngeal neuroanatomy and be able to recognize symptoms of vocal fold paresis and paralysis. Neuropraxia may occur even with excellent surgical technique. Patients should be counseled appropriately, particularly if they are professional voice users. Preoperative or early postoperative changes in voice, swallowing, and airway function should prompt immediate referral to an otolaryngologist. Early recognition and treatment may avoid the development of complications and improve patient quality of life.

References

[1] Poletto CJ, Verdun LP, Strominger R, et al. Correspondence between laryngeal vocal fold movement and muscle activity during speech and nonspeech gestures. J Appl Physiol 2004; 97:858–66.
[2] Eisele D. Intraoperative electrophysiologic monitoring of the recurrent laryngeal nerve. Laryngoscope 1996;106:443–9.
[3] Farrar W. Complications of thyroidectomy. Surg Clin North Am 1983;63(6):1353–61.
[4] Schroder DM. Operative strategy for thyroid cancer: is total thyroidectomy worth the price? Cancer 1986;58:2320–8.
[5] Crumley R. Repair of the recurrent laryngeal nerve. Otolaryngol Clin North Am 1990; 23(3):553–63.
[6] Hollinshead WH. Anatomy for surgeons: the head and neck. 3rd edition. Philadelphia: Harper & Row, Publishers; 1982.
[7] Wang C. The anatomic basis of parathyroid surgery. Ann Surg 1976;183(3):271–5.
[8] Wang C. The use of the inferior cornu of the thyroid cartilage in identifying the recurrent laryngeal nerve. Surg Gynecol Obstet 1975;140:91–4.
[9] Wheeler MH. Thyroid surgery and the recurrent laryngeal nerve. Br J Surg 1999;86(3): 291–2.
[10] Crumley RL. Unilateral recurrent laryngeal nerve paralysis. J Voice 1994;8(1):79–83.
[11] Kierner A, Aigner M, Burian M. The external branch of the superior laryngeal nerve: its topographical anatomy as related to surgery of the neck. Otolaryngology - HNS 1998; 124(3):301–3.
[12] Loré J. Thirty-eight-year evaluation of a surgical technique to protect the external branch of the superior laryngeal nerve during thyroidectomy. Ann Otol Rhinol Laryngol 1998;107: 1015–22.

[13] Jansson S, Tisell L, Hagne I, et al. Partial superior laryngeal nerve lesions before and after thyroid surgery. World J Surg 1988;12:522–7.

[14] Rubin A, Sataloff RT, Hawkshaw M, et al. Arytenoid cartilage dislocation: a 20-year experience. J Voice 2005;19(4):687–701.

[15] Bridge PM, Ball DJ, Mackinnon SE, et al. Nerve crush injuries—a model for axonotmesis. Exp Neurol 1994;127:284–90.

[16] Horn K, Crumley RL. The physiology of nerve injury and repair. Otolaryngol Clin North Am 1984;17(2):321–33.

[17] Shindo M, Herzon G, Hanson D, et al. Effects of denervation on laryngeal muscles: a canine model. Laryngoscope 1992;102:663–9.

[18] Flint P, Downs D, Coltrera M. Laryngeal synkinesis following reinnervation in the rat. Ann Otol Rhinol Laryngol 1991;100:797–806.

[19] Crumley R. Laryngeal synkinesis revisited. Ann Otol Rhinol Laryngol 2000;109:365–71.

[20] Bevan K, Griffiths MF, Morgan MH. Cricothyroid muscle paralysis: its recognition and diagnosis. J Laryngol Otol 1989;103:191–5.

[21] Eckley C, Sataloff R, Hawkshaw M, et al. Voice range in superior laryngeal nerve paresis and paralysis. J Voice 1998;12(3):340–8.

[22] Arnold GE. Physiology and pathology of the cricothyroid muscle. Laryngoscope 1961;71: 687–753.

[23] Rubin A, Sataloff R. Vocal fold paresis and paralysis. In: Sataloff R, editor. Professional voice: the science and art of clinical care. 3rd edition. San Diego (CA): Plural Publishing, Inc.; 2005. p. 881–7.

[24] Durson G, Sataloff RT, Spiegel J, et al. Superior laryngeal nerve paresis and paralysis. J Voice 1996;10(2):206–11.

[25] Halum S, Shemirani NL, Merati A, et al. Electromyography findings of the cricopharyngeus in association with ipsilateral pharyngeal and laryngeal muscles. Ann Otol Rhinol Laryngol 2006;115(4):312–6.

[26] Lee B, Woo P. Chronic cough as a sign of laryngeal sensory neuropathy: diagnosis and treatment. Ann Otol Rhinol Laryngol 2005;114(4):253–7.

[27] Bastian RW, Vaidya AM, Delsupehe KG. Sensory neuropathic cough: a common and treatable cause of chronic cough. Otolaryngol Head Neck Surg 2006;135(1):17–21.

[28] Chiang FY, Lin JC, Lee KW, et al. Thyroid tumors with preoperative recurrent laryngeal nerve palsy: clinicopathologic features and treatment outcome. Surgery 2006;140(3): 413–7.

[29] Slomka WS, Abedi E, Sismanis A, et al. Paralysis of the recurrent laryngeal nerve by an extracapsular thyroid adenoma. Ear Nose Throat J 1989;68(11):855–63.

[30] Jellish WS, Jensen RL, Anderson DE, et al. Intraoperative electromyographic assessment of recurrent laryngeal nerve stress and pharyngeal injury during anterior cervical spine surgery with Caspar instrumentation. J Neurosurg 1999;91:170–4.

[31] Johansson S, Lofroth PO, Denekamp J. Left sided vocal cord paralysis: a newly recognized late complication of mediastinal irradiation. Radiother Oncol 2001;58(3):287–94.

[32] Coover LR. Permanent iatrogenic vocal cord paralysis after I-131 therapy: a case report and literature review. Clin Nucl Med 2000;25(7):508–10.

[33] Benninger MS. Acyclovir for the treatment of idiopathic vocal fold paralysis. Ear Nose Throat J 1992;71(5):207–8.

[34] Rontal E, Rontal M, Wald J, et al. Botulinum toxin injection in the treatment of vocal fold paralysis associated with multiple sclerosis: a case report. J Voice 1999;13(2):274–9.

[35] Tyler HR. Neurology of the larynx. Otolaryngol Clin North Am 1984;17(1):75–9.

[36] Isozaki E, Osanai R, Horiguchi S, et al. Laryngeal electromyography with separated surface electrodes in patients with multiple system atrophy presenting with vocal cord paralysis. J Neurol 1994;241(9):551–6.

[37] Willis WH, Weaver DF. Syringomyelia with bilateral vocal cord paralysis. Report of a case. Arch Otolaryngol 1968;87(5):468–70.

[38] Cridge PB, Allegra J, Gerhard H. Myasthenic crisis presenting as isolated vocal cord paralysis. Am J Emerg Med 2000;18(2):232–3.

[39] Mao V, Spiegel JR, Mandel S, et al. Laryngeal myasthenia gravis: report of 40 cases. J Voice 2001;15(1):122–30.

[40] Yoskovitch A, Enepekides DJ, Hier MP, et al. Guillain-Barré syndrome presenting as bilateral vocal cord paralysis. Otolaryngol Head Neck Surg 2000;122(2):269–70.

[41] Plasse H, Lieberman A. Bilateral vocal cord paralysis in Parkinson's disease. Arch Otolaryngol 1981;107(4):252–3.

[42] Venketasubramanian N, Seshadri R, Chee N. Vocal cord paresis in acute ischemic stroke. Cerebrovasc Dis 1999;9(3):157–62.

[43] Ross DA, Ward PH. Central vocal cord paralysis and paresis presenting as laryngeal stridor in children. Laryngoscope 1990;100(1):10–3.

[44] Lacy PD, Hartley BE, Rutter MJ, et al. Familial bilateral vocal cord paralysis and Charcot-Marie-tooth disease type II-C. Arch Otolaryngol Head Neck Surg 2001;127(3): 322–4.

[45] Rosen CA, Thomas JP, Anderson D. Bilateral vocal fold paralysis caused by familial hypokalemic periodic paralysis. Otolaryngol Head Neck Surg 1999;120(5):785–6.

[46] Schroeter V, Belz GG, Blenk H. Paralysis of recurrent laryngeal nerve in Lyme disease. Lancet 1988;2(8622):1245.

[47] Maccioni A, Olcese A. Laryngeal paralysis caused by congenital neurosyphilis. Pediatria (Santiago) 1965;8(1):71–5.

[48] Feleppa AE. Vocal cord paralysis secondary to infectious mononucleosis. Trans Pa Acad Ophthalmol Otolaryngol 1981;34(1):56–9.

[49] Magnussen R, Patanella H. Herpes simplex virus and recurrent laryngeal nerve paralysis. Arch Intern Med 1979;139(12):1423–4.

[50] Sommer D, Freeman J. Bilateral vocal cord paralysis associated with diabetes mellitus: case reports. J Otolaryngol 1994;23(3):169–71.

[51] Kabadi U. Unilateral vocal cord palsy in a diabetic patient. Postgrad Med 1988;84(4):53–6.

[52] Imauchi Y, Urata Y, Abe K. Left vocal cord paralysis in cases of systemic lupus erythematosus. ORL J Otorhinolaryngol Relat Spec 2001;63(1):53–5.

[53] Conaghan P, Chung D, Vaughan R. Recurrent laryngeal nerve palsy associated with mediastinal amyloidosis. Thorax 2000;55(5):436–7.

[54] Fujiki N, Nakamura H, Nonomura M, et al. Bilateral vocal fold paralysis caused by polyarteritis nodosa. Am J Otolaryngol 1999;20(6):412–4.

[55] Eckel HE, Wittekindt C, Klussmann JP, et al. Management of bilateral arytenoid cartilage fixation versus recurrent laryngeal nerve paralysis. Ann Otol Rhinol Laryngol 2003;112(2): 103–8.

[56] Gardner GM. Posterior glottic stenosis and bilateral vocal fold immobility: diagnosis and treatment. Otolaryngol Clin North Am 2000;33(4):855–78.

[57] Cohen SM, Garrett CG, Netterville JL, et al. Laryngoscopy in bilateral vocal fold immobility: can you make a diagnosis? Ann Otol Rhinol Laryngol 2006;115(6):439–43.

[58] Rubin AD. Neurolaryngologic evaluation of the performer. Otolaryngol Clin North Am 2007;40(5):971–89.

[59] Rubin A, Praneetvatakul V, Heman-Ackah Y, et al. Repetitive phonatory tasks for identifying vocal fold paresis. J Voice 2005;19(4):679–86.

[60] Heman-Ackah YD, Barr A. Mild vocal fold paresis: understanding clinical presentation and electromyographic findings. J Voice 2006;20(2):269–81.

[61] Heman-Ackah YD, Barr A. The value of laryngeal electromyography in the evaluation of laryngeal motion abnormalities. J Voice 2005;20(3):452–60.

[62] Sataloff RT, Mandel S, Heman-Ackah Y, et al. Laryngeal electromyography. 2nd edition. San Diego (CA): Plural Publishing; 2006.

[63] Munin MC, Rosen CA, Zullot T. Utility of laryngeal electromyography in predicting recovery after vocal fold paralysis. Arch Phys Med Rehabil 2003;84(8):1150–3.

[64] Heuer R, Sataloff RT, Rulnick R, et al. Unilateral recurrent laryngeal nerve paralysis: the importance of preoperative voice therapy. J Voice 1998;11(1):88–94.

[65] Aronson AE. Clinical voice disorders. 3rd edition. New York: Thieme Medical Publishers, Inc.; 1990. p. 339–45.

[66] Greene MCL, Mathieson L. The voice and its disorders. 5th edition. London: Whurr Publishers; 1989. p. 305–6.

[67] O'Leary MA, Grillone GA. Injection laryngoplasty. Otolaryngol Clin North Am 2006; 39(1):43–54.

[68] Dedo HH. Injection and removal of Teflon for unilateral vocal cord paralysis. Ann Otol Rhinol Laryngol 1992;101(1):81–6.

[69] Dedo HH, Urrea RD, Lawson L. Intracordal injection of Teflon in the treatment of 135 patients with dysphonia. Ann Otol Rhinol Laryngol 1973;82(5):661–7.

[70] Coskun HH, Rosen CA. Gelfoam injection as a treatment for temporary vocal fold paralysis. Ear Nose Throat J 2003;82(5):352–3.

[71] Schramm VL, May M, Lavorato AS. Gelfoam paste injection for vocal cord paralysis: temporary rehabilitation of glottic incompetence. Laryngoscope 1978;88(8 Pt 1):1268–73.

[72] Shindo ML, Zaretsky LS, Rice DH. Autologous fat injection for unilateral vocal fold paralysis. Ann Otol Rhinol Laryngol 1996;105(8):602–6.

[73] Sataloff RT, Hawkshaw M, Shaw A. Autologous fat injection: the intraoperative endpoint. Ear Nose Throat J 1999;78(8):534.

[74] Remacle M, Lawson G, Keghian J, et al. Use of injectable autologous collagen for correcting glottic gaps: initial results. J Voice 1999;13(2):280–8.

[75] Milstein CF, Akst LM, Hicks MD, et al. Long-term effects of micronized Alloderm injection for unilateral vocal fold paralysis. Laryngoscope 2005;115(9):1691–6.

[76] Rosen CA, Gartner-Schmidt J, Casiano R, et al. Vocal fold augmentation with calcium hydroxylapatite (CaHA). Otolaryngol Head Neck Surg 2007;136(2):198–204.

[77] Hughes RG, Morrison M. Vocal cord medialization by transcutaneous injection of calcium hydroxylapatite. J Voice 2005;19(4):674–8.

[78] Hertegard S, Hallen L, Laurent C, et al. Cross-linked hyaluronan versus collagen for injection treatment of glottal insufficiency: 2-year follow-up. Acta Otolaryngol 2004;124(10): 1208–14.

[79] Hertegard S, Hallen L, Laurent C, et al. Cross-linked hyaluronan used as augmentation substance for treatment of glottal insufficiency: safety aspects and vocal fold function. Laryngoscope 2002;112(12):2211–9.

[80] Heman-Ackah YD. How I do it: miniplate reconstruction of the lateral thyroid lamina: one-stage restoration of voice after Teflon granuloma resection. J Voice 2005;19(3): 504–9.

[81] Netterville JL, Coleman JR, Chang S, et al. Lateral laryngotomy for the removal of Teflon granuloma. Ann Otol Rhinol Laryngol 1998;107(9 Pt 1):735–44.

[82] Isshiki N, Morita H, Okamura H. Thyroplasty as a new phonosurgical technique. Acta Otolaryngol 1974;78:451–7.

[83] Isshiki N, Tanabe M, Sawada M. Arytenoid adduction for unilateral vocal cord paralysis. Arch Otolaryngol 1978;104:555–8.

[84] Selber J, Sataloff R, Spiegel J, et al. Gore-Tex medialization thyroplasty: objective and subjective evaluation. J Voice 2003;17(1):88–95.

[85] Zeitels SM, Mauri M, Dailey SH. Adduction arytenopexy for vocal fold paralysis: indications and technique. J Laryngol Otol 2004;118(7):508–16.

[86] Gacek M, Gacek RR. Cricoarytenoid joint mobility after chronic vocal cord paralysis. Laryngoscope 1996;106(12 pt 1):1528–30.

[87] Colman MF, Schwartz I. The effect of vocal cord paralysis on the cricoarytenoid joint. Otolaryngol Head Neck Surg 1981;89(3 Pt 1):419–22.

[88] Crumley R. Update: ansa cervicalis to recurrent laryngeal nerve anastomosis for unilateral laryngeal paralysis. Laryngoscope 1991;101(4 pt 1):384–7.

[89] Baldissera F, Tredeci G, Marini S, et al. Innervation of the paralyzed laryngeal muscles by phrenic motoneurons. A quantitative study by light and electron microscopy. Laryngoscope 1992;102:907–16.

[90] Baldissera F, Cantarella G, Marini G, et al. Recovery of inspiratory abduction of the paralyzed vocal cords after bilateral reinnervation of the cricoarytenoid muscles by one single branch of the phrenic nerve. Laryngoscope 1989;99:1286–92.

[91] Jacobs I, Sanders I, Wu B, et al. Reinnervation of the canine posterior cricoarytenoid muscle with sympathetic preganglionic neurons. Ann Otol Rhinol Laryngol 1990;99: 167–74.

[92] Paniello R, Lee P, Dahm D. Hypoglossal nerve transfer for laryngeal reinnervation: a preliminary study. Ann Otol Rhinol Laryngol 1999;108:239–44.

[93] Tucker H. Long-term results of nerve-muscle pedicle reinnervation for laryngeal paralysis. Ann Otol Rhinol Laryngol 1989;98:674–6.

[94] Goding G. Nerve-muscle pedicle reinnervation of the paralyzed vocal cord. Otolaryngol Clin North Am 1991;24(5):1239–51.

[95] Secarz J, Nguyen L, Nasri S, et al. Physiologic motion after laryngeal nerve reinnervation: a new method. Otolaryngol Head Neck Surg 1997;116(4):466–74.

[96] Van Lith-Bijl J, Stolk R, Tonnaer J, et al. Selective laryngeal reinnervation with separate phrenic and ansa cervicalis nerve transfers. Arch Otolaryngol Head Neck Surg 1997;123: 406–11.

[97] Hogikyan N, Johns M, Kileny P, et al. Motion specific laryngeal reinnervation using muscle-nerve-muscle neurotization. Laryngoscope 2001;110(9):801–10.

[98] Tucker H. Long-term preservation of voice improvement following surgical medialization and reinnervation for unilateral vocal fold paralysis. J Voice 1999;13(2):251–6.

[99] Ossoff R, Duncavage J, Shapshay S, et al. Endoscopic laser arytenoidectomy revisited. Ann Otol Rhinol Laryngol 1990;99(10 part1):764–71.

[100] Segas J, Stavroulakis P, Manolopoulos L, et al. Management of bilateral vocal fold paralysis: experience at the University of Athens. Otolaryngol Head Neck Surg 2001;124(1): 68–71.

[101] Cummings C, Redd E, Westra W, et al. Minimally invasive device to effect vocal fold lateralization. Ann Otol Rhinol Laryngol 1999;108(9):833–6.

[102] Cohen S, Thompson J, Camilon FS. Botulinum toxin for relief of bilateral abductor paralysis of the larynx: histologic study in an animal model. Ann Otol Rhinol Laryngol 1989; 98(3):213–6.

[103] Cohen S, Thompson JW. Use of botulinum toxin to lateralize true vocal cords: a biochemical method to relieve bilateral abductor vocal cord paralysis. Ann Otol Rhinol Laryngol 1987;96(5):534–41.

[104] Broniatowski M, Tucker H, Nose Y. The future of electronic pacing in laryngeal rehabilitation. Am J Otolaryngol 1990;11(1):51–62.

[105] Bergmann K, Warzel H, Eckhardt H, et al. Long-term implantation of a system of electrical stimulation of paralyzed laryngeal muscles in dogs. Laryngoscope 1988;98(4):455–9.

[106] Goldfarb D, Keane W, Lowry L. Laryngeal pacing as a treatment for vocal fold paralysis. J Voice 1994;8(2):179–85.

[107] Kano S, Sasaki C. Pacing parameters of the canine posterior cricoarytenoid muscle. Ann Otol Rhinol Laryngol 1991;100(7):584–8.

[108] Kojima H, Omori K, Nonomura M, et al. Electrical pacing for dynamic treatment of unilateral vocal cord paralysis. Ann Otol Rhinol Laryngol 1991;100(1):15–8.

[109] Broniatowski M, Vito K, Shah B, et al. Contraction patterns of intrinsic laryngeal muscles induced by orderly recruitment in the canine. Laryngoscope 1996;106(12 Pt 1):1510–5.

[110] Lundy D, Casiano R, Landy H, et al. Effects of vagal nerve stimulation on laryngeal function. J Voice 1993;7(4):359–64.

[111] Billante CR, Zealear DL, Courey MS, et al. Effects of chronic electric stimulation of laryngeal muscle on voice. Ann Otol Rhinol Laryngol 2002;111(4):328–32.

[112] Zealear DL, Swelstad MR, Sant'Anna GD, et al. Determination of the optimal conditions for laryngeal pacing with the Itrel II implantable stimulator. Otolaryngol Head Neck Surg 2001;125(3):183–92.

[113] Hillel A, Benninger M, Blitzer A, et al. Evaluation and management of bilateral vocal cord immobility. Otolaryngol Head Neck Surg 1999;121(6):760–5.

[114] Shiotani A, O'Malley BW Jr, Coleman ME, et al. Human insulinlike growth factor 1 gene transfer into paralyzed rat larynx: single vs multiple injection. Arch Otolaryngol Head Neck Surg 1999;125:555–60.

[115] Rubin A, Hogikyan N, Sullivan K, et al. Remote delivery of rAAV-GFP to the rat brainstem via the recurrent laryngeal nerve. Laryngoscope 2001;111:2041–5.

[116] Rubin A, Mobley B, Hogikyan N, et al. Delivery of an adenoviral vector to the crushed recurrent laryngeal nerve. Laryngoscope 2003;113(6):985–9.

ELSEVIER
SAUNDERS

Surg Oncol Clin N Am
17 (2008) 197–218

SURGICAL
ONCOLOGY CLINICS
OF NORTH AMERICA

Postoperative Management of Thyroid Carcinoma

Timothy A. Manzone, MD, JD[a,*],
Hung Q. Dam, MD[a,b,c], Charles M. Intenzo, MD[d],
Vidya V. Sagar, MD[a], Charles J. Schneider, MD[e,f],
Prakash Seshadri, MD[g]

[a]Section of Nuclear Medicine, Department of Medicine, Christiana Care Health System/Helen F. Graham Cancer Center, 4755 Ogletown-Stanton Road, Newark, DE 19718, USA
[b]Nuclear Medicine Service, Department of Medicine, Wilmington Veterans' Affairs Medical Center, 1601 Kirkwood Highway, Wilmington, DE 19805, USA
[c]Division of Nuclear Medicine, Department of Radiology, Thomas Jefferson University, 132 S. 10th St., Philadelphia, PA 19107, USA
[d]Division of Nuclear Medicine and PET, Department of Radiology, Thomas Jefferson University, 132 S. 10th St., Philadelphia, PA 19107, USA
[e]Section of Oncology, Department of Medicine, Christiana Care Health System/Helen F. Graham Cancer Center, 4701 Ogletown-Stanton Road Suite 2200, Newark, DE 19713-2055, USA
[f]Department of Medicine, Thomas Jefferson University, 1025 Walnut Street, Philadelphia, PA 19107, USA
[g]Section of Endocrinology, Department of Medicine, Diabetes and Metabolic Diseases Center at Christiana, Christiana Care Health System, PMRI, 3506 Kennett Pike, Wilmington, DE 19807, USA

Although the primary treatment for thyroid cancer is surgery, postsurgical management has a major impact on morbidity and recurrence-free survival. The "good prognosis" generally attributed to thyroid cancer presupposes effective postoperative management after appropriate surgery. Survival from differentiated thyroid cancer (DTC) is good, with 10-year survival rates of 93% for papillary and 85% for follicular types [1]. On the other hand, disease recurrence (most often in thyroid bed or cervical nodes) is relatively common and may occur in up to 20% to 30% of patients [2]. The primary goals of postoperative management are to (1) minimize the likelihood of recurrence and (2) perform optimal surveillance so that recurrence may be managed swiftly.

* Corresponding author.
E-mail address: tmanzone@christianacare.org (T.A. Manzone).

1055-3207/08/$ - see front matter © 2008 Elsevier Inc. All rights reserved.
doi:10.1016/j.soc.2007.10.003

This article on postoperative management focuses on adult DTC, which comprises most thyroid cancers. Conventional chemotherapy has almost no role in DTC. The unique ability of differentiated thyroid cells to concentrate iodine, together with their exquisite sensitivity to hormonal manipulation, presents a unique cancer management situation and an unparalleled opportunity to exploit hormonal therapy and "targeted" radiotherapy. Postoperative evaluation and treatment of DTC are generally performed by endocrinologists and nuclear medicine physicians, often as members of a multidisciplinary team. Endocrinologists manage thyroid hormone replacement/thyroid-stimulating hormone (TSH) suppression, monitor endocrinologic markers, and coordinate surveillance. Nuclear medicine physicians evaluate patients who have thyroid cancer with imaging studies and administer targeted therapy with radioactive iodine (^{131}I).

This article gives an overview of postoperative management of adult DTC, including initial patient evaluation and risk stratification, treatment with thyroid remnant ablation (TRA), TSH manipulation, and surveillance for disease recurrence. We note some special issues in pediatric patients who have DTC. Finally, we briefly review postoperative management of medullary thyroid cancer (MTC) and anaplastic thyroid cancer (ATC); the entirely different biology of these diseases mandates completely different approaches to evaluation and treatment.

Initial evaluation and risk stratification

After the surgeon has completed a near-total thyroidectomy, the patient is generally evaluated by an endocrinologist. Almost all patients who have DTC have good prospects for long-term survival but are at risk for having recurrence of disease, most often locally. Because the goal of postoperative management is to extend recurrence-free survival, assessment of risk for recurrence is the foundation for patient management. Each patient's risk is assessed based on age, tumor histology (papillary cancer has best prognosis, followed by follicular, Hürthle cell, and so forth), tumor size, completeness of resection, and involvement of lymph nodes. Approximately one third of differentiated (follicular and papillary) thyroid cancers recur, and approximately 20% have distant metastases [3]. The risk of recurrence is best predicted by tumor stage and tumor histology. Much of the discussion regarding recurrence centers on what staging system is used and the stage of disease within this system. Because of its relative ease of use and predictability, the American Thyroid Association 2006 management guidelines for DTC [4] endorse the TNM model created by the American Joint Commission on Cancer [5]. Age is the greatest predictor of recurrence in the American Joint Commission on Cancer model. Patients who have DTC and are younger than 45 years are classified as stage I unless there are distant metastases; metastatic disease raises young patients only to stage II [5]. DTC tends to recur in patients diagnosed early (<15 years) and late (>65 years) in life and usually takes place within the first 5 years of diagnosis [2]. Recurrence is more common in tumors that initially present with local invasion, lymph node metastases, and larger tumor size [2]. A detailed analysis of risk factors for recurrence forms the basis for the National Comprehensive Cancer Network guidelines for DTC issued in 2006 (Table 1) [6].

Risk assessment centers on the pathology of the tumor and the extent to which it has been removed. One large multicenter study showed that residual tumor remained in 10.7% of papillary, 8.0% of follicular, and 10.5% of Hürthle cell neoplasms [7]; however, in this series, papillary thyroid cancers had only 4.8% vascular invasion versus follicular at 28.7% and Hürthle cell at 25.4% [7]. Reoperation was also more common in Hürthle cell cancers in another surgical series [8].

Risk assessment also must take into account the prevalence of incidental small thyroid carcinomas in the thyroidectomy specimen. The frequency of these microcarcinomas (<1 cm) has been shown in one autopsy series to be twice that of macrocarcinomas [9]. The American Thyroid Association has not defined how to evaluate these patients; however, patients with aggressive histology or capsular or vascular invasion in incidental microcarcinomas

Table 1
Risk stratification variables influencing differentiated thyroid cancer recurrence and cancer death

Factors predictive of high risk	Factors predictive of moderate to low risk
Patient variables	
Age <15 or >45 y	Age 15–45 y
Male sex	Female sex
Family history of thyroid cancer	No family history of thyroid cancer
Tumor variables	
Tumor >4 cm in diameter	Tumor <4 cm in diameter
Bilateral disease	Unilateral disease
Extrathyroidal extension	No extrathyroidal extension
Vascular invasion (papillary and follicular types)	Absence of vascular invasion
Cervical or mediastinal lymph node metastases	No lymph node metastases
Certain cell types: Hürthle cell, columnar cell, tall cell, diffuse sclerosis, insular variants	Encapsulated papillary thyroid carcinoma, papillary microcarcinoma, cystic papillary thyroid carcinoma
Marked nuclear atypia, necrosis, vascular invasion (ie, histologic grade)	Absence of nuclear atypia, tumor necrosis, and vascular invasion
Tumors or metastases that concentrate iodine poorly or not at all	Tumors or metastases that concentrate iodine well
Distant metastases	No distant metastases

From Mazzaferri EL, Kloos RT. Clinical report 128: current approaches to primary therapy for papillary and follicular thyroid cancer. J Clin Endocrinol Metab 2001;86(4):1449; with permission. Copyright © 2001, The Endocrine Society.

should be considered at higher risk [4]. In aggressive histologies and invasion, treatment of micropapillary thyroid carcinoma should proceed as for larger tumors.

Postoperative DTC treatment seeks to minimize each patient's risk of disease recurrence. Recurrence-free survival in DTC is maximized by total thyroidectomy, followed by TRA with radioactive iodine, and long-term thyroid hormone supplementation sufficient to produce TSH suppression [2].

Preparation for thyroid remnant ablation

TRA with ^{131}I is recommended in most cases, because TRA significantly lowers the recurrence rate. The goal of TRA is to destroy any residual thyroid cancer cells in the thyroid bed or in metastatic sites and remove any remaining normal thyroid tissue. The rationale behind destroying the latter includes the following: (1) serum thyroglobulin (Tg) measurement is the most sensitive indicator of cancer recurrence when there is no normal thyroid tissue present, (2) destruction of residual normal thyroid cells eliminates the possibility that they could later transform into occult malignancy, and (3) destroying the thyroid remnant increases the sensitivity and specificity of radioiodine scanning for the detection of recurrent or metastatic disease [10].

Ablation of remnant thyroid tissue with ^{131}I is most effective under stimulation by elevated TSH, because iodine uptake by thyroid cells is directly proportional to the serum TSH level. TSH elevation is achieved through thyroid hormone withdrawal, which raises serum TSH through negative feedback as the patient becomes hypothyroid. The standard of care is elevation of TSH level to at least 30 µIU/mL. After thyroidectomy, hypothyroidism is readily achieved by simply withholding thyroid hormone replacement. Depending on the size of the remnant, a TSH level of 30 µIU/mL is reached approximately 3 to 6 weeks after total thyroidectomy. For comfort reasons, patients are often supplemented for 1 month after surgery with liothyronine (Cytomel) and then taken off all thyroid medication for 2 weeks before ^{131}I TRA. Patients are warned that they will not feel well in those last 2 weeks but are reassured that their symptoms (eg, fatigue, constipation, edema, cold intolerance) should diminish soon after they start levothyroxine therapy. A potential alternative to thyroid hormone withdrawal is administration of exogenous TSH in the form of recombinant human TSH (rhTSH) or Thyrogen (Genzyme). Studies support the use of rhTSH for TRA [11]; however, this use of rhTSH does not yet have US Food and Drug Administration approval and is still deemed experimental by the American Thyroid Association [4].

For 2 weeks before TRA, patients should be placed on a low iodine diet. The typical American diet contains enough iodine to compete with the radioactive iodine for uptake in normal and malignant thyroid tissue. The low-iodine diet requires avoiding seafood, restaurant or packaged meals and snacks, dairy products, and iodized salt. Patients also should check product labels, because cough suppressants, nutritional supplements, and other over-the-counter products often contain considerable iodine. Some endocrinologists measure urinary iodine to ensure depletion of body iodine stores.

Targeted therapy

TRA with ^{131}I is a form of "targeted" radiotherapy that exploits the iodine avidity of thyroid cells to deliver a radiation dose from ^{131}I directly to the thyroid. ^{131}I, a radioactive isotope of iodine (half-life 8 days), is concentrated in the thyroid, where its radiation damages and destroys the cells. Because TRA efficacy depends on iodine uptake by thyroid cells, it is important to ensure that any thyroid cells are highly iodine avid. Before TRA, test results should confirm that the patient has serum TSH more than 30 µIU/ mL and has adhered to a low-iodine diet.

In most institutions worldwide, empiric fixed-activity levels of ^{131}I are administered. This approach is taken more often because of its simplicity. Thyroid remnants without local soft-tissue invasion are usually given 100 mCi (3700 MBq) of ^{131}I. For large tumors with soft-tissue invasion beyond the thyroid capsule, a higher dose of 150 to 200 mCi (5550–7400 MBq) is given. For cervical nodal disease, 150 to 175 mCi (5550–7350 MBq) is prescribed, depending on disease extent. Distant organ metastases (ie, lung, bone, and liver) are treated with 200 mCi (7400 MBq) or more [12]. An alternative to the fixed-activity method is the quantitative approach using ^{131}I dosimetry. The latter approach is more scientific because a calculated, patient-specific dose of ^{131}I is prescribed. Quantitative dosimetry involves one of two approaches—either calculation of the upper limits of a safe whole-body/blood level of radiation exposure from ^{131}I or calculation of the amount of radiation to be delivered to the target tissue. Dosimetry involves administering a small tracer dose of ^{131}I followed by scans and urine ^{131}I measurements performed over several days. Although ^{131}I dosimetry yields a calculated, patient-specific ^{131}I dosage, most medical centers use the fixed activity approach because it is less labor intensive and more convenient for patients. The optimal method of determining the ^{131}I TRA dose (ie, empiric activity versus individualized dosimetry) is controversial and remains a subject of ongoing research [2,4,13].

For many years, almost all patients who underwent TRA were admitted to the hospital for the procedure, unless the ^{131}I dose administered was less than 30 mCi. Some patients were treated with low doses to avoid admission. Since 1997, the Nuclear Regulatory Commission has allowed patients to be released after TRA provided that the total radiation exposure to any person in contact with the patient is anticipated to be less than a certain "maximum permissible dose" [14]. This anticipated exposure is determined by patient-specific calculations that take into account the prescribed ^{131}I dose, anticipated thyroid remnant uptake, and various "occupancy factors" that reflect the patient's transportation home after the procedure, level of independence in daily living, and availability of exclusive use of bathroom and sleeping facilities for one to two full nights. The patient must be given detailed instructions on social isolation and disposal of wastes, which must be followed for 2 to 3 days after treatment. As a practical matter, most TRA procedures are performed on an outpatient basis, which produces cost savings and increased patient convenience. Outpatient TRA cannot be performed in situations in which a patient (1) requires physical assistance for usual daily activities, (2) does not have exclusive bathroom and bedroom use for at least 24 hours, (3) lives in a nursing facility, or (4) is on dialysis [15]. Pregnancy is an absolute contraindication to ^{131}I treatment. A serum pregnancy test must be obtained before TRA for any woman of childbearing potential. American Thyroid Association guidelines recommend that women avoid becoming pregnant for at least 6 to 12 months after TRA, primarily in case a second TRA treatment is required.

After a nuclear medicine physician completes the required patient counseling and documentation, the ^{131}I dose is administered orally in the form of sodium iodide in either liquid or capsule form. TRA is well tolerated by most patients; however, there are several recognized complications. Nearly 50% of patients undergoing TRA experience radiation sialadenitis caused by ^{131}I uptake by the salivary glands. This complication usually manifests with discomfort, a metallic taste, lack of taste, or xerostomia at approximately 5 to 7 days after TRA. Symptoms usually resolve but are occasionally protracted or even permanent. The likelihood of sialadenitis is proportional to the ^{131}I dose given, so it is more common in patients who receive higher doses. Patients are advised to increase normal fluid intake and periodically stimulate the salivary glands with sour hard candy starting the day after treatment. The candy increases saliva secretion and decreases the residence time of ^{131}I in the salivary glands.

Another common acute side affect of TRA is radiation-induced gastritis, usually manifested by nausea, which is seen in at least one third of patients. It usually starts approximately 24 hours after treatment and lasts 1 or 2 days but occasionally is more delayed. Some facilities routinely prescribe antiemetic suppositories. Like sialadenitis, radiation gastritis is ^{131}I dose related and seems less frequent with vigorous oral hydration.

In general, late complications of ^{131}I therapy occur only after multiple cumulative doses of ^{131}I, including temporary bone marrow suppression, blood dyscrasias, and temporary (rarely permanent) male sterility. In cases of widespread pulmonary metastases, radiation-induced pulmonary fibrosis has been reported. Overall, late complications from ^{131}I therapy have been uncommon over the many decades that this highly effective targeted modality has been used, perhaps because only a few patients require multiple treatments.

The postablation scan

Routinely, approximately 1 week after ablation, an iodine whole-body scan (WBS) is obtained to image the photons emitted by the ablation dose. The scan shows ^{131}I uptake by thyroid tissue (normal and malignant), and visualization of remnant activity is a confirmation of TRA dose targeting (Fig. 1). In nearly 25% of cases, the postablation scan demonstrates additional lesions or metastases not detected by a diagnostic WBS, because the posttreatment scan provides imaging of a much higher amount of [131]I. As a result, the postablation scan can be an indicator of prognosis. In a few instances, the scan may change patient management; visualization of unexpected sites of iodine uptake may prompt other studies or a repeat diagnostic WBS earlier than anticipated (ie, at 6 months rather than 12 months). The postablation scan is also useful in situations in which a diagnostic WBS produces negative results but the serum Tg levels are elevated. In this setting, the postablation WBS performed after empiric TRA can confirm therapy targeting in the thyroid bed, in cervical nodes, or occasionally

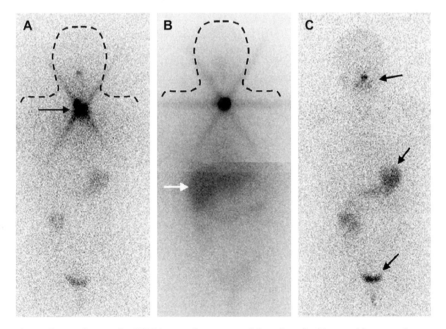

Fig. 1. Composite anterior WBS images from sequential studies of a 44-year-old woman 5 years after thyroidectomy for 3-cm papillary cancer with one positive node. TSH maximized at 10 μIU/mL despite thyroid hormone withdrawal. (*A*) Diagnostic ^{123}I WBS showed uptake in large functioning remnant (*arrow*). The dashed line outlines head and shoulders. (*B*) Postablation WBS 1 week after TRA with 155 mCi (5735 MBq) [131]I confirms TRA dose targeting; activity in the liver (*white arrow*) reflects metabolism of radioactive thyroglobulin (Tg). (*C*) Diagnostic ^{123}I WBS performed at 9 months shows normal uptake in mouth, stomach, and bladder (*arrows*) but no remnant activity or metastasis.

in pulmonary metastases. Whether a diagnostic WBS should be performed before TRA is controversial. Some centers obtain only a postablation WBS; however, a pre-TRA diagnostic WBS can change management in many patients (Fig. 2) [16].

Thyroid-stimulating hormone suppression therapy

Once ablation has been completed, TSH must be suppressed with levothyroxine to prevent thyroid cancer growth [2]. Typical replacement doses can be started on a weight basis at approximately 1.6 µg/kg/d. This dose gets a patient's TSH into the normal range. Patients considered at low risk (ie, small tumor size, no invasion or metastasis, non–high-risk pathology) should keep their TSH between 0.1 and 0.5 µIU/mL. High-risk patients should have their TSH below 0.1 µIU/mL as tolerated without hyperthyroid symptoms [4]. TSH can be followed every 6 weeks once levothyroxine is initiated to obtain the desired TSH level.

Thyroglobulin assay

In recent years, serum Tg measurement has become a mainstay of surveillance for DTC recurrence. Tg is the major protein product of thyroid cell function and is not produced by other cells in the body. If all thyroid cells have been eliminated, serum Tg should be negligibly low. Elevated serum Tg level (> 2 ng/mL) is highly sensitive and specific for DTC recurrence after

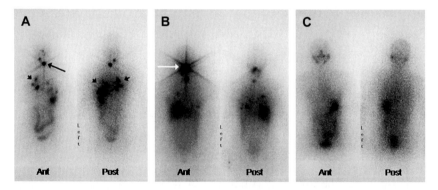

Fig. 2. Sequential studies from 55-year-old woman who has papillary thyroid carcinoma who presented 8 weeks after total thyroidectomy. (*A*) WBS performed 48 hours after the oral administration of 5 mCi (185 MBq) [131]I shows a functioning remnant (*long arrow*), a probable metastatic node in the right neck, and metastases in the lower chest bilaterally (*short arrows*). The patient received 250 mCi (9250 MBq) of [131]I. (*B*) Postablation WBS obtained at 1 week confirms TRA targeting. "Star" artifact (*white arrow*) is from high-energy ^{131}I photons. (*C*) One-year follow-up ^{131}I WBS shows complete resolution of all of the lesions.

TRA [4]. Serum anti-Tg antibodies also must be measured at the time of each Tg test, because presence of Tg antibodies (more frequently positive in patients who have DTC than the general population) invalidates the Tg assay [17]. The sensitivity of the Tg assay for DTC recurrence greatly increases when obtained as a "stimulated Tg" (ie, blood drawn when the patient's TSH is elevated). TSH stimulation is accomplished by either thyroid hormone withdrawal or rhTSH (Thyrogen). (TSH stimulation is also required for the iodine WBS, so the two tests are usually done together.) American Thyroid Association guidelines suggest baseline Tg and Tg antibody tests just before TRA. Although Tg is almost always detectable in the presence of any functioning thyroid remnant, high levels may suggest residual or metastatic malignancy [4].

Radioactive iodine (^{131}I or ^{123}I) whole-body scan

The radioactive iodine WBS has long been a diagnostic workhorse in DTC management, although its role has diminished with the availability of the Tg assay. Functioning thyroid cells appear on the WBS because they concentrate the radioactive iodine tracer. Two radioactive isotopes (^{131}I and ^{123}I) may be used. [131]I, the same isotope used for therapy, has been used for many years. Although ^{131}I is sensitive and specific, this radionuclide has drawbacks: the ^{131}I photon energy (364 kV) is not optimal for standard nuclear medicine imaging equipment and ^{131}I emits beta particles, which are more damaging to tissue than other radiation forms. This fact raises the controversial issue of thyroid "stunning." "Stunning" refers to the concern that the radiation from a diagnostic WBS ^{131}I dose impairs thyroid cells' absorption of iodine, which potentially decreases the efficacy of a subsequent therapeutic iodine dose. Although stunning is a real phenomenon, it may not actually impair therapeutic efficacy [18]; however, the problem can be avoided entirely by performing the WBS with [123]I. [123]I is more expensive and has a short half-life (13 hours) but produces excellent images and has no beta emissions. Studies have indicated that a ^{123}I WBS has diagnostic accuracy comparable to [131]I [19]. As a result, ^{123}I has replaced ^{131}I for WBS in many facilities.

The first surveillance ^{123}I WBS is typically performed for patients who have low risk of recurrence approximately 6 to 12 months after TRA. Because iodine uptake is TSH dependent, the WBS requires elevated serum TSH, which can be done by withdrawal of thyroid hormone as described for the initial ablation or by injection of rhTSH (Thyrogen) [20]. For Thyrogen studies, the patient receives rhTSH, 0.9 mg, intramuscularly daily for 2 days followed by ^{123}I administration on day 3 and imaging on day 4. By allowing patients to achieve TSH stimulation without symptomatic hypothyroidism, rhTSH improves quality of life; however, it is prudent to use thyroid hormone withdrawal if there is any anticipation that ^{131}I treatment will be required. rhTSH use is often reserved for low-risk patients. The WBS is also optimized by a 2-week low-iodine diet.

Positron emission tomography

Positron emission tomography (PET) using ^{18}F-fluorodeoxyglucose (FDG) is a functional imaging modality that can detect malignant tissue based on cellular glucose use. Many malignant cells have elevated glycolytic activity that results in high avidity for FDG; PET shows FDG uptake to differentiate between malignant and benign tissues. In early 2005, the Centers for Medicare and Medicaid Services approved the use of FDG PET for evaluation of patients who have DTC with (1) previous thyroidectomy and TRA, (2) negative iodine WBS, and (3) serum Tg more than 10 ng/mL.

Although early studies were variable, FDG PET is currently recognized as highly sensitive (93.7%) and highly specific (77.8%) in DTC evaluation [21]. The diagnostic yield from FDG PET increases with increased serum Tg [22], which is not surprising, because higher Tg indicates larger bulk of disease. Also not surprising are laboratory and clinical data that support the use of TSH stimulation before scanning with PET. PET scans of the same DTC patients under euthyroid and hypothyroid states showed an increase in tumor-to-background ratio and improved lesion detection when PET was performed when TSH was elevated [23,24]. TSH stimulation can be performed with either thyroid hormone withdrawal or rhTSH [25]. Many institutions currently perform FDG PET studies for DTC exclusively under TSH stimulation.

Interpretation of PET images requires correlation with anatomic findings, usually provided by CT. Formerly, this required careful visual image comparison; however, integrated PET/CT scanners are available that combine PET and CT devices in a single machine. PET/CT acquires anatomic and metabolic data simultaneously, which provides more accurate lesion localization, reduced scan times, and improved image quality. PET/CT is highly sensitive for thyroid carcinoma, with increased sensitivity at higher Tg levels [26]. One recent study showed a diagnostic accuracy of 93% for PET/CT compared with 78% for PET alone [27]. PET/CT findings change patient management in a significant number of patients who have DTC (Fig. 3) [27,28].

The combination of ^{131}I WBS and ^{18}F-FDG PET gives a sensitivity of 95% for recurrent DTC [29]. Some authors have reported an inverse relationship ("flipflop" pattern) between iodine uptake on WBS and FDG uptake on PET in which lesions negative on WBS are positive on PET and vice versa [30,31]. The superior spatial resolution of PET over ^{131}I may explain its ability to detect lesions that are not visualized on WBS. The "flipflop" pattern is probably best explained by the tendency of some DTC lesions to de-differentiate and progressively lose ability to concentrate iodine in up to 20% of cases, however [31,32]. Iodine uptake in DTC lesions indicates a high level of differentiation. On the other hand, markedly increased FDG uptake often indicates more poorly differentiated disease [33]. A single DTC lesion may contain poorly and well-differentiated components [33].

Because less well-differentiated DTC has higher mortality [34], the level of FDG uptake on PET is a strong predictor of survival in DTC and can help risk stratify patients and guide the aggressiveness of therapy [31,35]. Markedly hypermetabolic FDG uptake on PET or PET/CT predicts more aggressive tumor behavior and unfavorable prognosis [36].

PET or PET/CT may be useful in evaluating the "iodine-negative, Tg-positive" patient (ie, a patient with a negative WBS despite elevated serum Tg) (Fig. 4). One study of the use of PET in this clinical setting found that PET identified disease in 19 of 27 patients [37]. Empiric treatment with ^{131}I is sometimes recommended for PET-positive recurrent DTC; however, Wang and colleagues [38] showed that high-dose ^{131}I therapy has little or no effect on PET-positive (but iodine-negative) DTC lesions.

PET and PET/CT may be particularly useful in Hürthle cell carcinoma, an uncommon and aggressive form of DTC that often has low avidity for radioactive iodine. Pryma and colleagues [39] showed that PET had a sensitivity of 95.8% and specificity of 95% for Hürthle cell carcinoma and provided incremental improvement in accuracy over CT and WBS.

Surveillance for differentiated thyroid cancer recurrence

The long-term follow up of DTC is based on the initial pathology, metastasis (vascular invasion, lymph nodes, distant metastases), and patient age. An iodine WBS is performed for low-risk patients and an ultrasound for high-risk patients. The reasoning is that ultrasound has greater sensitivity for neck metastasis and shows anatomy for possible surgical resection [4]. Ultrasound and Tg measurement are performed approximately 6 months after TRA while the patient is taking levothyroxine sufficient to suppress TSH. Positive ultrasound results require surgical intervention. Positive Tg results (Tg >1 ng/mL or <1 ng/mL with positive Tg antibodies) with negative ultrasound require further evaluation, which may include stimulated ^{123}I WBS, stimulated Tg measurement, CT scan of the chest, or FDG PET, depending on clinical circumstances [4].

A WBS and stimulated Tg measurement are typically performed for low-risk patients approximately 6 to 12 months after TRA [4]. These procedures can use either thyroid hormone withdrawal or rhTSH. Patients with known distant metastasis at the time of diagnosis who are ultrasound negative should undergo 6-month surveillance with withdrawal of thyroid hormone in the event that ^{131}I therapy is needed. If initial WBS and Tg are negative, surveillance with ultrasound and TSH-suppressed Tg can continue for 3 to 5 years on an annual basis depending on disease stage and clinical status [4].

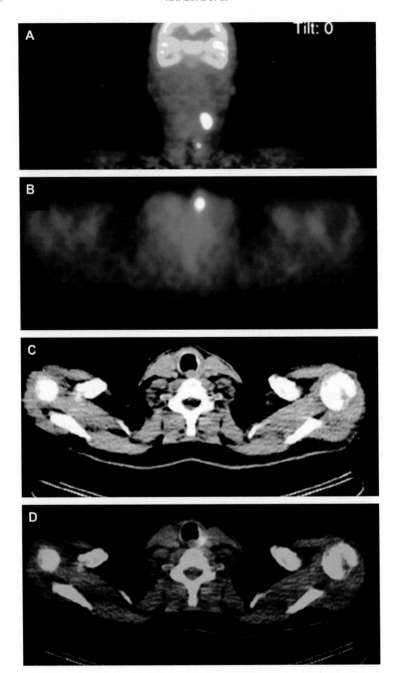

The follow-up interval may be extended to every other year or even longer if there is no evidence of recurrence. Positive results of ultrasound, Tg, or WBS at any point from initial TRA initiate more extensive evaluation.

Treatment of recurrence of differentiated thyroid cancer

In an analysis of 40 years of data, Mazzaferri and Kloos [2] found an overall recurrence rate of approximately 35% in patients who had DTC. Most of these recurrences occurred during the first decade after initial therapy. Local disease accounted for 68% of recurrences and was associated with a mortality rate of only 12%. In comparison, distant metastases (mostly to the lungs) comprised 32% of recurrences and led to a higher mortality rate of 43% [2].

In patients with gross locoregional metastases that are detected either clinically or by imaging, surgical resection is the preferred method of treatment [4,40]; up to half of these patients are disease free after surgery in the short-term [41]. Because imaging studies do not always reveal other smaller lymph node metastases, many surgeons advocate complete ipsilateral compartmental dissection rather than selective lymph node resection [42–45]. Locoregional metastases that are demonstrated on radioiodine scans are also amendable to ^{131}I therapy, which can be given adjunctively after surgery [4]. The ^{131}I therapy dose is determined using either the empiric activity or individualized dosimetry methods [2,4,13]. For patients with locoregional recurrence not detected clinically or by conventional imaging but only evident on ^{131}I WBS, surgery is not an option. These patients are typically treated by ^{131}I therapy alone. In patients who have non–iodine-avid DTC recurrence demonstrated by elevated Tg alone and a negative WBS, some authors advocate empiric ^{131}I therapy on the theory that micrometastases too small to be detected by low-dose WBS may still take up some iodine (such lesions are sometimes seen on posttherapy scans) [46,47]. This strategy is controversial, however, and its efficacy has been questioned [48–50].

Fig. 3. A 58-year-old patient (oxyphilic, follicular, pT3 N0 M0 G2) who underwent total thyroidectomy and TRA 2 years earlier presented with a markedly elevated Tg level but no iodine uptake on WBS. Sonography-guided fine-needle aspiration biopsy of a suspicious cervical lymph node revealed cells suggestive of tumor. Preoperative PET showed intense ^{18}F-FDG uptake in the known left cervical node, as shown on the coronal slice (A). PET also detected a second tumor focus located further caudally. For this second tumor, shown on transverse PET slice (B), no corresponding abnormality could be identified on CT images (C). Only by fusion of PET and CT images (D) could the second lesion be localized precisely (between esophagus and dorsolateral trachea) and removed surgically. Histopathology showed a 5-mm lymph node metastasis. Two years after surgery, the patient had no tumor recurrence. (*From* Palmedo H, Bucerius J, Joe A, et al. Integrated PET/CT in differentiated thyroid cancer: diagnostic accuracy and impact on patient management. J Nucl Med 2006;47(4):621;with permission from the Society of Nuclear Medicine.)

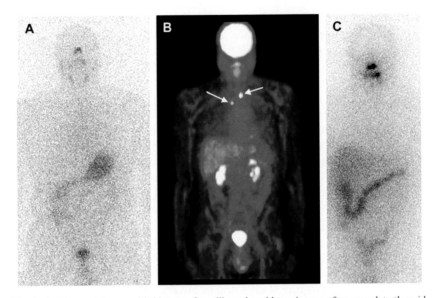

Fig. 4. A 66-year-old man with history of papillary thyroid carcinoma after complete thyroid-ectomy and ^{131}I TRA presented with elevated Tg, which suggested recurrence. (*A*) Anterior WBS performed 24 hours after the oral administration of ^{123}I was normal; however, subsequent neck dissection showed metastatic disease in 13 of 69 nodes. (*B*) A postoperative ^{18}F-FDG PET WBS performed after thyroid hormone withdrawal revealed two hypermetabolic foci in the left upper paratracheal and right paratracheal regions (*white arrows*) compatible with residual met-astatic disease. (The FDG activity in the brain, kidneys, and bladder is normal FDG distribu-tion.) (*C*) The patient was empirically treated with 200 mCi (7400 MBq) [131]I, but the postablation scan is normal, showing that the metastases are not iodine avid.

The most common sites of distant metastases from DTC are the lungs, bone, and central nervous system. For patients with iodine-avid pulmonary metastases, particularly young patients, ^{131}I therapy should be used and repeated as long as there is an objective response; some of these patients may show a complete response [4]. Pulmonary fibrosis is an uncommon side effect of high-dose ^{131}I therapy and may be monitored with serial pul-monary function tests and CT scans. Patients with non–iodine-avid pulmo-nary metastases may have slowly progressive disease. Because no specific therapy has demonstrated significant benefit in these patients, they may be managed conservatively with TSH suppression alone as long as their symp-toms and imaging studies show minimal progression [4].

In patients with iodine-avid bone metastases, ^{131}I therapy should be used because it is associated with prolonged survival [51,52]. In the setting of a single painful osseous metastasis, surgical resection may be able to palliate and improve survival and should be considered [52]. External beam radia-tion may benefit patients with unresectable gross disease or bone metastases that are painful or at risk of fracture [53,54]. In patients with central nervous system metastases, surgical resection is recommended because it can prolong survival [55]. External beam radiation also may benefit patients with central nervous system metastases who are not candidates for surgery [4]. If central nervous system metastases are radioiodine avid, ^{131}I therapy also can be used. Treatment with steroids before ^{131}I therapy is highly recommended to limit inflammation from ^{131}I therapy and the increase in tumor size from TSH stimulation needed for the ^{131}I therapy [56]. These effects can lead to spinal cord or cerebral tissue compression.

Chemotherapy has a limited role in radioiodine-resistant recurrent or metastatic DTC. Single-agent doxorubicin has produced a response in up to 40% of patients, but few durable responses have been described [57]. There is no demonstrable additional benefit of combination therapy [58].

Pediatric thyroid carcinoma

Thyroid cancer in children is rare, accounting for only approximately 1.3% of new pediatric malignancies in the United States [59]. Treatment of juvenile DTC generally follows the same paradigm as DTC treatment in adults; however, several features distinguish juvenile DTC from its adult counterpart. Juvenile DTC tends to present with larger primary tumors and more frequent involvement of neck nodes; there is also more frequent metastatic disease at presentation, almost always to the lungs [60]. Despite these ominous features, however, prognosis for pediatric DTC is good—less than 10% of children and adolescents with thyroid cancer die of their disease [61]. As in adults, the primary treatment is surgical resection, typically with total or near-total thyroidectomy and, frequently, removal of local lymph nodes [60,62]. TRA with ^{131}I is important in children, and it reduces risk of death and local recurrence [61], which reflects the fact that pediatric DTC concentrates iodine more reliably than adult disease and generally responds well to ^{131}I therapy. Successful long-term management of juvenile DTC often can be accomplished with TSH suppression, periodic ^{131}I therapy for metastatic disease, and surgery for resectable local recurrence.

Medullary thyroid carcinoma

MTC is a rare endocrine tumor that originates from C cells of the thyroid. The mainstay of treatment for MTC is surgery, with the goal of complete removal of the primary tumor and any lymph node metastases. Local recurrence is often treated with surgical resection of gross tumor [63,64]. Radioactive iodine is not a treatment option for MTC because thyroid C cells do not concentrate iodine. External beam radiation is sometimes used after surgical resection to improve local control but has not been shown to improve survival [63]. Despite evaluation of multiple chemotherapeutic agents, no effective systemic treatment has been found for patients who have metastatic MTC [63].

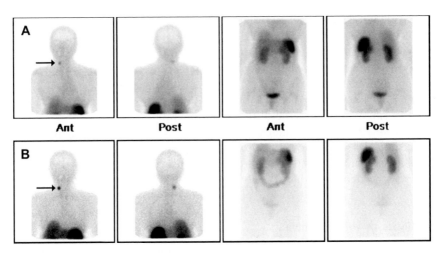

Fig. 5. Somatostatin receptor imaging study performed for a 67-year-old woman with a thyroid lesion. Anterior and posterior images were obtained 4 hours (*A*) and 24 hours (*B*) after intravenous administration of 6 mCi (222 MBq) ^{111}In pentetreotide (OctreoScan). The activity in the spleen, liver, kidneys, and gastrointestinal tract is the normal distribution of the agent. There is distinct focal tracer uptake in the neck just to the right of midline (*arrows*); this pattern is typical of medullary thyroid carcinoma. The thyroid C cells, which give rise to MTC, do not absorb iodine but frequently express somatostatin receptors, which can provide targeting for imaging and potentially for therapeutic agents.

Some MTC cells have somatostatin receptors on their surface, and somatostatin analogs have been evaluated in this disease. Somatostatin analogs inhibit neuroendocrine tumor cell growth by inhibiting the release of growth-promoting hormones, inhibiting angiogenesis, modulating immunologic activity, and exerting direct cytotoxic effects. Somatostatin analog therapy using octreotide has been investigated [63]. Octreotide may improve symptoms in some patients by reducing tumor hormone release, but it has not been shown to reduce tumor mass or improve survival [65]. The radiolabeled somatostatin analog Indium ^{111}In pentetreotide (OctreoScan) is used as an imaging agent to evaluate MTC, particularly metastatic disease (Fig. 5). The performance of OctreoScan in MTC varies; however, the agent has proved to be a valuable adjunct to anatomic imaging [66]. FDG PET is also useful in evaluating MTC. PET has greater sensitivity for MTC than CT, MRI, or other nuclear medicine studies [67]. PET seems to have the greatest accuracy when serum calcitonin exceeds 1000 pg/mL [68].

Because C cells express carcinoembryonic antigen (CEA), anti-CEA antibodies have been investigated as a therapeutic agent. The humanized anti-CEA antibody labetuzumab showed some promise in an early laboratory study but provided limited benefit as part of combination therapy for advanced MTC in a phase-1 trial [69]. Because mutations in the RET proto-oncogene are a component of hereditary MTC, the transmembrane tyrosine-kinase receptor RET product may be a potential treatment target.

Tyrosine-kinase receptor blockade or inhibition has been shown to induce apoptosis in MTC cells. Small molecule tyrosine-kinase inhibitors under study for MTC include ZD6474 (Zactima), sorafenib (Nexavar), sunitinib (Sutent), and imatinib mesylate (Gleevec) [70].

Anaplastic thyroid carcinoma

Because ATC is rare, treatment approaches are not standardized. Complete surgical resection has been shown to confer a survival benefit [71]. Total thyroidectomy and resection of cervical and mediastinal lymph node metastases with a goal of clear margins are justified if they can be accomplished with acceptable morbidity [72]. External beam radiation is the most commonly used form of palliative treatment for ATC [64]. ATC is relatively radioresistant, but radiation sometimes can palliate by preventing local progression of disease. Radiation achieves local control in 68% to 80% of patients; in some patients, external beam radiation combined with surgery or chemotherapy can improve short-term survival [72,73]. Multimodality therapy seems necessary to treat this condition. A common approach is neoadjuvant or adjuvant therapy with combined adriamycin and cisplatin, together with hyperfractionated radiation therapy [71,74].

ATC should be considered a systemic disease, even in patients whose measurable disease is limited to the neck. Chemotherapy agents with significant activity against ATC cell lines include doxorubicin, paclitaxel, vinorelbine, gemcitabine, bleomycin, cyclophosphamide, 5-fluorouracil, cisplatin, and mitoxantrone [71,75]. Monotherapy with doxorubicin demonstrates a response rate of approximately 20%. Combining doxorubicin with cisplatin or bleomycin yields little improvement over doxorubicin alone. The addition of paclitaxel showed some improvement in response but did not improve survival [72].

Additional agents are under study in ATC. Infusional taxol produced short-duration responses in 57% of patients in a phase 2 trial [76]. Because approximately 40% of ATC cases overexpress the epidermal growth factor receptor, it may be a promising target for ATC treatment [77]. In vitro and animal studies have suggested that the epidermal growth factor receptor blocker gefitinib (Iressa) may have potential against ATC [78]. Bortezomib (Velcade), a proteasome inhibitor that blocks the ubiquitin-proteasome pathway, has shown some promise in MTC and ATC cell lines in vitro and may be synergistic with doxorubicin [79].

Summary

Although postoperative treatment options for ATC and MTC are limited, these entities comprise only a small fraction of all thyroid malignancies. For the vast majority of thyroid cancer patients who present with DTC, postoperative management, which exploits DTC's properties of high sensitivity to TSH and avid concentration of iodine can have substantial benefit. A coordinated postoperative management approach that combines initial risk stratification, TRA with ^{131}I, TSH suppression, and periodic surveillance using serum Tg measurement and imaging studies is highly effective in maximizing recurrence-free survival.

Acknowledgments

Preparation of this article was supported by resources and use of facilities of the Veterans Affairs Medical Center, Wilmington, Delaware.

References

[1] Hundahl SA, Fleming ID, Frengen AM, et al. A National Cancer Data Base report on 53,856 cases of thyroid carcinoma treated in the US, 1985-1995. Cancer 1998;83:2638–48.

[2] Mazzaferri EL, Kloos RT. Clinical report 128: current approaches to primary therapy for papillary and follicular thyroid cancer. J Clin Endocrinol Metab 2001;86(4):1447–63.

[3] Sturgeon C, Angelos P. Identification and treatment of aggressive thyroid cancers. Part 2: risk assessment and treatment. Oncology 2006;20(4):397–404.

[4] Cooper DS, Doherty GM, Haugen BR, et al. The American Thyroid Association Guidelines Taskforce. Management guidelines for patients with thyroid nodules and differentiated thyroid cancer. Thyroid 2006;16(2):109–42.

[5] Greene FL, Page DL, Fleming ID, et al, editors. American Joint Committee on Cancer. AJCC cancer staging manual. 6th edition. New York: Springer-Verlag, Inc.; 2002.

[6] Sherman SI, Angelos P, Ball DW, et al. NCCN Thyroid Carcinoma Panel. The NCCN Thyroid Carcinoma Clinical Practice Guidelines in Oncology (Version 2.2007). Available at: http://www.nccn.org. Accessed April 30, 2007.

[7] Hundahl SA, Cady B, Cunningham MP, et al. Initial results from a prospective cohort study of 5583 cases of thyroid carcinoma treated in the United States during 1996. Cancer 2000; 89(1):202–17.

[8] Wu HS, Young MT, Ituarte PH, et al. Death from thyroid cancer of follicular cell origin. J Am Coll Surg 2000;191(6):600–6.

[9] Kovacs GL, Gonda G, Vadasz G, et al. Epidemiology of thyroid microcarcinoma found in autopsy series conducted in areas of different iodine intake. Thyroid 2005;15(2):152–7.

[10] Intenzo CM, Jabbour S, Dam HQ, et al. Changing concepts in the management of differentiated thyroid cancer. Semin Nucl Med 2005;35:257–65.

[11] Ladenson PW, Pacini F, Schlumberger M, et al. Randomized study of remnant ablation using recombinant human TSH versus thyroid hormone withdrawal. The Endocrine Society Abstract S35–1. New Orleans (LA): June 16–19, 2004.

[12] Amdur RJ, Mazzaferri EL. Choosing the activity of I-131 for therapy. In: Amdur RJ, Mazzaferri EL, editors. Essentials of thyroid cancer management. New York: Springer-Verlag, Inc; 2005. p. 169–75.

[13] Van Nostrand D, Atkins F, Yeganeh F, et al. Dosimetrically determined doses of radioiodine for the treatment of metastatic thyroid carcinoma. Thyroid 2002;12:121–34.

[14] US Nuclear Regulatory Commission Regulatory Guide 8.39. Release of patients administered radioactive materials. Washington, DC: U.S. Government Printing Office; 1997.

[15] Amdur RJ, Snyder G, Mazzaferri EL. Requirements for outpatient release following I-131 therapy. In: Amdur RJ, Mazzaferri EL, editors. Essentials of thyroid cancer management. New York: Springer-Verlag, Inc; 2005. p. 177–82.

[16] Van Nostrand D, Aiken M, Atkins F, et al. The utility of radioiodine whole body scans prior to 131-I ablation in patients with well-differentiated thyroid cancer. J Nucl Med 2007; 48(Suppl 2):15P.

[17] Mazzaferri EL. Follow-up of differentiated thyroid cancer using serum thyroglobulin measurements. In: Amdur RJ, Mazzaferri EL, editors. Essentials of thyroid cancer management. New York: Springer-Verlag, Inc; 2005. p. 295–301.

[18] Dam HQ, Lin HC, Kim SM, et al. [131]I therapeutic efficacy is not influenced by stunning after diagnostic whole body scanning. Radiology 2004;232(2):527–33.

[19] Mandel SJ, Shankar LK, Benard F, et al. Superiority of iodine-123 compared with iodine-131 scanning for thyroid remnants in patients with differentiated thyroid cancer. Clin Nucl Med 2001;26(1):6–9.

[20] Ladenson PW, Braverman LE, Mazzaferri EL, et al. Comparison of administration of recombinant human thyrotropin with withdrawal of thyroid hormone for radioactive iodine scanning in patients with thyroid carcinoma. N Engl J Med 1997;337:888–95.

[21] Choi MY, Chung JK, Lee HY, et al. The clinical impact of 18F-FDG PET in papillary thyroid carcinoma with a negative 131I whole body scan: a single-center study of 108 patients. Ann Nucl Med 2006;20(8):547–52.

[22] Schluter B, Bohuslavizki KH, Beyer W, et al. Impact of FDG PET on patients with differentiated thyroid cancer who present with elevated thyroglobulin and negative 131I scan. J Nucl Med 2001;42(1):71–6.

[23] Moog F, Linke R, Manthey N, et al. Influence of thyroid-stimulating hormone levels on uptake of FDG in recurrent and metastatic differentiated thyroid carcinoma. J Nucl Med 2000;41(12):1989–95.

[24] van Tol KM, Jager PL, Piers DA, et al. Better yield of (18)fluorodeoxyglucose-positron emission tomography in patients with metastatic differentiated thyroid carcinoma during thyrotropin stimulation. Thyroid 2002;12(5):381–7.

[25] Petrich T, Borner AR, Otto D, et al. Influence of rhTSH on [(18)F]fluorodeoxyglucose uptake by differentiated thyroid carcinoma. Eur J Nucl Med Mol Imaging 2002;29(5): 641–7, Epub 2002 Feb 27.

[26] Shammas A, Degirmenci B, Mountz JM, et al. 18F-FDG PET/CT in patients with suspected recurrent or metastatic well-differentiated thyroid cancer. J Nucl Med 2007;48(2):221–6, Erratum in: J Nucl Med 2007;48(3):412.

[27] Palmedo H, Bucerius J, Joe A, et al. Integrated PET/CT in differentiated thyroid cancer: diagnostic accuracy and impact on patient management. J Nucl Med 2006;47(4): 616–24.

[28] Zoller M, Kohlfuerst S, Igerc I, et al. Combined PET/CT in the follow-up of differentiated thyroid carcinoma: what is the impact of each modality? Eur J Nucl Med Mol Imaging 2007; 34(4):487–95.

[29] Feine U, Lietzenmayer R, Hanke JP, et al. Fluorine-18-FDG and iodine-131-iodide uptake in thyroid cancer. J Nucl Med 1996;37(9):1468–72.

[30] Feine U, Lietzenmayer R, Hanke JP, et al. [18FDG whole-body PET in differentiated thyroid carcinoma: flipflop in uptake patterns of 18FDG and 131I]. Nuklearmedizin 1995; 34(4):127–34 [in German].

[31] Wang W, Larson SM, Fazzari M, et al. Prognostic value of [18F]fluorodeoxyglucose positron emission tomographic scanning in patients with thyroid cancer. J Clin Endocrinol Metab 2000;85(3):1107–13.

[32] Wang W, Macapinlac H, Larson SM, et al. [18F]-2-fluoro-2-deoxy-D-glucose positron emission tomography localizes residual thyroid cancer in patients with negative diagnostic (131)I whole body scans and elevated serum thyroglobulin levels. J Clin Endocrinol Metab 1999; 84(7):2291–302.

[33] Grunwald F, Schomburg A, Bender H, et al. Fluorine-18 fluorodeoxyglucose positron emission tomography in the follow-up of differentiated thyroid cancer. Eur J Nucl Med 1996; 23(3):312–9.

[34] Mazzaferri EL, Jhiang SM. Long-term impact of initial surgical and medical therapy on papillary and follicular thyroid cancer. Am J Med 1994;97:418–28.

[35] Robbins RJ, Wan Q, Grewal RK, et al. Real-time prognosis for metastatic thyroid carcinoma based on 2-[18F]fluoro-2-deoxy-D-glucose-positron emission tomography scanning. J Clin Endocrinol Metab 2006;91(2):498–505.

[36] Schonberger J, Ruschoff J, Grimm D, et al. Glucose transporter 1 gene expression is related to thyroid neoplasms with an unfavorable prognosis: an immunohistochemical study. Thyroid 2002;12(9):747–54.

[37] Helal BO, Merlet P, Toubert ME, et al. Clinical impact of (18)F-FDG PET in thyroid carcinoma patients with elevated thyroglobulin levels and negative (131)I scanning results after therapy. J Nucl Med 2001;42(10):1464–9.

[38] Wang W, Larson SM, Tuttle RM, et al. Resistance of [18F]-fluorodeoxyglucose-avid metastatic thyroid cancer lesions to treatment with high-dose radioactive iodine. Thyroid 2001; 11(12):1169–75.

[39] Pryma DA, Schoder H, Gonen M, et al. Diagnostic accuracy and prognostic value of 18F-FDG PET in Hurthle cell thyroid cancer patients. J Nucl Med 2006;47(8):1260–6.

[40] Cohen EG, Tuttle M, Kraus DH. Postoperative management of differentiated thyroid cancer. Otolaryngol Clin North Am 2003;36:129–57.

[41] Kloos RT, Mazzaferri EL. A single recombinant human thyrotrophin-stimulated serum thyroglobulin measurement predicts differentiated thyroid carcinoma metastases three to five years later. J Clin Endocrinol Metab 2005;90:5047–57.

[42] Kupferman ME, Patterson DM, Mandel SJ, et al. Safety of modified radical neck dissection for differentiated thyroid carcinoma. Laryngoscope 2004;114:403–6.

[43] Uchino S, Noguchi S, Yamashita H, et al. Modified radical neck dissection for differentiated thyroid cancer: operative technique. World J Surg 2004;28:1199–203.

[44] Noguchi S, Yamashita H, Murakami N, et al. Small carcinomas of the thyroid: a long-term follow-up of 867 patients. Arch Surg 1996;131:187–91.

[45] Marchesi M, Biffoni M, Biancari A, et al. Predictors of outcome for patients with differentiated and aggressive thyroid carcinoma. Eur J Surg Suppl 2003;588:46–50.

[46] Pineda JD, Lee T, Ain K, et al. Iodine-131 therapy for thyroid cancer patients with elevated thyroglobulin and negative scan. J Clin Endocrinol Metab 1995;80:1488–92.

[47] Clark OH, Hoelting T. Management of patients with differentiated thyroid cancer who have positive thyroglobulin levels and negative radioiodine scans. Thyroid 1994;4:501–5.

[48] McDougall IR. I-131 treatment of I-131 negative whole body scan, and positive thyroglobulin in differentiated thyroid carcinoma: what is being treated? Thyroid 1997; 7:69–72.

[49] Mazzaferri EL. Treating high thyroglobulin with radioiodine: a magic bullet or a shot in the dark? J Clin Endocrinol Metab 1995;80:1485–7.

[50] Fatourechi V, Hay ID. Treating the patient with differentiated thyroid cancer with thyroglobulin-positive iodine-131 diagnostic scan-negative metastases: including comments on the role of serum thyroglobulin monitoring in tumor surveillance. Semin Nucl Med 2000; 30:107–14.

[51] Bernier MO, Leenhardt L, Hoang C, et al. Survival and therapeutic modalities in patients with bone metastases of differentiated thyroid carcinomas. J Clin Endocrinol Metab 2001; 86:1568–73.

[52] Schlumberger M, Challeton C, De Vathaire F, et al. Radioactive iodine treatment and external radiotherapy for lung and bone metastases from thyroid carcinoma. J Nucl Med 1996;37: 598–605.

[53] Tsang RW, Brierley JD, Simpson WJ, et al. The effects of surgery, radioiodine, and external radiation therapy on the clinical outcome of patients with differentiated thyroid carcinoma. Cancer 1998;82:375–88.

[54] Brierley JD, Tsang RW. External-beam radiation therapy in the treatment of differentiated thyroid cancer. Semin Surg Oncol 1999;16:42–9.

[55] Chiu AC, Delpassand ES, Sherman SI. Prognosis and treatment of brain metastases in thyroid carcinoma. J Clin Endocrinol Metab 1997;84:3867–71.

[56] Luster M, Lippi F, Jarzab B, et al. rhTSH-aided radioiodine ablation and treatment of differentiated thyroid carcinoma: a comprehensive review. Endocr Relat Cancer 2005;12:49–64.

[57] Gottlieb JA, Hill CS Jr, Ibanez ML, et al. Chemotherapy of thyroid cancer: an evaluation of experience with 37 patients. Cancer 1992;30:848–53.

[58] Haugen BR. Management of the patients with progressive radioiodine non-responsive disease. Semin Surg Oncol 1999;16:34–41.

[59] Miller RW, Young JL, Novakovic B. Childhood cancer. Cancer 1995;75:177–783.

[60] Jarzab B, Handkiewicz-Junak D, Wloch J. Juvenile differentiated thyroid carcinoma and the role of radioiodine in its management: a qualitative review. Endocr Relat Cancer 2005;12: 773–803.

[61] Bauer AJ, Poth M. Papillary cancer: special aspects in children. In: Wartofsky L, VanNostrand D, editors. Thyroid cancer: a comprehensive guide to clinical management. 2nd edition. Totowa (NJ): Humana Press; 2006. p. 377–86.

[62] Hung W, Sarlis NJ. Current controversies in the management of pediatric patients with well-differentiated nonmedullary thyroid cancer: a review. Thyroid 2002;12:683–702.

[63] Moley JF, Fialkowski EA. Evidence-based approach to the management of sporadic medullary thyroid carcinoma. World J Surg 2007;31:946–56.

[64] Nix PA, Nicolaides A, Coatesworth AP. Thyroid cancer review 3: management of medullary and undifferentiated thyroid cancer. Int J Clin Pract 2006;60(1):80–4.

[65] Cohen R, Quidville V, Bihan H. Medullary carcinoma and hormones. Ann Med Interne 2003;154(2):109–16.

[66] Esposito G. Radionuclide imaging of medullary carcinoma. In: Wartofsky L, VanNostrand D, editors. Thyroid cancer: a comprehensive guide to clinical management. 2nd edition. Totowa (NJ): Humana Press; 2006. p. 597–602.

[67] Diehl M, Risse JH, Brandt-Mainz K, et al. Fluorine-18 fluorodeoxyglucose positron emission tomography in medullary thyroid cancer: results of a multicentre study. Eur J Nucl Med 2001;28(11):1671–6.

[68] Ong SC, Schoder H, Patel SG, et al. Diagnostic accuracy of 18F-FDG PET in restaging patients with medullary thyroid carcinoma and elevated calcitonin levels. J Nucl Med 2007;48(4):501–7.

[69] Sharkey RM, Hajjar G, Yeldell D, et al. A phase I trial combining high-dose 90Y-labelled humanized anti-CEA monoclonal antibody with doxorubicin and peripheral blood stem-cell rescue in advanced medullary thyroid cancer. J Nucl Med 2005;46:620–33.

[70] Ball DW. Medullary thyroid cancer: therapeutic targets and molecular markers. Curr Opin Oncol 2007;1:18–23.

[71] Veness MJ, Porter GS, Morgan GJ. Anaplastic thyroid carcinoma: dismal outcome despite current treatment approach. Aust N Z J Surg 2004;74:559–62.

[72] Patel KN, Shaha AR. Poorly differentiated and anaplastic thyroid cancer. Cancer Control 2006;13(2):119–28.

[73] Haigh PI, Ituarte PH, Wu HS, et al. Completely resected anaplastic thyroid carcinoma combined with adjuvant chemotherapy and irradiation is associated with prolonged survival. Cancer 2001;91:2335–42.

[74] Chang HS, Nam KH, Chung WY, et al. Anaplastic thyroid carcinoma: a therapeutic dilemma. Yonsei Med J 2005;46(6):759–64.

[75] Voigt W, Kegel T, Weis M, et al. Potential activity of paclitaxel, vinorelbine and gemcitabine in anaplastic thyroid carcinoma. J Cancer Res Clin Oncol 2005;131:585–90.

[76] Ain KB, Egorin MJ, DeSimone PA. Treatment of anaplastic thyroid carcinoma with paclitaxel: phase 2 trial using ninety-six hour infusion: Collaborative Anaplastic Thyroid Cancer Health Intervention Trials (CATCHIT) Group. Thyroid 2000;10:587–94.

[77] Ensinger C, Spizzo G, Moser P, et al. Epidermal growth factor receptor as a novel therapeutic target in anaplastic thyroid carcinomas. Ann N Y Acad Sci 2004;1030:69–77.

[78] Schiff BA, McMurphy AB, Jassar SA, et al. Epidermal growth factor receptor (EGFR) is overexpressed in anaplastic thyroid cancer, and the EGFR inhibitor gefitinib inhibits the growth of anaplastic thyroid cancer. Clin Cancer Res 2004;10:8594–602.
[79] Mitsiades CS, McMillin D, Kotoula V, et al. Antitumor effects of the proteasome inhibitor bortezomib in medullary and anaplastic thyroid carcinoma cells in vitro. J Clin Endocrinol Metab 2006;91:4013–21.

ELSEVIER
SAUNDERS

Surg Oncol Clin N Am
17 (2008) 219–232

SURGICAL
ONCOLOGY CLINICS
OF NORTH AMERICA

The Role of Radiation Therapy in the Management of Thyroid Cancer

Jon F. Strasser, MD, Adam Raben, MD*,
Chris Koprowski, MD

Department of Radiation Oncology, Helen F. Graham Cancer Center, Christiana Care Health Systems, 4701 Ogletown-Stanton Rd, Newark, DE 19713, USA

Malignancies of the thyroid comprise a broad array of neoplasms, with different natural histories and treatments. Although papillary carcinomas tend to behave indolently, are amenable to multiple forms of therapy, and frequently may be managed like chronic disease, anaplastic tumors are aggressive and often incurable, even with multimodality treatment. External beam radiotherapy (EBRT) plays a limited but important role in the management of thyroid carcinomas. This article discusses the role of modern external beam radiation in the management of this diverse class of tumors.

Well-differentiated malignancies: papillary, follicular thyroid cancer, Hürthle cell carcinoma

Treatment of thyroid cancer depends on the histology of the neoplasm, extent of surgical resection, and presence of high-risk features. Surgical management and histology are discussed elsewhere in this issue. Histologic classification is relevant for the use of radiation therapy, however. Well-differentiated tumors include papillary tumors, which comprise approximately 70% to 80% of thyroid tumors, follicular tumors, which comprise approximately 10% of thyroid malignancies, and Hürthle cell tumors, which comprise 2% to 3% of thyroid malignancies [1]. These malignancies have similar natural histories and similarly concentrate iodine and recur locally and distantly with similar frequencies.

Surgical management of thyroid cancer remains the primary modality in diagnosis and therapy of thyroid cancer. In situations in which surgery is

* Corresponding author.
E-mail address: araben@christianacare.org (A. Raben).

1055-3207/08/$ - see front matter © 2008 Elsevier Inc. All rights reserved.
doi:10.1016/j.soc.2007.10.005

not possible, gross total removal is not feasible, or microscopic residual disease remains, however, other modalities help to reduce local and distant failures. Although adjuvant radioiodine ablation is considered standard in well-differentiated cancers and has a demonstrated role in eradicating residual normal thyroid gland and residual tumor, the role of EBRT after radioiodine remains somewhat controversial. Many studies in the literature address this topic; however, the retrospective nature of these studies limits the ability to draw definitive conclusions, even when comparing directly patients who receive radioiodine alone with patients who also received EBRT. Because most patients referred for EBRT present with unfavorable clinical characteristics, it is difficult to draw firm inferences if no clear-cut benefit is demonstrated. Equivalency in both groups may suggest a benefit to the addition of external beam, given the poorer prognosis of these individuals.

Sheline and colleagues [2] reported one of the earliest experiences with EBRT for thyroid malignancies. This retrospective series of well-differentiated thyroid cancer evaluated the role of 30- to 50-Gy external beam irradiation administered to 58 patients treated from 1935 to 1964 without radioiodine ablation. Follow-up in this series ranged from 2 to 14 years. Of the 58 patients treated in this series, 44 patients underwent surgery, with 25 having residual microscopic disease and 19 having gross residual tumor. Fourteen patients were unresectable at presentation. Even with potentially suboptimal radiation therapy doses, they noted complete responses in several patients with gross residual disease postoperatively, which suggested a potential role of EBRT in controlling gross residual and microscopic disease.

O'Connell and colleagues [3] reported on the Royal Marsden experience of 113 patients with well-differentiated thyroid carcinoma treated from 1969 to 1991 with a median follow-up of 49 months. Patients received an EBRT dose of 60 Gy in 30 fractions to the thyroid, both necks, and upper mediastinum. Seventy-four patients received radioiodine, and all had a suppressive dose of thyroid hormone. In patients with probable or definitive microscopic residual disease ($n = 53$), the local recurrence rate was 19%; in patients with gross residual disease ($n = 49$), 37.5% had a complete regression of tumor and 25% had a partial regression of disease. Overall survival rate at 5 years was 85% for patients with residual microscopic disease but 27% for patients with gross disease. Of note, one third of all patients who died in this series died of nonthyroid cancer causes.

One of the largest series that evaluated the role of adjuvant EBRT is from Canada. Simpson and colleagues [4] reviewed the Canadian experience of 1578 patients with papillary and follicular thyroid cancers. Surgical resection was performed in most patients, and EBRT ($n = 201$), radioactive iodine ablation ($n = 214$), or both ($n = 107$) were used in patients who were deemed high risk based on previously identified high-risk prognostic factors [5]. In patients with no residual disease, there was no benefit to any adjuvant radiation, either external or radioiodine. In patients who had papillary histology and microscopic residual disease (margins within 2 mm) or gross residual disease, however, adjuvant treatment with any radiation technique significantly improved local control from 82% to 90%, compared with surgery and hormone suppression alone (26%; $P = .00001$). In patients who had follicular histology there was a trend of a benefit to adjuvant radiation on local control: 53% to 77% versus 38% ($P = .079$).

Another large series from France evaluated 539 patients who had differentiated thyroid cancer that was treated before 1976. Tubiana and colleagues [6] reported results in 97 patients with incomplete surgical resection treated with EBRT. Local recurrence rates at 15 years with adequate radiotherapy doses (defined as 50 Gy or more) were 11% versus 23% treated without radiation. This study also demonstrated a dose response effect on local recurrence with doses more than 50 Gy: 10% versus 15%.

Several smaller series have examined the role of additional radiotherapy after iodine ablation. Mazzaferri and colleagues [7] looked at a set of 576 patients, in which 28 patients were treated with EBRT. Although most tumors were small (<1.5 cm) with no extrathyroid extension, 75% of patients had lymph node involvement. Radiation doses of 10 to 70 Gy were used; however, only 5 patients had doses of 50 to 70 Gy. As expected (given the radiation details), no benefit for external radiotherapy was identified; however, there seemed to be a higher rate of recurrence in patients treated (16.7% versus 2.3%). The small sample size and potential biases (ie, patients who had EBRT may have had unfavorable prognostic factors) could easily explain the controversial results. Benker and colleagues [8] also reported on 932 patients with follicular and papillary thyroid cancer treated in Germany between 1970 and 1986. EBRT to a dose of 40 to 60 Gy was delivered to 346 patients and failed to show a significant benefit to radiotherapy on survival; however, there was a trend toward significance in older patients (48% versus 58%; $P = .09$). Of note, almost two thirds of patients in this series had T1 or T2 disease, which diluted the potential overall benefit.

More recent series looking at high-risk patients suggested an advantage to EBRT with radioiodine. Farahati [9] updated the German experience looking at 238 patients with differentiated papillary and follicular thyroid cancer treated between 1979 and 1992 with pathologic T4 disease. One hundred sixty-nine patients received surgery, radioiodine, and TSH suppression, of whom 99 received external radiation to doses of 50 to 60 Gy. External radiation was identified as a predictive factor for improvement of local recurrence ($P = .004$) and locoregional and distant failure ($P = .0003$). Subgroup analysis demonstrated that the effects of radiotherapy on time to locoregional and distant failure were significant in patients with papillary histology, lymph node involvement, and age older than 40.

Tsang and colleagues [10] reported on the Princess Margaret experience of 382 patients treated with surgery, radioiodine, and EBRT in 262 patients with papillary cancer and 120 patients with follicular cancer treated from

1958 to 1985. With a median follow-up of 10.8 years, 155 patients with papillary histology and microscopic residuum had a better 10-year cause-specific
survival rate (100% versus 95%; $P = .038$) and local relapse-free rate (93%
versus 78%; $P = .01$). Multivariate analysis demonstrated that age older
than 60, tumor size larger than 4 cm, multifocality, postoperative residuum,
lymph node involvement, less extensive surgery (less than near-total thyroidectomy), and lack of use of radioiodine were significant factors for local
failure.

Chow and colleagues [11] reviewed the Hong Kong experience of 842 patients who had papillary thyroid cancer treated at Queen's Hospital from
1960 to 1997 with a mean follow-up of 9.2 years (10 EBRT was delivered
to 105 patients. EBRT was effective at controlling residual disease in patients with gross postoperative neck disease, with a 10-year local control
rate in EBRT (56.2%) versus no radiotherapy (24%) ($P \le .001$). There
was no survival benefit to radiotherapy, as in prior studies. Although
EBRT was associated with an overall worse prognosis on multivariable
analysis in this study, as was advancing age, locoregional residual disease,
distant metastases, and absence of radioiodine ablation, EBRT was only
given to patients with advanced disease, which confounded the analysis.

Numerous risk factors in well-differentiated thyroid cancer have been evaluated for significance on local control and survival. Tsang and colleagues
identified several factors for local recurrence. Passler and colleagues [12] found
similar results, demonstrating age older than 45, positive lymph nodes, and increasing tumor size to be associated with poor prognosis. Other groups have
looked at histologic vascular invasion and tumor capsular invasion, which
have been shown not to be adverse prognostic factors for local recurrence
or survival [13,14]. Shaha and colleagues [15] retrospectively reviewed 1038
patients with well-differentiated thyroid cancer treated at Memorial Sloan-
Kettering Cancer Center from 1930 to 1985 with a mean follow-up of 20 years.
This analysis identified advancing age (>45), presence of distant metastases,
extrathyroidal extension, size larger than 4 cm, and high grade to be associated
with poor prognosis. They identified risk criteria associated with significant
decrements in survival. Persons in the low-risk category had a 20-year overall
survival rate of 99%, whereas persons in intermediate and high-risk categories
had survival rates of 87% and 46%, respectively.

The role of EBRT in papillary and follicular thyroid cancer remains controversial. Although the literature demonstrates mixed success, it is difficult
to draw conclusions from individual studies because of the retrospective
nature and inherent biases of these trials. The role of external radiation
therapy in these differentiated cancers should be individualized on a case-
by-case basis. In practice, patients who have favorable cancers and have
undergone complete surgical resection and radioiodine ablation with no
evidence of residual uptake likely do not benefit from external radiotherapy;
standard practice is to not treat these patients. Lymph node involvement by
itself does not necessarily increase the local recurrence risk. In patients with

bulky gross residual disease, it is unlikely that radioiodine ablation would be completely effective, and adjuvant EBRT is indicated. The previous data from Sheline [2], O'Connell [3], Simpson [4], Tubiana [6], Tsang [10], and Chow [11] demonstrate a role for postoperative radiotherapy in improving local control.

In patients with microscopic residual disease, the role of adjuvant EBRT is less certain and limits the ability to draw accurate conclusions with the data presented. Data from Princess Margaret Hospital suggest that high-risk patients seem to derive the most benefit from treatment [10]. Many studies have suggested possible high-risk features, including increasing age, large tumors, multifocal disease, clear postoperative residuum, nodal involvement, and lack of radioiodine, to be significant [5,11–15]. The role of EBRT can only be elucidated clearly in a prospective, randomized trial controlling for each variable. In the absence of such data, however, one needs to weigh these features and risk of recurrence with the potential side effects of treatment.

At our institution, we consider EBRT after radioiodine ablation in patients older than age 45 with probable or definite microscopic disease (<2-mm margins) or invasion into surrounding structures, such as the trachea, in which a clean surgical margin after thyroidectomy is not feasible or in recurrent disease that shows no iodine uptake. In patients with extensive nodal involvement with high-risk features, such as advanced age, multifocal disease, or large tumor, we also consider adding adjuvant external radiation therapy after radioiodine ablation in a multidisciplinary format. In patients with unresectable disease, we recommend EBRT along with radioiodine ablation if there is uptake. Patients who have Hürthle cell carcinoma, which is considered to be a variant of follicular carcinoma, tend to have worse prognoses than patients with standard well-differentiated tumors, probably because of their low radioiodine uptake. These patients are treated in a similar fashion to patients with well-differentiated histologies. These recommendations are similar to the National Comprehensive Cancer Network guidelines. In the postoperative setting we recommend a dose of 45 to 50 Gy for microscopic disease and 54 to 60 Gy for gross residual disease using three-dimensional conformal radiation therapy or intensity-modulated radiation therapy (IMRT) with image-guided radiation therapy.

Medullary thyroid carcinoma

Medullary thyroid cancer represents a small subset of thyroid cancer arising from the parafolliclular C cells of the thyroid gland. This variant can arise sporadically within the gland or in familial lines because of genetic aberrations associated with type II multiple endocrine neoplasia. Medullary thyroid cancers have a relatively high propensity for nodal involvement (approximately 40%) [16]. Although C cells are not iodine concentrating, radioiodine has been used postoperatively in local disease because residual follicular cells can absorb iodine and theoretically radiate the neighboring C cells [17,18]. As is the case with well-differentiated histologies, complete surgical extirpation remains the standard treatment, and the limited data on adjuvant EBRT are retrospective in nature and controversial.

Several early retrospective reviews suggested a role for EBRT in medullary thyroid carcinoma [19–21]. In the late 1980s, Samaan and colleagues [22] published an MD Anderson experience of 202 patients with medullary thyroid cancer treated from 1943 to 1987. In their analysis, they matched patients who received EBRT to those who did not receive EBRT by age, extent of disease, and surgery and found that patients who had radiotherapy had a worse survival ($P < .05$). In comparison, Fife and colleagues [23] published a report on a cohort of patients who received 60 Gy of conventional fractionated external radiotherapy and found an improvement in local control on univariate analysis, with 100% local control at 5 years in the absence of residual disease, dropping to 65% with microscopic residual disease and 24% with gross disease.

Rougier and colleagues [24] reviewed the Institut Gustave-Roussy experience of 75 patients treated from 1932 to 1979. Six patients were treated with definitive radiotherapy for inoperable disease, and 29 patients had surgery and external radiotherapy for high-risk features (eg, residual disease or cervical lymph node involvement). Although these 29 patients had more extensive local disease than 27 patients in the study treated with surgery alone, the patients who received radiation therapy had a slightly better survival than patients treated with surgery alone ($P < .05$), which suggested a benefit to adjuvant EBRT in eradicating small foci of residual disease. Of 6 patients with inoperable disease, 4 remained in clinical remission with 4 years of follow-up.

Fifty-nine patients with medullary thyroid cancer treated with postoperative radiation therapy between 1971 and 1989 at the Institut Jean-Gordinot in France were reported by Nguyen and colleagues [25]. Most patients had a total thyroidectomy (55/59); however, 11 patients had residual disease, and 44 patients had involved cervical lymph nodes. Patients received 54 Gy of radiation therapy to the whole neck and upper mediastinum, with a reported local control rate of 70%.

Brierly and colleagues [26] reported a similar improvement in local control with the use of EBRT in the Princess Margaret series of 73 patients with medullary thyroid cancer treated from 1954 to 1992. Three quarters of patients had lymph node involvement, 56% had extraglandular extension, and 41 underwent near total thyroidectomy. Forty-six patients received radiation therapy to a median dose of 40 Gy (range 20–75.5 Gy). Multivariate analysis for cause-specific survival demonstrated extraglandular invasion and postoperative gross residual disease to be negative prognostic factors. Overall, there was no benefit to radiation, but on a subgroup analysis of 40 patients with high-risk features (ie, microscopic residual disease, extraglandular invasion, or lymph node involvement), patients who received radiation ($n = 25$) had a local/regional relapse-free rate of 86% at 10 years, compared with 52% in patients who had no radiation ($n = 15$) ($P = .049$).

Similar to well-differentiated cancers, the data on medullary thyroid cancers are retrospective and controversial. The preponderance of the data suggests that adjuvant radiation is potentially capable of sterilizing microscopic and gross disease and improving local control [19–21,23–26]. Unfortunately, many patients present with advanced disease because of the early metastatic involvement of regional nodes and likely have occult metastatic systemic disease, which limits the benefit of radiotherapy. In the absence of a prospective, randomized trial, our institutional bias is to proceed with surgical resection and lymph node dissection and systemic staging with imaging (CT/MRI) and serum calcitonin measurements. In patients with no evidence of systemic metastasis but microscopic residual, extrathyroidal extension (T4), or lymph node metastases, we recommend postoperative radiation therapy to the locoregional bed to a dose of 45 to 50 Gy. In patients with gross residual disease or inoperable disease, we recommend a dose of 45 to 50 Gy to sites of microscopic disease and 54 to 60 Gy to sites of gross involvement. The logistics of EBRT are similar for patients with well-differentiated tumors, using either three-dimensional conformal radiation therapy or IMRT/image-guided radiation therapy.

Anaplastic carcinoma

Anaplastic carcinoma of the thyroid gland is an uncommon but extremely aggressive variant of thyroid cancer. Approximately 2% of patients with thyroid cancer have this histology, with half of patients presenting with systemic metastases, and median survival even with aggressive treatment is often limited to months [27]. Although surgery is the initial first line of therapy, only a minority are ever surgically approachable. In patients eligible for surgery, the local recurrence rate is high, and the 5-year survival rate for all patients is less than 10%, with median survivals of 2 to 12 months [28–40]. Surgery remains important in multimodality management, with adjuvant doxorubicin-based chemotherapy and radiation therapy being used to improve on this poor prognosis [38,39]. Although radical resection over a more limited surgery does not seem to improve on outcomes, patients who have surgery have better outcomes [29,30,40].

Levendag and colleagues [28] retrospectively reviewed the outcomes of 51 patients with anaplastic thyroid cancer who were treated from 1970 to 1986 in the Netherlands with EBRT. Most patients died within 1 year, with almost half presenting with distant metastasis. In patients who had no residual disease at the end of treatment, the median survival was 8 months; however, in patients who had residual local regional disease, the median survival was 1.6 months, and all patients died within 8 months. The outcomes of 91 patients treated with surgery and radiation therapy from 1961 to 1986 in

Glasgow demonstrated that surgery improved local control rates to 39%; however, the 2-year survival rate was still only 11% [33].

Kim and colleagues [39] published on the prospective Memorial Sloan-Kettering Cancer Center experience of 41 patients treated from 1979 to 1989 with sensitizing doxorubicin and radiation therapy. Nineteen patients had spindle or anaplastic histologies, which were treated with a combination of low-dose (10 mg/m^2) doxorubicin-based chemotherapy and concurrent hyperfractionated EBRT to a dose of 57.6 Gy (1.6 Gy twice daily for 3 days per week). Initial response rates and local control at 2 years were 84% and 68%, respectively. Median survival was 1 year, with most patients developing and succumbing to distant metastatic disease. The only patients who had survivals longer than 1 year had radical surgery with minimal residual disease before commencing chemoradiotherapy.

The Swedish experience examined multimodality treatment with surgery, hyperfractionated radiation therapy, and concurrent doxorubicin in 55 patients treated between 1984 and 1999 with daily hyperfractionated radiation therapy on three protocols [38]. In the first arm (patients treated from 1984–1988), patients received 30 Gy of preoperative chemoradiotherapy using 1 Gy twice-daily fractionation, with an additional 16 Gy given postoperatively with a similar fractionation. In the second arm (patients from 1989–1992), patients received 30 Gy of preoperative chemoradiotherapy using 1.3 Gy twice-daily fractionation, with an additional 16 Gy given postoperatively with a similar fractionation. From 1992 onward, patients received preoperative chemoradiotherapy to 46 Gy using 1.6 Gy twice-daily fractionation. Weekly doxorubicin at 20 mg/m^2 was delivered during radiation therapy. Forty patients were ultimately surgically resectable. Overall, local failure occurred in 24% of patients. In patients who underwent surgery, local control was seen in 56% of the first arm, 79% of the second arm, and 100% of the third arm ($P = .005$). Only 9% of patients lived more than 2 years, however, which demonstrated the high rate of distant metastatic disease.

Heron and colleagues [27] reviewed the Pittsburgh experience of 32 patients treated from 1952 to 1999 who received hyperfractionated chemoradiotherapy. Nine patients treated from 1952 to 1980 received once-daily radiotherapy without chemotherapy, and 23 patients treated from 1981 to 1999 received twice-daily radiotherapy and chemotherapy. Various radiotherapy techniques and chemotherapy regimens (doxorubicin, palliate, incrusting, capsulation) were used in this subgroup, which limited the conclusions. Overall survival rates for the two groups were 44% and 52%, respectively; however, progression-free survival was worse in the twice-daily concurrent regimen: 53% versus 38%. Ten patients survived longer than 10 years.

Prognostic factors in this disease have been evaluated in many series [28–40]. Kebebew and colleagues [36] analyzed prognostic factors and treatment outcomes from the SEER database. They identified 517 patients treated between 1973 and 2000. Multivariable modeling demonstrated that age less than 60, tumor confined to the thyroid, and the combined use of surgery and EBRT were identified as independent predictors of lower cause-specific mortality. Given the continued poor outcomes in this disease and high rates of distant and local recurrence, continued management with multimodality treatment with surgery, chemotherapy, and radiation therapy is considered standard of care. At our institution we recommend doxorubicin-based chemotherapy with daily radiation therapy to doses of 60 Gy with three-dimensional conformal radiotherapy or IMRT. Care is taken to keep critical tissues, such as the spinal cord, within their tolerances. Further progress must be made on randomized trials to evaluate more intensive radiation and chemotherapy regimens.

Techniques of radiotherapy

The last decade has brought significant paradigm changes in how EBRT is delivered. Up until the early 1990s, radiation therapy was delivered with two-dimensional treatment planning, using fluoroscopy to identify bony landmarks. With the widespread availability of CT, radiation therapy planning went from two-dimensional bony anatomic imaging to three-dimensional soft-tissue anatomic imaging, which allowed for more accurate field delineation based on actual structures, including surgical beds, lymph node beds, and normal critical structures and facilitated three-dimensional conformal planning (three-dimensional conformal radiation therapy). Over the last decade, the treatment planning systems and delivery systems have become more sophisticated. With the proliferation of multi-leaf collimation systems, radiation fluences could be developed to deliver highly conformal radiation beams with varying intensities. This technique is called IMRT, which allows for dose shaping around critical structures (ie, spinal cord, parotid gland), with convex and concave isodose distributions (Fig. 1). With IMRT, crucial structures, such as the spinal cord and parotid glands, can be physically adjacent to a high-dose region and yet only receive a small fraction of the dose because of the steep drop off of the dose gradient.

For the last 5 years, treatment delivery units have had capabilities of on-board imaging using orthogonal kilovoltage radiographs for daily portal imaging and for kilovoltage cone beam imaging. Some linear accelerators are able to use the primary radiation beam to generate a CT quality image using megavoltage radiation. The ability to do daily imaging for localization and guidance in a real-time setting allows for precise daily set up, otherwise called image-guided radiation therapy. Set up and positioning errors can be virtually eliminated, leaving organ motion as the only uncertainty in radiation treatment delivery. This process allows for safety in the delivery of highly focused radiation treatments with IMRT, ensuring that the target receives the dose prescribed to it. It also ensures that set-up error is eliminated,

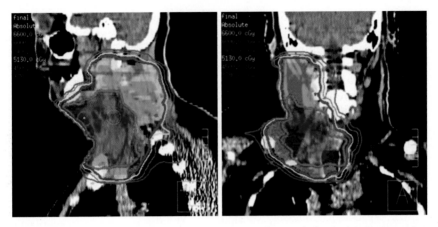

Fig. 1. IMRT plan on a patient with high-risk features after surgical resection. Isodose color-wash shows concurrent differential dose distributions with tight dose gradients to spare normal tissue.

which reduces the chance that a critical structure, such as the spinal cord, will fall within the high-dose gradient.

For the most part, radiation is delivered to the primary tumor bed and regional lymphatics to a dose of 45 to 60 Gy, depending on the pathologic findings and degree of resection. Treatments are delivered in 1.8 to 2.0 Gy per fraction, once a day, 5 days per week. Dose to the spinal cord is generally kept below 45 Gy. With three-dimensional conformal treatment, the dose is frequently delivered with an anterior posterior/posterior anterior portal arrangement, with an off cord boost delivered with oblique fields occurring at approximately 40 Gy.

With IMRT, there are no standard radiation portals. Using CT-based planning, targets, including the primary tumor, postoperative bed, and regional lymphatics, are identified on the treatment planning system. Critical structures, such as the spinal cord and parotid glands, are also identified on the planning system. Dose limits are input to the system for the target (45–60 Gy) and to limit the spinal cord to 45 Gy and the mean parotid dose to less than 26 Gy to limit long-term xerostomia [41]. The treatment planning system determines the appropriate fluence from multiple gantry angles, typically a combination of anterior posterior/posterior anterior, lateral, and oblique fields, to achieve an adequate dose distribution. To achieve adequate coverage, the plan depends on the physician carefully contouring out all structures in the planning system to avoid geographic misses. With IMRT, differential dose painting to treat the primary tumor to a higher dose than the lymphatics is possible either with consecutive boosts or a simultaneous integrated boost that delivers a slightly different daily dose to the respective sites (ie, 1.7–2.1 Gy/d).

Head and neck cancers are an ideal site for IMRT because numerous critical tissues are unable to tolerate the high doses of radiation needed to eradicate a tumor. The critical issues in IMRT/image-guided radiation therapy treatment delivery are consistent, reproducible immobilization and accurate delineation and identification of high-risk volumes of interest and critical structures. Because there is little organ motion (other than swallowing), precise treatments can be delivered to head and neck structures with relative safety and minimal error.

Side effects of radiotherapy

Radiation side effects can be classified as acute effects, which occur during or within the first few months of completion of treatment, or late effects, which occur months to years after treatment. Toxicities are amplified in the setting of concurrent treatments, such as with adriamycin use in anaplastic tumors. In general, side effects are limited to tissues irradiated, with the exception of fatigue. Acute effects tend to resolve within 2 to 4 weeks of treatment. If only the thyroid bed is irradiated, patients can get acute skin erythema, hyperpigmentation or desquamative changes, esophagitis, tracheitis, laryngitis, and a low risk of Lhermitte's syndrome. When patients are also irradiated to the neck because of nodal risks, the acute side effects also can include acute mucositis within the pharynx and irradiated oral mucosa, xerostomia (if the upper necks are irradiated), alopecia, and acute pneumonitis.

Over the long-term, patients are at increased risk of permanent skin discoloration or sensitivity, telangiectasias, low risk of skin necrosis, esophageal strictures, chronic laryngeal edema, chronic xerostomia, permanent alopecia, scarring of the neck musculature, early atherosclerotic changes to blood vessels, chronic scarring of the apices of the lungs, and a low risk of injury to the spinal cord (when doses in excess of 45–50 Gy are used).

To reduce acute and long-term toxicities and improve patient quality of life, many investigators are evaluating the role of pharmacologic modulators, including ethyol (MedImmune) and palifermin (Amgen), and more conformal treatment delivery techniques. Ethyol is a scavenger of oxygen-derived free radicals and a hydrogen donor, capable of reducing acute DNA damage from radiation therapy. It is perhaps the most widely used radioprotectant to reduce the acute and late risks of xerostomia. In the head and neck literature, data from multiple trials, including prospective, randomized trials, demonstrated a significant improvement in late xerostomia without any detriment to local control or survival [42–45]. Palifermin, a keratinocyte growth factor, is a new agent currently under investigation as a protectant against mucositis. Results from the bone marrow transplant literature suggest that palifermin can reduce the duration and severity of acute mucositis in patients undergoing high-dose chemotherapy for transplantation, and it is approved by the US Food and Drug Administration for this use [46]. Several ongoing randomized trials are investigating the effectiveness of palifermin in reducing acute radiation mucositis and whether it offers any tumor protection.

IMRT and image-guided radiation therapy have been widely accepted in the head and neck radiation armamentarium. These techniques allow more precise shaping of radiation fields, potentially sparing critical normal tissues from high doses of radiation therapy. In particular, IMRT can allow for sparing of parotid gland and the spinal cord from receiving potentially injurious doses of radiation therapy while allowing the high-risk sites to receive adequate doses of radiation that are capable of sterilizing microscopic or gross disease. These are complicated techniques for delivery, and a center should have experience in this technology before making these their standard modalities.

Summary

Malignancies of the thyroid represent a diverse range of neoplasms. Surgery is the mainstay of management, but patients are treated in a multimodality fashion, which may include surgery, radioiodine ablation, EBRT, and chemotherapy. In well-differentiated malignancies and medullary thyroid cancer, the published data are controversial because of their retrospective nature, but most studies support some benefit for adjuvant EBRT to improve local control in selected patients. In anaplastic thyroid cancer, multimodality management with EBRT is standard, but overall outcomes remain poor.

References

[1] Goldman ND, Coniglio JU, Falk SA. Thyroid cancers. I. Papillary, follicular, and Hürthle cell. Otolaryngol Clin North Am 1996;29(4):593–609.

[2] Sheline GE. Radiation therapy in the control of persistent thyroid cancer. Am J Roentgenol Radium Ther Nucl Med 1966;97(4):923–30.

[3] O'Connell ME. Results of external beam radiotherapy in differentiated thyroid carcinoma: a retrospective study from the Royal Marsden Hospital. Eur J Cancer 1994;30A(6):733–9.

[4] Simpson WJ, Panzarella T, Carruthers JS, et al. Papillary and follicular thyroid cancer: impact of treatment in 1578 patients. Int J Radiat Oncol Biol Phys 1988;14(6):1063–75.

[5] Simpson WJ, McKinney SE, Carruthers JS, et al. Papillary and follicular thyroid cancer: prognostic factors in 1578 patients. Am J Med 1987;83(3):479–88.

[6] Tubiana M, Haddad E, Schlumberger M, et al. External radiotherapy in thyroid cancers. Cancer 1985;55:2062–71.

[7] Mazzaferri EL, Young RL. Papillary thyroid carcinoma: a 10-year follow-up report of the impact of therapy in 576 patients. Am J Med 1981;70:511–7.

[8] Benker G, Olbricht T, Reinwein D, et al. Survival rates in patients with differentiated thyroid carcinoma: influence of postoperative external radiotherapy. Cancer 1990;65:1517–20.

[9] Farahati J, Reinders C, Stuschke M, et al. Differentiated thyroid cancer: impact of adjuvant external radiotherapy with perithyroidal tumor infiltration (stage pT4). Cancer 1996;77(1): 172–80.

[10] Tsang RW, Brierly JD, Simpson WJ, et al. The effects of surgery, radioiodine, and external radiation therapy on the clinical outcome of patients with differentiated thyroid carcinoma. Cancer 1998;82(2):375–88.

[11] Chow SM, Law SC, Mendenhall WM, et al. Papillary thyroid carcinoma: prognostic factors and the role of radioiodine and external radiotherapy. Int J Radiat Oncol Biol Phys 2002;52: 784–95.

[12] Passler C, Scheuba C, Prager G, et al. Prognostic factors of papillary and follicular thyroid cancer: differences in an iodine-replete endemic goiter region. Endocr Relat Cancer 2004; 11(1):131–9.

[13] Furlan JC, Bedard YC, Rosen IB. Clinicopathologic significance of histologic vascular invasion in papillary and follicular thyroid carcinomas. J Am Coll Surg 2004;198(3): 341–8.

[14] Furlan JC, Bedard YC, Rosen IB. Significance of tumor capsular invasion in well-differentiated thyroid carcinomas. Am Surg 2007;73(5):484–91.

[15] Shaha AR. Implications of prognostic factors and risk groups in the management of differentiated thyroid cancer. Laryngoscope 2004;114:393–402.

[16] Saad M, Ordonez N, Rashid R, et al. Medullary carcinoma of the thyroid: a study of the clinical features and prognostic factors in 161 patients. Medicine 1984;63:319–42.

[17] Deftos LJ, Stein MF. Radioiodine as an adjunct to the surgical treatment of medullary thyroid carcinoma. J Clin Endocrinol Metab 1980;50:967–8.

[18] Hellman DE, Kartchner M, Van Antwerp JD, et al. Radioiodine in the treatment of medullary carcinoma of the thyroid. J Clin Endocrinol Metab 1979;48:451–5.

[19] Halnan KE. The non-surgical treatment of thyroid cancer. Br J Surg 1975;62:769–71.

[20] Steindfeld AD. The role of radiation therapy in medullary carcinoma of the thyroid. Radiology 1977;123:745–6.

[21] Simpson WJ, Palmer JA, Rosen IB, et al. Management of medullary carcinoma of the thyroid. Am J Surg 1982;144:420–2.

[22] Samaan NA, Schultz PN, Hickey RC. Medullary thyroid carcinoma: prognosis of familial versus sporadic disease and the role of radiotherapy. J Clin Endocrinol Metab 1988;67: 801–5.

[23] Fife KM, Bower M, Harmer CL. Medullary thyroid cancer: the role of radiotherapy in local control. Eur J Surg Oncol 1996;22:588–91.

[24] Rougier P, Parmentier C, Laplanche A, et al. Medullary thyroid carcinoma: prognostic factors and treatment. Int J Radiat Oncol Biol Phys 1983;9:161–9.

[25] Nguyen TD, Chassard JL, Lagarde P, et al. Results of postoperative radiation therapy in medullary carcinoma of the thyroid: a retrospective study by the French Federation of Cancer Institutes–the Radiotherapy Cooperative Group. Radiother Oncol 1992;23: 1–5.

[26] Brierley J, Tsang R, Simpson WJ, et al. Medullary thyroid cancer: analyses of survival and prognostic factors and the role of radiation therapy in local control. Thyroid 1996;6: 305–10.

[27] Heron DE, Karimpour S, Grigsby W. Anaplastic thyroid carcinoma: comparison of conventional radiotherapy and hyperfractionation chemoradiotherapy in two groups. Am J Clin Oncol 2002;25:442–6.

[28] Levendag PC, De Porre PM, van Putten WL. Anaplastic carcinoma of the thyroid gland treated by radiation therapy. Int J Radiat Oncol Biol Phys 1993;26:125–8.

[29] Venkatesh YS, Ordonez NG, Schultz PN, et al. Anaplastic carcinoma of the thyroid: a clinicopathologic study of 121 cases. Cancer 1990;66:321–30.

[30] Nel CJ, van Heerden JA, Goellner JR, et al. Anaplastic carcinoma of the thyroid: a clinicopathologic study of 82 cases. Mayo Clin Proc 1985;60:51–8.

[31] Kobayashi T, Asakawa H, Umeshita K, et al. Treatment of 37 patients with anaplastic carcinoma of the thyroid. Head Neck 1996;18:36–41.

[32] Demeter JG, De Jong SA, Lawrence AM, et al. Anaplastic thyroid carcinoma: risk factors and outcome. Surgery 1991;110:956–61.

[33] Junor EJ, Paul J, Reed NS. Anaplastic thyroid carcinoma: 91 patients treated by surgery and radiotherapy. Eur J Surg Oncol 1992;18:83–8.

[34] Voutilainen PE, Multanen M, Haapiainen RK, et al. Anaplastic thyroid carcinoma survival. World J Surg 1999;23:975–8.

[35] Brignardello E, Gallo M, Baldi I, et al. Anaplastic thyroid carcinoma: clinical outcome of 30 consecutive patients referred to a single institution in the past 5 years. Eur J Endocrinol 2007; 156:425–30.

[36] Kebebew E, Greenspan FS, Clark Oh, et al. Anaplastic thyroid carcinoma: treatment outcome and prognostic factors. Cancer 2005;103:1330–5.

[37] Heron DE, Karimpour S, Grigsby PW. Anaplastic thyroid carcinoma: comparison of conventional radiotherapy and hyperfractionation in two groups. Am J Clin Oncol 2002;25: 442–6.

[38] Tennvall J, Lundell G, Wahlberg P, et al. Anaplastic thyroid carcinoma: three protocols combining doxorubicin, hyperfractionated radiotherapy, and surgery. Br J Cancer 2002; 86:1848–53.

[39] Kim JH, Leeper RD. Treatment of locally advanced thyroid carcinoma with combination doxorubicin and radiation therapy. Cancer 1987;60:2372–5.

[40] Lang BH, Lo CY. Surgical options in undifferentiated thyroid carcinoma. World J Surg 2007;31:969–77.

[41] Eisbruch A, Ten Haken RK, Kim HM, et al. Dose, volume and function relationships in parotid salivary glands following conformal and intensity-modulated irradiation of head and neck cancer. Int J Radiat Oncol Biol Phys 1999;45:577–87.

[42] Brizel DM, Wesserman TH, Henke M, et al. Phase III randomized trial of amifostine as a radioprotector in head and neck cancer. J Clin Oncol 2000;18:3339–45.

[43] Wasserman TH, Brizel DM, Henke M, et al. Influence of intravenous amifostine on xerostomic tumor control, and survival after radiotherapy for head-and-neck cancer: 2-year follow up of prospective, randomized phase III trial. Int J Radiat Oncol Biol Phys 2005;63: 985–90.

[44] Bardet E, Martin L, Calais G, et al. Subcutaneous (SbQ) versus intravenous (IV) administration of amifostine for head and neck (HN) cancer patients receiving radiotherapy (RT): preliminary results of the GORTEC 2000–02 randomized trial [abstract 211]. Presented at the 47th Annual Meeting of the American Society for Therapeutic Radiology and Oncology. Denver (CO), October 16–20, 2005.

[45] Boccia R, Anne PR, Bourhis J, et al. Assessment and management of cutaneous reactions with amifostine administration: findings of the ethyol (amifostine) cutaneous treatment advisory panel (ECTAP). Int J Radiat Oncol Biol Phys 2004;60:302–9.

[46] Spielberger R, Stiff P, Bensinger W, et al. Palifermin for oral mucositis after intensive therapy for hematologic cancers. N Engl J Med 2004;351:2590–8.

ELSEVIER
SAUNDERS

Surg Oncol Clin N Am
17 (2008) 233–248

SURGICAL
ONCOLOGY CLINICS
OF NORTH AMERICA

New Technologies in Thyroid Surgery

Adam M. Becker, MD[a],
Christine G. Gourin, MD, FACS[b],*

[a]Department of Otolaryngology- Head and Neck Surgery, Medical College of Georgia,
1120 15th Street, Augusta, GA 30912, USA
[b]Johns Hopkins University School of Medicine, 6210 JHOC, 601 N. Caroline Street,
Baltimore, MD 21287, USA

The practice of thyroidectomy has evolved significantly over the past century. Once thyroidectomy was a feared procedure with mortality rates approaching 60%. Today, more than 80,000 thyroidectomy procedures are performed each year in the United States [1]. The principal concerns following thyroidectomy include formation of neck hematoma, acute airway compromise, recurrent laryngeal nerve palsy, and symptomatic hypocalcemia. Independent predictors for these complications have been difficult to identify [2]. For these reasons, patients have traditionally been admitted for 48 to 72 hours after surgery for observation. Continued refinement in technique with the application of new technologies has allowed a paradigm shift toward outpatient and short-stay surgery. These technologies have led to the development of new devices for achieving hemostasis, the wider practice of intraoperative neurophysiologic monitoring, the use of surgeon-performed ultrasound, and an increasing number of applications for minimally invasive techniques.

Surgical instruments for improved hemostasis

One of the major concerns following thyroid surgery is the risk of life-threatening hematoma. With a hematoma incidence of 0.3% to 3%, many endocrine surgeons argue that a 23-hour postoperative observation period should be mandatory to allow prompt identification and treatment of postoperative hematoma [3–24]. Furthermore, it has been suggested that 23-hour observation may identify an additional 38% to 50% of complications

---

* Corresponding author.
E-mail address: cgourin@mcg.edu (C.G. Gourin).

1055-3207/08/$ - see front matter © 2008 Elsevier Inc. All rights reserved.
doi:10.1016/j.soc.2007.10.001

that would be otherwise missed in outpatient procedures [25,26]. The use of a drain is often employed in patients who undergo total thyroidectomy, concomitant neck dissection, or resection of a large or substernal goiter. Such patients often require admission for drain management, but this is a topic of debate [27].

Several randomized clinical studies have documented that the presence of a drain has no effect on the incidence of hematoma formation [28,29]. In addition, the argument has been made that because most significant neck hematomas manifest either immediately following extubation or early in the postoperative period, routine hospital admission may not be justified. Delayed hematoma formation may occur as late as 2 to 3 days after surgery and is usually not clinically significant [30]. Schwartz and colleagues [26] speculate that one factor potentially contributing to poor outcomes in cases of neck hematoma might be the extent to which the strap muscles are closed. By reapproximating only the upper portions of the strap muscles, they propose that any bleeding can escape the confines of the thyroid compartment, and will allow earlier presentation and prevents compressive symptoms.

Evolutions in technology have allowed surgeons to achieve a better balance between hemostasis and tissue preservation. Accurate control of vascular structures is paramount in the safe performance of thyroid surgery. Several adjuncts are available to assist in maintaining hemostasis, and these devices are essential for minimally invasive approaches. The Harmonic Scalpel (Ethicon Endo-Surgery, Cincinnati, Ohio) offers the ability to cut and cauterize while reducing injury to collateral tissue. The harmonic blade vibrates longitudinally at 55,500 times per second, which transfers frictional energy to the tissues, resulting in protein denaturation by cleaving hydrogen bonds at temperatures in the range of 60°C to 80°C. Pressure exerted on the tissue by the blade causes surface blood vessels to collapse and allows the coagulum to form a hemostatic seal. Only mechanical vibration at the distal end is used to form the coagulum, with no electrical current transmitted to the patient. As a result, thermal injury to the surrounding tissue is minimized, which makes the Harmonic Scalpel well suited for thyroid surgery, where protection of nerve function is especially important. Nicastri and colleagues [31] demonstrated that the Harmonic Scalpel was 100% effective in ligating arteries 5 mm or less and veins 7 mm or less. Several investigators have reported a reduction in operative time for thyroidectomy using the Harmonic Scalpel [32–34].

The LigaSure System (Tyco Healthcare, Boulder, Colorado) incorporates a feedback-controlled response system that determines the nature of the tissues between the jaws and transfers radio frequency energy to tissues through a bipolar device, creating a coagulum capable of sealing vessels up to 7 mm in diameter. Several investigators have demonstrated a significant decrease in operative times when this device is used in thyroid surgery [35–37].

Intraoperative nerve monitoring

To avoid injury to the recurrent laryngeal nerve (RLN), surgeons are increasingly using nerve monitoring. The reported incidence of temporary RLN paresis is 1% to 5% with permanent paralysis occurring in less than 1% of cases in experienced hands [38–48]. Factors associated with higher rates of nerve injury include surgeon experience, the extent of resection, presence of malignancy, the presence of substernal goiter, and reoperative cases [8,11,15,17,48,49]. The surgeon should also be cognizant of variations in RLN anatomy. Right-sided nonrecurrent laryngeal nerves have been reported in 0.5% of patients and are seen in association with abnormal subclavian artery development [50–52]. Approximately 0.2% of patients have simultaneous right-sided recurrent and nonrecurrent laryngeal nerves in which a small-diameter RLN merges into a larger nonrecurrent nerve [53]. A left-sided nonrecurrent RLN is particularly rare, occurring on only 0.04% of patients [54]. The presence of a tubercle of Zückerkandl can help in the identification of the RLN, but can also cause the RLN to be displaced laterally when enlarged [55].

Head and neck surgeons have used electrophysiologic monitoring routinely for decades. The earliest attempts at RLN "monitoring" involved palpation of the posterior cricoarytenoid muscle while electrically stimulating the ipsilateral RLN. Currently, 29% of thyroid and parathyroid surgeons use laryngeal nerve monitoring in the United States [56]. Monitoring can be performed with invasive needle electrodes or surface electrodes. Invasive methods employ monopolar or bipolar needle electrodes, placed either laryngoscopically or transcricoid into the thyroarytenoid muscle. Alternatively, surface electrodes contacting either the posterior cricoarytenoid muscle or thyroarytenoid muscle can be used. Intramuscular electrodes have been shown to be more sensitive than surface electrodes, but have the disadvantage of increased procedure time related to electrode placement [57]. More recently, endotracheal tubes with integrated surface electrodes for RLN monitoring have been developed. These allow noninvasive intraoperative RLN monitoring.

Little objective data exists to support the routine use of RLN monitoring. Shindo and Chheda [58] investigated the incidence of postoperative vocal cord paresis or paralysis in a cohort of patients who underwent thyroidectomy with and without continuous RLN monitoring. The incidence of unexpected unilateral vocal cord paresis based on RLNs at risk was 2.09% in the monitored group and 2.96% in the unmonitored group, a difference that was not statistically significant. The incidence of unexpected complete unilateral vocal cord paralysis was 1.6% in each group, leading the investigators to conclude that monitoring did not appear to reduce the incidence of RLN paresis. The lack of a statistically significant difference in RLN injury may be in part due to its low overall incidence. Additionally, published reports generally stem from high-volume practices where surgery is performed by experienced surgeons, which is why several investigators have suggested that low-volume thyroid surgeons may benefit from RLN monitoring. Others have found RLN monitoring useful to closely gauge trauma to the nerve and increase surgeon confidence [11,59–62]. RLN monitoring is still not a substitute for systematic nerve identification and careful dissection.

Recently, Lamade and colleagues [63] described a new tripolar cuff electrode that can be placed around the vagus nerve. This technique has the obvious disadvantage of requiring identification and dissection of the vagus nerve, which adds to the length and extent of the procedure and may limit its routine use in thyroid surgery.

Assessment of hypocalcemia

The most common complication following thyroid surgery is transient hypocalcemia, with an incidence ranging from 2% to 30% [1,64–69]. Hypocalcemia has many possible causes, with parathyroid gland injury the most common. Increased preoperative free T4 levels, reduced stores of vitamin D, hemodilution, carcinoma, thyrotoxic osteodystrophy, and the presence of substernal thyroid extension have also been found to play a role [70,71]. In seeking ways to reduce hospital stays, many investigators have attempted to identify risk factors for the development of postoperative hypocalcemia. However, identification of these patients remains difficult [64,65,70–72].

In the past, several investigators have advocated routine admission to monitor patients at risk for postthyroidectomy hypocalcemia [68,72]. In his review of "outpatient" thyroid surgery, McHenry [70] defined at-risk patients as patients undergoing reoperative thyroidectomy, patients with an elevated preoperative free T4, patients with thyroid cancer or substernal goiter treated by more extensive bilateral thyroidectomy, and patients with known parathyroid devascularization. Patients meeting any of these criteria were observed and underwent measurement of serum calcium on the morning following surgery. Patients were extensively counseled regarding the signs of hypocalcemia. In the event symptoms developed, they were instructed to notify the surgeon and to begin 1000 mg of elemental calcium every 6 hours. In McHenry's review, all patients with hypocalcemia were treated successfully on an outpatient basis with no adverse sequelae, though it should be mentioned that "outpatients" in this group included those high-risk patients admitted for overnight observation.

In the absence of reliable predictors of hypocalcemia, investigators have relied on serum calcium measurements to direct early treatment [64–66,72]. Several investigators have shown that an up-sloping curve derived from serum calcium levels obtained at several intervals postoperatively can predict normocalcemia [67,73]. These results, however, take nearly 24 hours to obtain. Adams and colleagues [64] retrospectively reviewed postoperative calcium levels in 128 patients who underwent either parathyroid surgery or nonparathyroid operations, including total thyroidectomy, completion thyroidectomy, and "other" operations where the parathyroid glands were at risk. The slope of the curve of two sequential serum ionized calcium levels obtained in the first 12 hours after surgery was plotted as a function of time. An initial positive slope was 100% predictive of normocalcemia, while patients with a negative sloping curve but a calcium within the low-normal range had an 85% chance of remaining normocalcemic. This study was limited because of small numbers and a lack of standardized postoperative timing for blood draws. In a follow-up study, investigators attempted to identify an algorithm that would predict patients at risk for hypocalcemia using ionized calcium levels drawn preoperatively and 2 hours postoperatively [72]. Although they were unable to find a statistically significant difference between preoperative and 2-hour calcium levels, they found that patients who became hypocalcemic had an average decline in ionized calcium of 1.671% per hour ($P = .006$).

Husein and colleagues [66] prospectively enrolled 68 patients who underwent total thyroidectomy. Corrected serum calcium levels were drawn at 6, 12, and 20 hours after thyroidectomy and then twice daily. Transient hypocalcemia was seen in 21% of patients and permanent hypocalcemia in 6%. They found that patients who exhibited a positive slope between 6- and 12-hour calcium levels remained normocalcemic with a positive predictive value of 85.7%. When plotting the slope, they found that an increase of 0.02 or more was associated with normocalcemia 97% of the time. When applying this algorithm to patient care, they were able to discharge patients 1 day earlier on average. Bentrem and colleagues [65] conducted a similar study using total and ionized calcium levels collected at 8, 16, and 22 hours postoperatively. Ionized calcium levels obtained at 16 hours allowed identification of patients who would eventually develop hypocalcemia 94.4% of the time. They also found that ionized calcium levels more accurately correlated with symptomatic hypocalcemia than total calcium and allowed identification of more patients at risk for significant hypoparathyroidism. Based on this data, they advocate 23-hour hospital admission to safely monitor patients undergoing parathyroidectomy, total thyroidectomy, or near-total thyroidectomy.

The obvious disadvantage of using postoperative calcium monitoring in the prediction of hypocalcemia is the requirement for extended hospital stay. It has been reported that early serum calcium monitoring is only reliable when measurements are performed on the morning after surgery [74]. Furthermore, calcium levels can take up to 48 hours to decline and postoperative calcium decline within 24 hours has been demonstrated in operations outside the cervical area despite normal parathyroid hormone (PTH) levels [75].

Because of the problems inherent to calcium monitoring, several investigators have explored the use of intraoperative PTH (iPTH) as an alternative method of predicting hypocalcemia in the immediate postoperative period. Lo and colleagues [74] sought to examine the utility of iPTH levels drawn at 10 minutes following removal of the thyroid gland. In their series, a decline in iPTH of more than 75% correlated with the development of hypocalcemia with 100% sensitivity and 72% specificity. In addition, all patients with normal iPTH after thyroidectomy remained normocalcemic during the postoperative period. Lo and colleagues concluded that by facilitating early discharge and reducing the need for additional calcium testing, iPTH can avoid the costs of additional serum calcium monitoring. Lombardi and colleagues [76] reviewed 53 consecutive patients who underwent total or completion thyroidectomy. iPTH was measured at induction of anesthesia, at skin closure, and at 2, 4, 6, 24, and 48 hours after surgery. They found that postoperative iPTH levels were reduced (<10 pg/mL) in hypocalcemic patients at the end of the operation and 2, 4, 6, 24, and 48 hours postoperatively. All normocalcemic patients had perioperative iPTH levels within the normal range. iPTH levels less than 10 pg/mL at 4 and 6 hours were predictive of hypocalcemia with 100% specificity and 94% sensitivity, whereas iPTH measurements obtained earlier were less accurate in predicting hypocalcemia. These findings have been confirmed by other investigators [67,77].

Prediction of hypocalcemia with iPTH may be useful in reoperative cases. To determine the relationship between perioperative changes in PTH levels and the likelihood of post-thyroidectomy hypocalcemia, Scurry and colleagues [78] prospectively reviewed 63 patients who underwent either total or completion thyroidectomy. PTH levels were obtained preoperatively and then intraoperatively 10 minutes after removal of the gland. In their series, 23.8% of patients developed hypocalcemia, including 6 of 13 patients who underwent completion thyroidectomy and 9 of 50 patients who underwent total thyroidectomy. There was no significant difference in preoperative iPTH levels between normo- and hypocalcemic patients. Patients with hypocalcemia exhibited lower postoperative iPTH levels than normocalcemic patients (10.0 pg/mL versus 23.3 pg/mL, $P = .0086$). Using receiver operator characteristics curves, Scurry and colleagues concluded that a change of 75% in iPTH resulted in maximum sensitivity and specificity for predicting hypocalcemia. They determined that an absolute PTH level of 7 pg/mL was the most sensitive and specific indicator for predicting hypocalcemia. In their series, patients undergoing completion thyroidectomy were at greater risk of developing hypocalcemia than patients undergoing total thyroidectomy ($P = .030$). The major limitation to widespread use of the PTH assay is the added costs, which often exceed the costs of additional serum calcium monitoring in high-risk patients.

Ultrasound

The use of ultrasound in the evaluation of thyroid disorders is well established but has only recently been embraced by surgeons as part of the preoperative and intraoperative evaluation of patients with thyroid disease.

Ultrasound is relatively inexpensive and has the advantage of providing real-time information without subjecting patients to ionizing radiation. Conversely, there is a high degree of operator dependence. In many centers, ultrasound is performed by technicians who may be unfamiliar with cervical anatomy, with the radiologist interpreting only the static images. Increasingly, surgeon-performed ultrasound is being incorporated into surgical practice and the American College of Surgeons now offers an ultrasound course for surgeons that provides training in basic ultrasound techniques.

Ultrasound evaluation of the thyroid gland is optimized by using a high-frequency linear transducer in the range of 7 to 12 MHz with the neck extended [79]. Patients with thick, obese necks or large thyroid glands may require a lower frequency 5-MHz transducer with a larger footprint for penetration. However this results in a compensatory decrease in resolution [80]. Imaging in the transverse plane provides an axial view of the thyroid gland and its relationships to the carotid sheath, strap muscles, trachea, and esophagus. Longitudinal images allow visualization of the thyroid gland in a cranio-caudal direction and differentiation of the thyroid from vascular structures and the esophagus. Transverse and longitudinal scanning are both required for accurate three-dimensional imaging. The trachea is a useful reference point by virtue of its size, consistent anechoic interior, and midline position.

Thyroid nodules are common and as many as 70% of patients examined by ultrasound have small nodules (<1 cm) not suspected clinically [79]. Nodules are usually multiple in number and generally encapsulated with cystic areas [81]. Simple cysts appear anechoic while complex cysts appear hypoechoic and solid nodules hyperechoic. The incidence of malignancy is approximately 5% in hyperechoic nodules and 26% in hypoechoic nodules [79]. Hypoechogenicity alone, however, is inaccurate in predicting malignancy, with poor specificity and a low positive predictive value [79]. Nodules with a large cystic component usually represent benign cysts that have undergone hemorrhage or cystic degeneration. A peripheral halo with decreased echogenicity is seen surrounding hypoechoic or isoechoic nodules and represents either the capsule of the nodule or compressed thyroid tissue. The absence of such a halo is associated with an increased incidence of malignancy [79]. The comet tail sign within a thyroid nodule is associated with the presence of colloid in a benign nodule. Calcifications appear as echogenic foci. Punctate calcifications that do not exhibit shadowing are associated with papillary carcinoma, whereas larger areas of calcification with dense posterior shadowing secondary to acoustical impedance mismatch are more commonly benign.

The use of color flow Doppler imaging in ultrasound has several advantages. Patients with thyroiditis show marked diffuse glandular vascularity. Benign hyperplastic nodules are associated with an absence of flow within the nodule or exclusively perinodular flow signals. Marked intranodular flow is associated with an increased likelihood of malignancy [79]. Inability to visualize the thyroid gland by ultrasound in the absence of a history of prior thyroidectomy should alert the examiner to the possibility of an ectopic gland, either mediastinal, which is beyond the reach of ultrasound imaging, or a lingual thyroid. Color Doppler ultrasound has been shown to be superior to standard ultrasound in detection of lingual thyroid glands [82].

Surgeon-performed ultrasound is gaining recognition as an important part of the preoperative and intraoperative management of the patient with thyroid disease. Ultrasound allows recognition of the extent and spread of disease and permits a tailored surgical approach to thyroidectomy [83]. In a series of 72 patients with thyroid cancer, Solorzano and colleagues [84] reported that surgeon-performed ultrasound resulted in a change in management in 57% of cases. The acquisition of familiarity and skill with this technology is becoming increasingly important for the modern thyroid surgeon.

Endoscopic techniques

The application of endoscopic visualization to thyroid surgery has allowed surgeons to perform thyroidectomy through minimal incisions, thus minimizing the extent of dissection and improving cosmesis. Several approaches have been proposed in the application of endoscopic thyroidectomy. In 2002, Bellantone and colleagues [85] proposed a technique that uses a minimal central neck incision to gain access to the thyroid compartment with the use of video endoscopes to aid in visualization. In a review of this endoscopically assisted approach, Terris and colleagues [86] reported that the most compelling benefit noted was superior visualization afforded by the endoscopic magnification (up to 20×). Additionally, they proposed that tissue trauma and, as a result, wound healing is more rapid as a result of reduced dissection. In their technique, no subplatysmal flaps are raised and no muscles are divided, resulting in reduced tissue edema compared with conventional surgery. Patients may also achieve a cosmetic benefit from a smaller incision. The procedure has complication rates equivalent to those for conventional approaches. Drains are generally not required and the patient can be discharged several hours after surgery. One disadvantage of this technique is the requirement for additional surgical assistants: one to provide retraction for the operative surgeon, and a second assistant to maneuver the endoscope.

Palazzo and colleagues [87] described an endoscopic lateral cervical approach to the thyroid gland in 2006. In their technique used for hemithyroidectomy, two 2.5-mm trocars and one 10-mm trocar are inserted along the anterior border of the sternocleidomastoid muscle on the ipsilateral side. Using endoscopic instruments specifically designed for this procedure, dissection then proceeds from the lateral aspect of the thyroid gland medially with identification of the RLN, superior and inferior parathyroid glands, and skeletonization of the superior and inferior pole vessels. Following this, the trocars are removed, the thyroid gland is extracted through the main incision, and the skeletonized vessels and thyroid isthmus divided using a harmonic scalpel. In their series of 38 patients, identification and preservation of the RLN was achieved in all patients. The superior parathyroid gland was preserved in 36 patients and inferior parathyroid gland preserved in 33 patients. Because of difficulty of dissection, 2 patients required open conversion by extending the main trocar incision. Palazzo and colleagues reported that an additional advantage of their technique over endoscopically assisted midline techniques was that no additional assistants were required to hold retractors. Their technique has the disadvantage of being limited to hemithyroidectomy, and requires a lateral approach that may be unfamiliar to many thyroid surgeons.

Several investigators have described totally endoscopic approaches to the thyroid compartment [88–94]. Early totally endoscopic approaches described by Ikeda and colleagues [88] used three ports located in the axillary region with low-pressure insufflation. Although cosmetic results are excellent in this technique, others noted that the location of the ports in such a narrow area resulted in frequent interference of the surgical instruments [88]. In addition, only the ipsilateral hemithyroid can be addressed in this manner. Ohgami and colleagues [95] used two circumareolar incisions in addition to a suprasternal incision in a breast approach to the thyroid. This improved the narrow angle enforced on instrumentation by the axillary approach, but resulted in an incision on the anterior chest, an area prone to hypertrophy. To avoid a chest-wall incision, the axillo-breast approach was subsequently developed by placing two circumareolar trochars and a single trochar in the ipsilateral axilla [93]. This approach was later modified by using bilateral axillary ports to allow for adequate exposure to address both sides of the thyroid compartment [90]. In a study comparing the bilateral axillo-breast approach (BABA) to standard open thyroidectomy, Chung and colleagues [92] showed similar results in terms of transient hypocalcemia, bleeding, permanent RLN paralysis, and length of hospital stay. Whereas applicability of the endoscopic-assisted approach is limited by the size of the gland, the investigators noted that this constraint does not exist for BABA, as even large glands are easily retrieved through the axillary port. The disadvantages reported for BABA are a significant increase in the rate of transient RLN injury (2.5% versus 25.2%) and significantly longer surgical times [92].

Disadvantages of endoscopic thyroidectomy include the requirement for additional equipment, namely high-resolution endoscopes and monitors for endoscopic-assisted techniques and insufflation units for purely endoscopic cases. In addition, there is a distinct learning curve, which is more pronounced with purely endoscopic approaches. While endoscopic-assisted techniques clearly result in limited surgical dissection, purely endoscopic approaches, by virtue of their remote approaches, result in an equivalent amount of dissection. Because of this, most descriptions include the routine use of drains, which may increase the length of hospitalization. Furthermore, the increased chest-wall dissection can result in hypoesthesia in this area, and cases of pneumothorax have been described [89]. Finally, operative times for endoscopic or endoscopically assisted procedures may be up to 30% longer than they are for traditional open approaches [86].

Future directions

While conventional endoscopic techniques have revolutionized minimally invasive surgical procedures in areas with well-defined anatomic cavities, the application of such techniques in neck surgery has been underdeveloped. Insufficient maneuverable space and the lack of a well-defined cavity limit endoscopic neck surgery. As previously mentioned, evolution in surgical techniques has allowed surgeons to apply conventional endoscopic techniques to the thyroid compartment. As surgical robotic technology continues to evolve, the restrictions of conventional instruments, namely limited range of motion, reversed hand-eye coordination, and problems with depth perception, are being reduced.

The earliest surgical application of robotics was the Application of Automated Endoscopic System for Optimal Positioning (AESOP; Computer Motion, Goleta, California). AESOP is a robotic laparoscopic camera holder controlled by the surgeon and used in many general surgical, gynecologic, and urologic procedures [96]. The successful application of AESOP led to the development of the first telerobotic systems. The Zeus robot surgical system (Computer Motion) and the da Vinci surgical system (Intuitive Surgical, Sunnyvale, California) each consists of a surgical workstation containing a three-dimensional imaging system at which the surgeon is seated. The Zeus system uses three robotic arms: one that holds the camera and two that hold instruments. The newest models of the da Vinci system include four robotic arms. The robot is positioned at the patient's bedside with the surgeon's workstation located at a remote console. One of the main differences between the two devices is that the Zeus system uses a video monitor that displays a composite three-dimensional image viewed by the surgeon through polarized glasses. The da Vinci system, by comparison, uses a stereoscopic image viewed through binocular telescopes, which gives the illusion that the surgeon is in front of the patient. In addition, the da Vinci system incorporates an articulated wrist with seven degrees of freedom and 90° of articulation. The da Vinci has largely supplanted the Zeus surgical robotic system, which is no longer commercially available.

The da Vinci robotic system has been approved by the US Food and Drug Administration (FDA) for adult and pediatric use in urologic, general, and gynecologic laparoscopic surgical procedures, in noncardiovascular thorascopic surgical procedures, and in thorascopically assisted cardiotomy procedures. The da Vinci System may also be employed with adjunctive mediastinotomy to perform coronary anastomosis during cardiac revascularization. While there are currently no FDA-approved applications in the head and neck, research models have been developed in the bovine, canine, and human cadaveric models for neck, oral cavity, oropharyngeal, and laryngeal applications [97–102]. Terris and colleagues [97,98], in the first reports on the use of telerobotics in otolaryngology, found that surgical times for removal of the submandibular gland and selective neck dissection were similar to those with conventional endoscopic techniques.

In the only report to date of the application of robotics in endocrine surgery, Tanna and colleagues [103] in 2006 reviewed their experience with two cases of robot-assisted endocrine surgery. In the first case, the da Vinci robot was used in the excision of a mediastinal parathyroid gland, with the thoracic surgeons providing mediastinal access and the otolaryngologist removing the adenoma. The second case involved a patient with a multinodular goiter and a large substernal component. Again, thoracic surgeons provided exposure for the otolaryngologist to address the mediastinal component via a transthoracic approach. The remainder of the thyroid gland was excised via a standard transcervical approach. The robot facilitated a minimally invasive thoracic approach as opposed to conventional sternotomy.

Advantages of robot-assisted surgery over conventional endoscopic techniques include the improved range of motion and added safety afforded by the three-dimensional imaging system [97,98]. Limitations include interference of the surgical arms with one another during neck surgery, resulting from the narrow operative area [98]. This can be significantly alleviated by increasing the distance of the camera port and the instrument port from 4 to 5 cm and switching from a 0° to a 30° endoscope, which alters the angle of the camera's arm. The second major limitation is the lack of tactile feedback and proprioception, which is an area of active investigation [98]. The development of microrobotic technology with enhanced directional ability may expand the applications of robotic technology to the thyroid compartment.

Summary

A number of recent innovations facilitate new approaches to surgery of the thyroid gland. Technologic advancements have led to improved instrumentation for maintaining meticulous hemostasis. These devices have been instrumental in the development of minimally invasive approaches and have the added advantage of allowing the surgeon to avoid drains, thus facilitating outpatient surgery. Laryngeal nerve monitoring may be a useful adjunct in identifying the RLN, particularly for the low-volume endocrine surgeon. Endoscopic surgical techniques allow improved visualization and permit thyroidectomy to be performed through small incisions, often less than 3 cm, which may improve cosmetic outcomes. Finally, the evolution of surgical robotics holds the promise of further enhancing visualization and surgeon dexterity in comparison with traditional endoscopic approaches, and may have future applications to thyroid surgery.

References

[1] Higgins KM, Mandell DL, Govindaraj S, et al. The role of intraoperative rapid parathyroid hormone monitoring for predicting thyroidectomy-related hypocalcemia. Arch Otolaryngol Head Neck Surg 2004;130(1):63–7.

[2] Avvas G, Dubner S, Heller KS. Re-operation for bleeding after thyroidectomy and parathyroidectomy. Head Neck 2001;23(7):544–6.

[3] Spanknebel K, Chabot JA, DiGiorgi M, et al. Thyroidectomy using monitored local or conventional general anesthesia: an analysis of outpatient surgery, outcome and cost in 1,194 consecutive cases. World J Surg 2006;30:1–12.

[4] Torre G, Borgonovo G, Amato A, et al. Surgical management of substernal goiter: analysis of 237 patients. Am Surg 1995;61:826–31.

[5] Shaha AR, Jaffe BM. Practical management of post-thyroidectomy hematoma. J Surg Oncol 1994;57:235–8.

[6] Shaha AR, Jaffe BM. Selective use of drains in thyroid surgery. J Surg Oncol 1993;52:241–3.

[7] Matory YL, Spiro RH. Wound bleeding after head and neck surgery. J Surg Oncol 1993;53:17–9.

[8] Bergamaschi R, Becouarn G, Ronceray J, et al. Morbidity of thyroid surgery. Am J Surg 1998;176:71–5.

[9] Ruark DS, Abdel-Misih RZ. Thyroid and parathyroid surgery without drains. Head Neck 1992;14:285–7.

[10] Ayyash K, Khammash M, Tibblin S. Drain vs. no drain in primary thyroid and parathyroid surgery. Eur J Surg 1991;157:113–4.

[11] Sosa JA, Bowman HM, Tielsch JM, et al. The importance of surgeon experience for clinical and economic outcomes from thyroidectomy. Ann Surg 1998;228:320–30.

[12] Max MH, Scherm M, Bland KI. Early and late complications after thyroid surgery. South Med J 1983;76:977–80.

[13] Menegaux F, Turpin G, Dahman M, et al. Secondary thyroidectomy in patients with prior thyroid surgery for benign disease: a study of 203 cases. Surgery 1999;125:479–83.

[14] Chao T, Jeng L, Lin J, et al. Reoperative thyroid surgery. World J Surg 1997;21:644–7.

[15] Harness JK, Fung L, Thompson NW, et al. Total thyroidectomy: complications and technique. World J Surg 1986;10:781–6.

[16] Flynn MB, Lyons KJ, Tarter JW, et al. Local complications after surgical resection for thyroid carcinoma. Am J Surg 1994;168:404–7.

[17] Levin KE, Clark AH, Duh Q, et al. Reoperative thyroid surgery. Surgery 1992;111:604–9.

[18] Pezzullo L, Delrio P, Losito NS, et al. Post-operative complications after completion thyroidectomy for differentiated thyroid carcinoma. Eur J Surg Oncol 1997;23:215–8.

[19] Cusick EL, Krukowski ZH, Matheson NA. Outcome of surgery for Grave's disease reexamined. Br J Surg 1987;74:780–3.

[20] Lennquist S, Jortso E, Anderberg B, et al. Betablockers compared with antithyroid drugs as preoperative treatment in hyperthyroidism: drug tolerance, complications, and postoperative thyroid function. Surgery 1985;98:1141–6.

[21] Andaker L, Johansson K, Smeds S, et al. Surgery for hyperthyroidism: hemithyroidectomy plus contralateral resection or bilateral resection? A prospective randomized study of postoperative complications and long-term results. World J Surg 1992;16:765–9.

[22] Ryan JA Jr, Lee F. Effectiveness and safety of 100 consecutive parathyroidectomies. Am J Surg 1997;173:441–4.

[23] Punch JD, Thompson NW, Merion RM. Subtotal parathyroidectomy in dialysis and postrenal transplant patients. Arch Surg 1995;130:538–43.

[24] Croyle PH, Oldroyd JJ. Incidental parathyroidectomy during thyroid surgery. Am Surg 1978;44:559–63.

[25] Burkey SH, Van Heerden JA, Thompson GB, et al. Reexploration for symptomatic hematomas after cervical exploration. Surgery 2001;130(6):914–20.

[26] Schwartz AE, Clark OH, Ituarte P, et al. Therapeutic controversy: thyroid surgery—the choice. J Clin Endocrinol Metab 1998;83(4):1097–105.

[27] Kristoffersson A, Sandzen B, Jarhult J. Drainage in uncomplicated thyroid and parathyroid surgery. Br J Surg 1986;73(2):121–2.

[28] Corsten M, Johnson S, Alherabi A. Is suction drainage an effective means of preventing hematoma in thyroid surgery? A meta-analysis. J Otolaryngol 2005;34(6):415–7.

[29] Potheir DD. The use of drains following thyroid and parathyroid surgery: a meta-analysis. J Laryngol Otol 2005;119(9):669–71.

[30] McHenry CR. "Same day" thyroid surgery: an analysis of safety, cost savings, and outcome. Am Surg 1997;63(7):586–9.

[31] Nicastri DG, Wu M, Yun J, et al. Evaluation of efficacy of an ultrasonic scalpel for pulmonary vascular ligation in an animal model. J Thorac Cardiovasc Surg 2007;134(1):160–4.

[32] Kilic M, Keskek M, Ertan T, et al. A prospective randomized trial comparing the harmonic scalpel with conventional knot tying in thyroidectomy. Adv Ther 2007;24(3):632–8.

[33] Koutsoumanis K, Koutras AS, Drimousis PG, et al. The use of a harmonic scalpel in thyroid surgery: report of a 3-year experience. Am J Surg 2007;193(6):693–6.

[34] Cordón C, Fajardo R, Ramírez J, et al. A randomized, prospective, parallel group study comparing the harmonic scalpel to electrocautery in thyroidectomy. Surgery 2005;137(3):337–41.

[35] Saint Marc O, Cogliandolo A, Piquard A, et al. LigaSure vs clamp-and-tie technique to achieve hemostasis in total thyroidectomy for benign multinodular goiter: a prospective randomized study. Arch Surg 2007;142(2):150–6.

[36] Franko J, Kish KJ, Pezzi CM, et al. Safely increasing the efficiency of thyroidectomy using a new bipolar electrosealing device (LigaSure) versus conventional clamp-and-tie technique. Am Surg 2006;72(2):132–6.

[37] Kirdak T, Korun N, Ozguc H. Use of LigaSure in thyroidectomy procedures: results of a prospective comparative study. World J Surg 2005;29(6):771–4.

[38] Chiang F, Wang L, Huang Y, et al. Recurrent laryngeal nerve palsy after thyroidectomy with routine identification of the recurrent laryngeal nerve. Surgery 2005;137:342–7.

[39] Ozbas S, Kocak S, Aydintug S, et al. Comparison of the complications of subtotal, near total and total thyroidectomy in the surgical management of multinodular goitre. Endocr J 2005;52:199–205.

[40] Filho JG, Kowalski LP. Surgical complications after thyroid surgery performed in a cancer hospital. Otolaryngol Head Neck Surg 2005;132:490–4.

[41] Rosato L, Avenia N, Bernante P, et al. Complications of thyroid surgery: analysis of a multicentric study on 14,934 patients operated on in Italy over 5 years. World J Surg 2004;28:271–6.

[42] Bron LP, O'Brien CJ. Total thyroidectomy for clinically benign disease of the thyroid gland. Br J Surg 2004;91:569–74.

[43] Friguglietti CU, Lin CS, Kulcsar MA. Total thyroidectomy for benign thyroid disease. Laryngoscope 2003;113:1820–6.

[44] Bellantone R, Lombardi CP, Bossola M, et al. Total thyroidectomy for management of benign thyroid disease: review of 526 cases. World J Surg 2002;26:1468–71.

[45] Hermann M, Alk G, Roka R, et al. Laryngeal recurrent nerve injury in surgery for benign thyroid disease. Effect of nerve dissection and impact of individual surgeon in more than 27,000 nerves at risk. Ann Surg 2002;235:261–8.

[46] Prim MP, De Diego JI, Hardisson D, et al. Factors related to nerve injury and hypocalcemia in thyroid gland surgery. Otolaryngol Head Neck Surg 2001;124:111–4.

[47] Lo C, Kwok K, Yuen P. A prospective evaluation of recurrent laryngeal nerve paralysis during thyroidectomy. Arch Surg 2000;135:204–7.

[48] Moulton-Barrett R, Crumley R, Jalilie S, et al. Complications of thyroid surgery. Int Surg 1997;82:63–6.

[49] Falk SA, McCaffrey TV. Management of the recurrent laryngeal nerve in suspected and proven thyroid cancer. Otolaryngol Head Neck Surg 1995;113:42–8.

[50] Srinivasan V, Premachandra DJ. Non-recurrent laryngeal nerve: identification during thyroid surgery. Otorhinolaryngology 1997;59:57–9.

[51] Toniato A, Mazzarotto R, Piotto A, et al. Identification of the nonrecurrent laryngeal nerve during thyroid surgery: 20 year experience. World J Surg 2004;28:659–61.

[52] Hermans R, Dewandel P, Debruyne F, et al. Arteria lusoria identified on preoperative CT and nonrecurrent inferior laryngeal nerve during thyroidectomy: a prospective study. Head Neck 2003;25:113–7.

[53] Proye CAG, Carnaille BM, Goropoulos A. Nonrecurrent and recurrent inferior laryngeal nerve: a surgical pitfall in cervical exploration. Am J Surg 1991;162:495–6.

[54] Henry JF, Audiffret J, Denizot A, et al. The nonrecurrent inferior laryngeal nerve: review of 33 cases, including two on the left side. Surgery 1988;104:977–84.

[55] Gauger PG, Delbridge LW, Thompson NW, et al. Incidence and importance of the tubercle of Zuckerkandl in thyroid surgery. Eur J Surg 2001;167(4):249–54.

[56] Horne SK, Gal TJ, Brennan JA. Prevalence and patterns of intraoperative nerve monitoring for thyroidectomy. Otolaryngol Head Neck Surg 2007;136(6):952–6.

[57] Tschopp KP, Gottardo C. Comparison of various methods of electromyographic monitoring of the recurrent laryngeal nerve in thyroid surgery. Ann Otol Rhinol Laryngol 2002; 111(9):811–6.

[58] Shindo M, Chheda N. Incidence of vocal cord paralysis with and without recurrent laryngeal nerve monitoring during thyroidectomy. Arch Otolaryngol Head Neck Surg 2007; 133(5):481–5.

[59] Dralle H, Sekulla C, Haerting J, et al. Risk factors of paralysis and functional outcome after recurrent laryngeal nerve monitoring in thyroid surgery. Surgery 2004;136:1310–22.

[60] Timon CI, Rafferty M. Nerve monitoring in thyroid surgery: is it worthwhile? Clin Otolaryngol Allied Sci 1999;24(6):487–90.

[61] Song P, Shemen L. Electrophysiologic laryngeal nerve monitoring in high-risk thyroid surgery. Ear Nose Throat J 2005;84(6):378–81.

[62] Bailleux S, Bozec A, Castillo L, et al. Thyroid surgery and recurrent laryngeal nerve monitoring. J Laryngol Otol 2006;120(7):566–9.

[63] Lamade W, Ulmer C, Seimer A, et al. A new system for continuous recurrent laryngeal nerve monitoring. Minim Invasive Ther Allied Technol 2007;16(3):149–54.

[64] Adams J, Andersen P, Everts E, et al. Early postoperative calcium levels as predictors of hypocalcemia. Laryngoscope 1998;108(12):1829–31.

[65] Bentrem DJ, Rademaker A, Angelos P. Evaluation of serum calcium levels in predicting hypoparathyroidism after total/near-total thyroidectomy or parathyroidectomy. Am Surg 2001;67(3):249–51.

[66] Husein M, Hier MP, Al-Abdulhadi K, et al. Predicting calcium status post thyroidectomy with early calcium levels. Otolaryngol Head Neck Surg 2002;127(4):289–93.

[67] Lam A, Kerr PD. Parathyroid hormone: an early predictor of postthyroidectomy hypocalcemia. Laryngoscope 2003;113(12):2196–200.

[68] LoGerfo P, Gates R, Gasetas P. Outpatient and short-stay thyroid surgery. Head Neck 1991;13(2):97–101.

[69] Warren FM, Andersen PE, Wax MK, et al. Intraoperative parathyroid hormone levels in thyroid and parathyroid surgery. Laryngoscope 2002;112(10):1866–70.

[70] McHenry CR, Speroff T, Wentworth D, et al. Risk factors for post-thyroidectomy hypocalcemia. Surgery 1994;116(4):641–8.

[71] Moore C, Lampe H, Agrawal S. Predictability of hypocalcemia using early postoperative serum calcium levels. J Otolaryngol 2001;30(5):266–70.

[72] Luu Q, Andersen PE, Adams J, et al. The predictive value of perioperative calcium levels after thyroid/parathyroid surgery. Head Neck 2002;24(1):63–7.

[73] Marohn MR, LaCivita KA. Evaluation of total/near-total thyroidectomy in a short stay hospitalization. Surgery 1995;118(6):943–7.

[74] Lo CY, Luk JM, Tam SC. Applicability of intraoperative parathyroid hormone assay during thyroidectomy. Ann Surg 2002;236(5):564–9.

[75] Demeester-Mirkine N, Hooghe L, Van Geertruyden J, et al. Hypocalcemia after thyroidectomy. Arch Surg 1992;127(7):845–58.

[76] Lombardi CP, Raffaelli M, Princi P, et al. Early prediction of postthyroidectomy hypocalcemia by one single iPTH measurement. Surgery 2004;136(6):1236–41.

[77] Quiros RM, Pesce CE, Wilhelm SM, et al. Intraoperative parathyroid hormone levels in thyroid surgery are predictive of postoperative hypoparathyroidism and need for vitamin D supplementation. Am J Surg 2005;189(3):306–9.

[78] Scurry WC, Beus KS, Hollenbeak CS, et al. Perioperative parathyroid hormone assay for diagnosis and management of postthyroidectomy hypocalcemia. Laryngoscope 2005; 115(8):1362–6.

[79] Wong KT, Ahuja AT. Ultrasound of thyroid cancer. Cancer Imaging 2005;5:167–76.

[80] Khati N, Adamson T, Johnson KS, et al. Ultrasound of the thyroid and parathyroid glands. Ultrasound Q 2003;19:162–76.

[81] McCaffrey TV. Evaluation of the thyroid nodule. Cancer Control 2000;7:223–8.

[82] Ohnishi H, Sato H, Noda H, et al. Color Doppler ultrasonography: diagnosis of ectopic thyroid gland in patients with congenital hypothyroidism caused by thyroid dysgenesis. J Clin Endocrinol Metab 2003;88:5145–9.

[83] Slough CM, Randolph GW. Workup of well-differentiated thyroid carcinoma. Cancer Control 2006;13(2):99–105.

[84] Solorzano CC, Carneiro DM, Ramirez M, et al. Surgeon-performed ultrasound in the management of thyroid malignancy. Am Surg 2004;70(7):576–80.

[85] Bellantone R, Lombardi CP, Raffaelli M, et al. Video-assisted thyroidectomy. J Am Coll Surg 2002;194:610–4.

[86] Terris DJ, Chin E. Clinical implementation of endoscopic thyroidectomy in selected patients. Laryngoscope 2006;116(10):1745–8.

[87] Palazzo FF, Sebag F, Henry JF. Endocrine surgical technique: endoscopic thyroidectomy via the lateral approach. Surg Endosc 2006;20:339–42.

[88] Ikeda Y, Takami H, Sasaki Y, et al. Clinical benefits in endoscopic thyroidectomy by the axillary approach. J Am Coll Surg 2003;196:189–95.

[89] Choe JH, Kim SW, Chung KW, et al. Endoscopic thyroidectomy using a new bilateral axillo-breast approach. World J Surg 2007;31(3):601–6.

[90] Cho YU, Park IJ, Choi KH, et al. Gasless endoscopic thyroidectomy via an anterior chest wall approach using a flap-lifting system. Yonsei Med J 2007;48(3):480–7.

[91] Yoon JH, Park CH, Chung WY. Gasless endoscopic thyroidectomy via an axillary approach: experience of 30 cases. Surg Laparosc Endosc Percutan Tech 2006;16(4):226–31.

[92] Chung YS, Choe JH, Kang KH, et al. Endoscopic thyroidectomy for thyroid malignancies: comparison with conventional open thyroidectomy. World J Surg 2007 [Epub ahead of print].

[93] Barlehner E, Benhidjeb T. Cervical scarless endoscopic thyroidectomy: axillo-bilateral-breast approach (ABBA). Surg Endosc 2007 [Epub ahead of print].

[94] Duncan TD, Rashid Q, Speights F, et al. Endoscopic transaxillary approach to the thyroid gland: our early experience. Surg Endosc 2007 [Epub ahead of print].

[95] Ohgami M, Ishii S, Arisawa Y, et al. Scarless endoscopic thyroidectomy: breast approach for better cosmesis. Surg Laparosc Endosc Percutan Tech 2000;10(1):1–4.

[96] Gourin CG, Terris DJ. Surgical robotics in otolaryngology: expanding the technology envelope. Curr Opin Otolaryngol Head Neck Surg 2004;12(3):204–8.

[97] Terris DJ, Haus BM, Gourin CG, et al. Endo-robotic resection of the submandibular gland in a cadaver model. Head Neck 2005;27(11):946–51.

[98] Haus BM, Kambham N, Le D, et al. Surgical robotic applications in otolaryngology-Laryngoscope 2003;113(7):1139–44.

[99] Weinstein GS, O'Malley BW Jr, Snyder W, et al. Transoral robotic surgery: supraglottic partial laryngectomy. Ann Otol Rhinol Laryngol 2007;116(1):19–23.

[100] O'Malley BW Jr, Weinstein GS, Snyder W, et al. Transoral robotic surgery (TORS) for base of tongue neoplasms. Laryngoscope 2006;116(8):1465–72.

[101] Weinstein GS, O'malley BW Jr, Hockstein NG. Transoral robotic surgery: supraglottic laryngectomy in a canine model. Laryngoscope 2005;115(7):1315–9.

[102] Hockstein NG, Nolan JP, O'Malley BW Jr, et al. Robot-assisted pharyngeal and laryngeal microsurgery: results of robotic cadaver dissections. Laryngoscope 2005;115(6):1003–8.

[103] Tanna N, Joshi AS, Glade RS, et al. Da Vinci robot-assisted endocrine surgery: novel applications in otolaryngology. Otolaryngol Head Neck Surg 2006;135(4):633–5.

**ELSEVIER
SAUNDERS**

Surg Oncol Clin N Am
17 (2008) 249–256

SURGICAL
ONCOLOGY CLINICS
OF NORTH AMERICA

Index

Note: Page numbers of article titles are in **boldface** type.

A

Ablation, thyroid remnant, preparation for, 198–199

Adjuvant therapy, for locally invasive well-differentiated cancer, 153

Adults, initial surgical management of differentiated thyroid cancer in, 81

AKT activation, in follicular thyroid carcinoma, 8–9

Anaplastic thyroid carcinoma, initial surgical management of, 85–87
  molecular analysis of, 13–17
    global genomic profile, 13–14
    individual genetic events, 14–17
      beta-catenin, 15–16
      other factors, 16–17
      p53 pathway, 14–15
      signaling pathways, 16–17
  pathology and cytology of, 65
  postoperative management of thyroid cancer in, 211
  radiation therapy for, 223–225

B

Beta-catenin, in poorly differentiated and anaplastic thyroid carcinoma, 15–16

C

Columnar cell variant, of papillary thyroid carcinoma, 62

Computed tomography (CT), for evaluation of thyroid nodules, 49–52
  in management of the neck in differentiated thyroid carcinoma, 161–162

Cribriform carcinoma, 63

Cytology, and pathology of thyroid cancer, **57–70**
  medullary thyroid carcinoma, 65–67
  metastatic tumors, 68

thyroid lymphomas, 67–68
tumors of follicular cell origin, 58–65
  anaplastic carcinoma, 65
  cribriform carcinoma, 63
  follicular carcinoma, 63–65
  papillary carcinoma, 58–62
  poorly differentiated carcinoma, 65

D

Diagnostics, molecular, clinical use in thyroid carcinomas, 17–19

Differentiated thyroid carcinoma, initial surgical management, during pregnancy, 81
    Hürthle cell carcinoma and other aggressive histologic subtypes, 82
    in elderly patients, 81–82
    in patients under 45, 81
    pediatric, 80–81
  management of the neck in, **157–173**
    effect of nodal metastasis on recurrence, 160
    effect of nodal metastasis on survival, 159–160
    operative, 163–170
    pattern of nodal metastasis, 158–159
    preoperative, 161–163
  poorly, molecular analysis of, 13–17
    global genomic profile, 13–14
    individual genetic events, 14–17
      beta-catenin, 15–16
      other factors, 16–17
      p53 pathway, 14–15
      signaling pathways, 16
  poorly, pathology and cytology of, 65
  well, locally invasive, **145–155**
    adjuvant treatment, 153
    evaluation of disease extent, 146–147
    histology, 147
    patterns of invasion, 147–148
    radiation therapy in, 217–221

1055-3207/08/$ - see front matter © 2008 Elsevier Inc. All rights reserved.
doi:10.1016/S1055-3207(07)00137-8

Differentiated (*continued*)
        surgical complications with,
                117–119
        surgical management, 148–153

E

Elderly patients, initial surgical
        management of differentiated thyroid
        cancer in, 81–82

Electormyography, laryngeal, in vocal fold
        paresis and paralysis after thyroid
        surgery, 180–182
        methods, for monitoring recurrent
                laryngeal nerve during
                thyroidectomy, 131–134
                sensitivity and specificity of,
                        134–135

Encapsulated variant, of papillary thyroid
        carcinoma, 62

Endoscopic techniques, use in thyroid
        surgery, 238–240
        in management of the neck in
                differentiated thyroid carcinoma,
                169–170

F

Fine needle aspiration, in management of
        the neck in differentiated thyroid
        carcinoma, 161
        ultrasound-guided, for evaluation of
                thyroid nodules, 43–49

Follicular cell origin, pathology and
        cytology of thyroid tumors with, 58–65
                anaplastic carcinoma, 65
                cribriform carcinoma, 63
                follicular carcinoma, 63–65
                papillary carcinoma, 58–62
                poorly differentiated carcinoma,
                        65

Follicular thyroid carcinoma, molecular
        analysis of, 4–9
                global genomic profile, 4–5
                individual genetic events, 5–9
                        AKT activation, 8–9
                        perioxisome proliferator-
                                activated receptor
                                gamma, 5–6
                        RAS mutation, 7–8
        pathology and cytology of, 63–65
                fine needle aspiration of, 65
                Hurtle cell, 64
                widely disseminated, 64
        radiation therapy for, 217–221
        thyroid lobectomy for low-risk, 76

Follicular variant, of papillary thyroid
        carcinoma, 61

G

Gene therapy, for vocal fold paresis and
        paralysis after thyroid surgery,
        188–189

Genomic profile, global, of follicular
        thyroid carcinoma, 4–5
        of papillary thyroid carcinoma, 13–14
        of poorly differentiated and anaplastic
                thyroid carcinoma, 13–14

Global genomic profile, of follicular thyroid
        carcinoma, 4–5
        of papillary thyroid carcinoma, 13–14
        of poorly differentiated and anaplastic
                thyroid carcinoma, 13–14

Goiter, large, with retrosternal extension,
        surgery for, 115

H

Hematoma, postoperative, after
        thyroidectomy for thyroid cancer,
        109–112

Hemorrhage, postoperative, after
        thyroidectomy for thyroid cancer,
        109–112

Hemostasis, in thyroid surgery, surgical
        instruments for improved, 231–232

Histology, of locally invasive
        well-differentiated cancer, 147

Hürthle cell follicular carcinoma, initial
        surgical management of, 82
        radiation therapy for, 217–221
        thyroid, pathology and cytology of, 64

Hypercalcemia, assessment of, after thyroid
        surgery, 234–236

Hyperparathyroidism, postoperative, after
        thyroidectomy for thyroid cancer,
        113–114

Hypocalcemia, postoperative, after
        thyroidectomy for thyroid cancer,
        113–114

I

Imaging, of thyroid nodules, **37–56**
        CT and MRI scans, 49–52
        radioisotope imaging, changing
                role of, 52–54
        ultrasound and fine needle
                aspiration, 43–49

Incidentalomas, thyroid nodule risk factors and, 42

Instruments, surgical, for improved hemostasis in thyroid surgery, 231–232

Intraoperative nerve monitoring. *See* Monitoring.

L

Laboratory tests, for evaluation of thyroid nodules, 42–43

Laryngeal electromyography, in vocal fold paresis and paralysis after thyroid surgery, 180–182

Laryngeal framework surgery, in vocal fold paresis and paralysis after thyroid surgery, 184

Laryngeal nerve, non-recurrent, as complication of thyroid surgery, 116–117
    recurrent, identifying and monitoring during thyroidectomy, **121–144,** 233–234
        anatomy, 122–127
        medicolegal implications, 137–140
        monitoring, evolution of, 127–134
        rationale for, 135–137
        sensitivity and specificity of modern monitoring devices, 134–135
    injury to, during thyroidectomy for thyroid cancer, 112–113

Laryngeal pacing, for vocal fold paresis and paralysis after thyroid surgery, 188

Legal issues, monitoring recurrent laryngeal nerve during thyroidectomy, 137–140

Lobectomy, thyroid, for low-risk follicular thyroid cancer, 76
    for low-risk papillary thyroid microcarcinoma, 75–76

Locally invasive thyroid cancer, well-differentiated, **145–155**
    adjuvant treatment, 153
    evaluation of disease extent, 146–147
    histology, 147
    patterns of invasion, 147–148
    surgical complications with, 117–119
    surgical management, 148–153

Lymphoma, thyroid, initial surgical management of, 87–88
    pathology and cytology of, 67–68

M

Magnetic resonance imaging (MRI), for evaluation of thyroid nodules, 49–52
    in management of the neck in differentiated thyroid carcinoma, 161–162

Medicolegal issues, monitoring recurrent laryngeal nerve during thyroidectomy, 137–140

Medullary thyroid carcinoma, initial surgical management of, 83–85
    pathology and cytology of, 65–67
    postoperative management of thyroid cancer in, 209–211
    radiation therapy for, 221–223

Metastases, nodal, in differentiated thyroid cancer, 158–160
        effect on recurrence, 160
        effect on survival, 159–160
        pattern of, 158–159
    to the thyroid, 68

Microcarcinoma, papillary thyroid, 62
    thyroid lobectomy for low-risk papillary thyroid, 75–76

Minimally invasive surgery, in management of the neck in differentiated thyroid carcinoma, 169–170

Molecular analysis, of thyroid cancer, clinical impact of, **1–35**
    clinical value of genetic aberrations in, 17–24
        molecular diagnostics, 17–19
        molecular staging, 19–21
        molecular therapeutics, 21–24
    follicular, 4–9
    papillary, 9–13
    poorly differentiated and anaplastic carcinomas, 13–17

Monitoring, of recurrent laryngeal nerve during thyroidectomy, **121–144,** 233–234
    anatomy, 122–127
    medicolegal implications, 137–140
    monitoring, evolution of, 127–134
        early technologies, 128–129
        electromyocardiographic, 131–134
        vocal fold visualization, 129–131
    rationale for, 135–137

Monitoring (*continued*)
    sensitivity and specificity of
        modern monitoring devices,
        134–135

N

Neck, management of, in differentiated
    thyroid cancer, **157–173**
        effect of nodal metastasis on
            recurrence, 160
        effect of nodal metastasis on
            survival, 159–160
        operative, 163–170
        pattern of nodal metastasis,
            158–159
        preoperative, 161–163

Nerves, recurrent laryngeal. *See* Recurrent
    laryngeal nerve.

Nodal metastases, in differentiated thyroid
    cancer, 158–160
        effect on recurrence, 160
        effect on survival, 159–160
        pattern of, 158–159

Nodules, thyroid, evaluation and imaging
    of, **37–56**
        CT and MRI scans, 49–52
        general considerations and risk
            factors, 39–42
        laboratory tests, 42–43
        radioisotope imaging, changing
            role of, 52–54
        risk factors and the
            "incidentaloma," 42
        ultrasound and fine needle
            aspiration, 43–49

P

p53 pathway, in poorly differentiated and
    anaplastic thyroid carcinoma, 14–15

Pacing, laryngeal, for vocal fold paresis and
    paralysis after thyroid surgery, 188

Papillary thyroid carcinoma, molecular
    analysis of, 9–13
        global genomic profile, 9
        individual genetic events, 9–13
            BRAF mutation, 12–13
            NTRK1 rearrangement, 12
            RET rearrangement, 9–11
        pathology and cytology of, 58–62
        variants of, 61–62
            columnar cell, 62
            diffuse sclerotic, 62
            encapsulated, 62
            follicular, 61–62

        microcarcinoma, 62
        tall cell, 62
    radiation therapy for, 217–221
    total thyroidectomy, for high-risk, 79
        for low-risk, 77–79

Pathology, and cytology of thyroid cancer,
    57–70
        medullary thyroid carcinoma,
            65–67
        metastatic tumors, 68
        thyroid lymphomas, 67–68
        tumors of follicular cell origin,
            58–65
            anaplastic carcinoma, 65
            cribriform carcinoma, 63
            follicular carcinoma, 63–65
            papillary carcinoma, 58–62
            poorly differentiated
                carcinoma, 65

Pediatrics, initial surgical management of
    differentiated thyroid cancer, 80–81
    postoperative management of thyroid
        cancer in, 209

Perioxisome proliferator-activated receptor
    gamma, in follicular thyroid
    carcinoma, 5–6

Poorly differentiated thyroid carcinoma,
    molecular analysis of, 13–17
        global genomic profile, 13–14
        individual genetic events, 14–17
            beta-catenin, 15–16
            other factors, 16–17
            p53 pathway, 14–15
            signaling pathways, 16
    pathology and cytology of, 65

Positron emission tomography, in
    management of the neck in
    differentiated thyroid carcinoma,
    161–162
    in postoperative management of
        thyroid cancer, 204–205

Postoperative management, of thyroid
    carcinoma, **197–218**
        anaplastic, 211–212
        initial evaluation and
            stratification, 196–198
        medullary, 209–211
        pediatric, 209
        positron emission tomography,
            204–205
        preparation for thyroid remnant
            ablation, 198–199
        radioactive iodine whole-body
            scan, 203–204
        recurrence of differentiated,
            207–209

surveillance for differentiated
thyroid cancer recurrence,
205–207
targeted therapy, 199–202
thyroglobulin assay, 202–203
thyroid-stimulating hormone
suppression therapy, 202

Pregnancy, initial surgical management of
differentiated thyroid cancer during, 81

R

Radiation therapy, role in thyroid cancer
management, **219–232**
in anaplastic carcinoma, 223–225
in medullary thyroid carcinoma,
221–223
in well-differentiated
malignancies, 217–221
side effects of, 227–228
techniques, 225–227

Radioactive iodine, whole-body scan, in
postoperative management of thyroid
cancer, 203–204

Radioisotope imaging, changing role of, for
evaluation of thyroid nodules, 52–54

RAS mutation, in follicular thyroid
carcinoma, 7–8

Recurrence, postoperative, of differentiated
thyroid cancer, surveillance for,
205–207
treatment of, 207–209

Recurrent laryngeal nerve, anatomy of,
174–175
identifying and monitoring during
thyroidectomy, **121–144,** 233–234
anatomy, 122–127
medicolegal implications,
137–140
monitoring, evolution of,
127–134
rationale for, 135–137
sensitivity and specificity of
modern monitoring devices,
134–135
injury to, during thyroidectomy for
thyroid cancer, 112–113

Reinnervation, in vocal fold paresis and
paralysis after thyroid surgery,
184–186

Remnants, of thyroid carcinoma, ablation
of, preparation for, 198–199

Risk factors, for thyroid nodules, 39–42
"incidentalomas" and, 42

S

Sentinel node biopsy, in management of the
neck in differentiated thyroid
carcinoma, 168–169

Signaling pathways, in poorly differentiated
and anaplastic thyroid carcinoma, 16

Staging, molecular, clinical use in thyroid
carcinomas, 19–21

Superior laryngeal nerve, 173, 175–176

Surgery, for thyroid cancer, **93–120**
large goiter and retrosternal
extension, 115–119
postoperative care and
management of
complications, 109–114
thyroidectomy, standard surgical
technique, 94–109
for thyroid cancer, new technologies
for, **233–248**
assessment of hypocalcemia,
234–236
endoscopic techniques,
238–240
future directions, 240–241
intraoperative nerve monitoring,
233–234
surgical instruments for
improved hemostasis,
231–233
ultrasound, 236–238
for vocal fold paresis and paralysis
after thyroid surgery, 183–186
laryngeal framework surgery, 184
reinnervation, 184–187
initial management of thyroid cancer,
71–91
extent of, for differentiated,
73–74
for anaplastic thyroid cancer,
85–87
for differentiated thyroid cancer,
during pregnancy, 81
Hürthle cell carcinoma and
other aggressive
histologic subtypes, 82
in elderly patients, 81–82
in patients under 45, 81
pediatric, 80–81
for medullary thyroid cancer,
83–85
for thyroid lymphoma, 87–88
thyroid lobectomy, for low-risk
follicular thyroid cancer, 76
for low-risk papillary
thyroid
microcarcinoma,
75–76

Surgery (*continued*)
  total thyroidectomy, for high-risk
    papillary thyroid cancer and
    invasive follicular thyroid
    cancer, 79
    for low-risk papillary
      thyroid cancer, 77–79

Surveillance, for postoperative recurrence of
  differentiated thyroid cancer, 205–207

T

Tall cell variant, of papillary thyroid
  carcinoma, 62

Targeted therapy, in postoperative
  management of thyroid cancer,
  199–202

Thyroglobulin assay, in postoperative
  management of thyroid cancer,
  202–203

Thyroid cancer, 1–246
  initial surgical management, **71–91**
    extent of, for differentiated,
      73–74
    for anaplastic thyroid cancer,
      85–87
    for differentiated thyroid cancer,
      during pregnancy, 81
      Hürthle cell carcinoma and
        other aggressive
        histologic subtypes, 82
      in elderly patients, 81–82
      in patients under 45, 81
      pediatric, 80–81
    for medullary thyroid cancer,
      83–85
    for thyroid lymphoma, 87–88
    thyroid lobectomy, for low-risk
      follicular thyroid cancer, 76
      for low-risk papillary
        thyroid
        microcarcinoma,
        75–76
    total thyroidectomy, for high-risk
      papillary thyroid cancer and
      invasive follicular thyroid
      cancer, 79
      for low-risk papillary
        thyroid cancer, 77–79
  locally invasive well-differentiated,
    145–155
    adjuvant treatment, 153
    evaluation of disease extent,
      146–147
    histology, 147
    patterns of invasion, 147–148
    surgical management, 148–153

molecular analysis, clinical impact of,
  1–35
    clinical value of genetic
      aberrations in, 17–24
      molecular diagnostics,
        17–19
      molecular staging, 19–21
      molecular therapeutics,
        21–24
    follicular, 4–9
    papillary, 9–13
    poorly differentiated and
      anaplastic carcinomas,
      13–17
  neck, management of, in
    differentiated, **157–173**
    effect of nodal metastasis on
      recurrence, 160
    effect of nodal metastasis on
      survival, 159–160
    operative, 163–170
    pattern of nodal metastasis,
      158–159
    preoperative, 161–163
  new technologies in surgery for,
    233–248
    assessment of hypocalcemia,
      234–236
    endoscopic techniques, 238–240
    future directions, 240–241
    intraoperative nerve monitoring,
      233–234
    surgical instruments for
      improved hemostasis,
      231–233
    ultrasound, 236–238
  nodules, evaluation and imaging of,
    37–56
    CT and MRI scans, 49–52
    general considerations and risk
      factors, 39–42
    laboratory tests, 42–43
    radioisotope imaging, changing
      role of, 52–54
    risk factors and the
      "incidentaloma," 42
    ultrasound and fine needle
      aspiration, 43–49
  pathology and cytology, **57–70**
    medullary thyroid carcinoma,
      65–67
    metastatic tumors, 68
    thyroid lymphomas, 67–68
    tumors of follicular cell origin,
      58–65
      anaplastic carcinoma, 65
      cribriform carcinoma, 63
      follicular carcinoma, 63–65
      papillary carcinoma, 58–62

poorly differentiated carcinoma, 65
postoperative management, **197–218**
  anaplastic, 211–212
  initial evaluation and stratification, 196–198
  medullary, 209–211
  pediatric, 209
  positron emission tomography, 204–205
  preparation for thyroid remnant ablation, 198–199
  radioactive iodine whole-body scan, 203–204
  recurrence of differentiated, 207–209
  surveillance for differentiated thyroid cancer recurrence, 205–207
  targeted therapy, 199–202
  thyroglobulin assay, 202–203
  thyroid-stimulating hormone suppression therapy, 202
radiation therapy for, **219–232**
  in anaplastic carcinoma, 223–225
  in medullary thyroid carcinoma, 221–223
  in well-differentiated malignancies, 217–221
  side effects of, 227–228
  techniques, 225–227
recurrent laryngeal nerve, identifying and monitoring during thyroidectomy, **121–144**
surgery for, **93–120**
  large goiter and retrosternal extension, 115–119
  postoperative care and management of complications, 109–114
  thyroidectomy, standard surgical technique, 94–109
vocal fold paresis and paralysis, **175–196**
  anatomy, 173–174
  bilateral, 187–188
  evaluation, 178–180
  gene therapy, 188–189
  laryngeal electromyography, 180–182
  laryngeal pacing, 188
  presentation, 176–177
  recurrent laryngeal nerve, 174–175
  superior laryngeal nerve, 173, 175–176
  surgical therapy, 183–186
    laryngeal framework surgery, 184

reinnervation, 184–187
treatment, 182
voice therapy, 182–183

Thyroid remnant ablation, preparation for, 198–199

Thyroid-stimulating hormone suppression therapy, in postoperative management of thyroid cancer, 202

Thyroidectomy, for thyroid cancer, postoperative care and management of complications, 109–114
  hemorrhage and hematoma, 109–112
  hypocalcemia and hypoparathyroidism, 113–114
  other sequelae, 114
  recurrent laryngeal nerve injury, 112–113
reoperation, 119
standard surgical technique, 94–109
  capsular dissection of thyroid lobe and preservation of parathyroid glands, 100–103
  development of cutaneous flaps, 96
  exposure and management of strap muscles, 96–98
  exposure of superior thyroid pole and preservation of superior laryngeal nerve, 98–100
  homeostasis, drains, and wound closure, 109
  identification of recurrent laryngeal nerve and its anatomic variations, 103–109
  positioning and draping, 94–96
  skin incision planning, 94
identifying and monitoring recurrent laryngeal nerve during, **121–144,** 233–234
  anatomy, 122–127
  medicolegal implications, 137–140
  monitoring, evolution of, 127–134
  rationale for, 135–137
  sensitivity and specificity of modern monitoring devices, 134–135

Thyroidectomy, total, for invasive follicular
　　thyroid cancer, 79
　　for papillary thyroid cancer, high
　　　　risk, 79
　　　　low risk, 77–79

U

Ultrasound, in management of the neck in
　　differentiated thyroid carcinoma,
　　161–162
　　use beefier and during thyroid surgery,
　　　　236–238
　　with fine needle aspiration for
　　　　evaluation of thyroid nodules,
　　　　43–49

V

Vocal fold paresis and paralysis, after
　　thyroid surgery, **175–196**
　　　　anatomy, 173–174
　　　　bilateral, 187–188
　　　　evaluation, 178–180
　　　　gene therapy, 188–189
　　　　laryngeal electromyography,
　　　　　　180–182
　　　　laryngeal pacing, 188
　　　　presentation, 176–177
　　　　recurrent laryngeal nerve,
　　　　　　174–175
　　　　superior laryngeal nerve, 173,
　　　　　　175–176

surgical therapy, 183–186
　　laryngeal framework
　　　　surgery, 184
　　reinnervation, 184–187
treatment, 182
voice therapy, 182–183

Vocal fold visualization, for monitoring
　　recurrent laryngeal nerve during
　　thyroidectomy, 129–131

Voice therapy, in vocal fold paresis and
　　paralysis after thyroid surgery,
　　182–183

W

Well-differentiated thyroid cancer, locally
　　invasive, **145–155**
　　adjuvant treatment, 153
　　evaluation of disease extent,
　　　　146–147
　　histology, 147
　　patterns of invasion, 147–148
　　radiation therapy in, 217–221
　　surgical complications with, 117–119
　　surgical management, 148–153

Whole-body scan, with radioactive iodine,
　　in postoperative management of
　　thyroid cancer, 203–204

Widely disseminated follicular carcinoma,
　　thyroid, pathology and cytology of, 64

Moving?

Make sure your subscription moves with you!

To notify us of your new address, find your **Clinics Account Number** (located on your mailing label above your name), and contact customer service at:

E-mail: elspcs@elsevier.com

800-654-2452 (subscribers in the U.S. & Canada)
407-345-4000 (subscribers outside of the U.S. & Canada)

Fax number: 407-363-9661

Elsevier Periodicals Customer Service
6277 Sea Harbor Drive
Orlando, FL 32887-4800

*To ensure uninterrupted delivery of your subscription, please notify us at least 4 weeks in advance of move.